Key Techniques in Orthopaedic Surgery

Key Techniques in Orthopaedic Surgery

Steven H. Stern, M.D.

Associate Professor of Clinical Orthopaedics

Department of Orthopaedics

Northwestern University

Chicago, Illinois

2001

Thieme

New York • Stuttgart

Thieme New York
333 Seventh Avenue
New York, NY 10001

Executive Editor: Jane Pennington, Ph.D.
Assistant Editor: Michelle Schmitt
Editorial Assistant: Todd Warnock
Production Editor: David Stewart
Director, Production and Manufacturing: Anne Vinnicombe
Marketing Director: Phyllis D. Gold
Sales Manager: Ross Lumpkin
Chief Financial Officer: Peter van Woerden
President: Brian D. Scanlan
Cover Design: Kevin Kall
Medical Illustrator: Anthony M. Pazos
Compositor: V&M Graphics
Printer: The Maple-Vail Book Manufacturing Group

Library of Congress Cataloging-in-Publication Data

Key techniques in orthopaedic surgery / [edited by] Steven H. Stern.
       p.   ;   cm.
    Includes bibliographical references and index.
    ISBN 0-86577-922-8 (hardcover) — ISBN 3131248513 (hardcover)
       1. Orthopedic surgery.   2. Musculoskeletal system—Diseases—Surgery. I.
Stern, Steven H., 1958–
    [DNLM: 1. Musculoskeletal Diseases—surgery.   2. Fractures—surgery.
3. Orthopedic Procedures—methods. WE 168 K44 2001]
    RD731.K49 2001
    617.4'7—dc21

                                                            00-059942

Important note: Medical knowledge is ever-changing. As new research and clinical experience
broaden our knowledge, changes in treatment and drug therapy may be required. The authors and
the editors of the material herein have consulted sources believed to be reliable in their efforts to
provide information that is complete and in accord with the standards accepted at the time of
publication. However, in view of the possibility of human error by the authors, editors, or publisher
of the work herein, or changes in medical knowledge, neither the authors, editors, publisher, nor
any other party who has been involved in the preparation of this work, warrants that the
information contained herein is in every respect accurate or complete, and they are not responsible
for any errors or omissions or for the results obtained from use of such information. Readers are
encouraged to confirm the information contained herein with other sources. For example, readers
are advised to check the product information sheet included in the package of each drug they plan
to use to be certain that the information contained in this publication is accurate and that changes
have not been made in the recommended doses or implant indications, or in the contraindications
for their use. This recommendation is of particular importance in connection with new or
infrequently used drugs or implants.

Some of the product names, patents, and registered designs referred to in this book are in fact
registered trademarks or proprietary names even though specific reference to this fact is not always
made in the text. Therefore, the appearance of a name without designation as proprietary is not to
be construed as a representation by the publisher that it is in the public domain.

Printed in the United States of America

5 4 3 2 1

TNY ISBN 0-86577-922-8
GTV ISBN 3-13-124851-3

Contents

To my wife Sharon,

my children Anna, Jacqueline, and Rebecca,

and my parents Martin and Marilyn,

all of whom have contributed and sacrificed endlessly to make my life meaningful

and to allow for a book like this to be written.

It is impossible to thank them enough.

Preface

Numerous orthopaedic textbooks are currently available that do an excellent job covering diverse topics in orthopaedics, ranging from cervical spine to foot surgery. Commonly, these texts draw liberally from the subspecialty expertise now widely available in almost all areas of orthopaedics. However, in some cases, the comprehensiveness of the text is somewhat foreboding and the task of reading individual chapters is daunting and time consuming. Despite the depth of detail in these books, specific information on the precise clinical steps that need to be followed in the operating room can be limited.

The idea for this text, *Key Techniques in Orthopaedic Surgery*, came directly as a response to these concerns. The specific goal of this book is to fill a void that the more comprehensive subspecialty texts may have created. The book is designed to cover the basic surgical aspects of common orthopaedic procedures in a straightforward and reproducible manner. It is hoped that its style will allow it to be easily read by practicing surgeons, resident physicians, and medical students. The chapters are designed to allow the reader to quickly review the basic steps and important issues associated with orthopaedic procedures. However, at its heart, this is a text focused on surgical technique and this section is the main focus of each chapter. Thus, it can serve as a handy reference that can be quickly reviewed just prior to performing an orthopaedic operation.

One of the keys to this book is the consistent organization of each chapter. Each chapter reviews a different surgical procedure in a concise, straightforward manner. The book employs a "cookbook" outline format, with the information in each section presented in a numbered fashion. This structure is designed to allow the reader to quickly read about an operative procedure and review the salient points associated with the procedure, with special emphasis on the operative technique.

Structurally each chapter conforms to a similar outline format and is divided into the following individual sections.

1. Indications: lists the common indications for the procedure.
2. Contraindications: lists the common contraindications for the procedure.
3. Preoperative Preparation, Special Instruments, Position, and Anesthesia: lists the common issues associated with these topics.
4. Tips and Pearls: lists special tips that the authors feel are especially helpful to remember in conjunction with the procedure.
5. What To Avoid: lists common pitfalls to try to avoid that are associated with the procedure.
6. Postoperative Care Issues: lists common issues in postsurgical care associated with the procedure.

7. Operative Technique: lists common basic steps necessary to perform the orthopaedic procedures; many procedures have optional or alternative steps that may be indicated or required depending on the clinical situation.

Each chapter is augmented by a number of illustrations. Because of the desire to make this a wide-ranging text that includes multiple common orthopaedic procedures, the number of illustrations that could be included was limited. Thus, the pictures attempt to augment the text by depicting the most salient points of the surgical procedures. The illustrations are all referenced in the text.

For many of the chapter authors, I have drawn liberally from my colleagues at Northwestern University. In general, the goal in selecting authors was to pick surgeons who have actual clinical experience performing the operative procedures. Hopefully, this allows for a more realistic description of surgical techniques that are currently being actively employed.

It must be remembered that orthopaedics is a surgical art that continues to change and evolve. Thus, the techniques in these chapters represent one method of performing each procedure at the time they were written. Many readers will employ their own appropriate variations to the listed steps in order to adapt them to their own surgical technique. The individual chapter authors will also modify and refine the techniques presented in this text as the field of orthopaedics evolves. Thus, these steps are not designed to be slavishly followed without regard for the clinical situation. Rather, they serve as a general outline or guidebook in performing these particular procedures. In no way do the authors or the text attempt to define the listed operative techniques as representative of the only, best, or standard way of performing surgery. In a similar manner, the other sections of the book should not be construed as representative of the only, best, or standard way of dealing with a particular clinical situation. As in all aspects of medicine, clinical judgement should always be employed in each individual situation.

Because the book is not designed to be all encompassing, I encourage readers to augment this book with subspecialty texts of their choosing. Furthermore, the book attempts to review common orthopaedic procedures that are employed to treat common orthopaedic problems. Therefore, the techniques listed may be less applicable to complex, revision, or other unusual cases.

Finally, I would like to suggest my own "pearl" that I think is applicable to almost all of the techniques in this book, and one that I have frequently told to residents and medical students. It has always been my thought that most orthopaedic procedures are relatively easy and straightforward, if appropriate visualization can be achieved. In fact, the most technically adept surgeons that I have ever worked with were those that were the most skilled in achieving excellent surgical exposure. Thus, I have always felt that (in most cases) "if you can see it, you can do it." It is hoped that the techniques in this book will aid the reader in achieving the necessary exposure and visualization, so they too can "see it" and "do it."

Steven H. Stern, M.D.

Acknowledgments

This book represents an accumulative amount of work by many authors, as well as many others behind the scenes. I would like to acknowledge some of those who have made this work possible.

I appreciate the time and effort that every author put into this project. Each author had to endure many phone calls from me as I pestered them to complete and optimize their chapters.

The credit for all of the book's illustrations goes to Tony Pazos. He was asked to undertake a vast project, requiring anatomical illustrations from the entire musculoskeletal system. His constant diligence to detail throughout the project has helped ensure that the graphical illustrations correspond as best as possible to the relevant clinical anatomy.

Specifically, I wish to acknowledge Jane Pennington. She provided the initial inspiration for this text, and I appreciate her invaluable advice and guidance in helping to define the exact scope and format of the book. It was her vision that commenced this project

There have been many people at Thieme who have been instrumental in helping to bring this project to fruition. Esther Gumpert was invaluable in ensuring that the final stages of this project went smoothly. Todd Warnock, the Editorial Assistant at Thieme for most of the project, was responsible for working with all of the authors and with the illustrator to coordinate their combined efforts. Furthermore, he had to put up with almost daily phone calls from me on the book's status. Finally, I would like to acknowledge David Stewart, Production Editor. David was in charge of the book's actual production from original manuscript to final bound book, and was responsible for the layout and design.

Thanks go to Carol Schreiber, Tina Blythe, Joyce Kelly, and Deanna Krolczyk. Their efforts in typing and editing the book's chapters were most appreciated.

I would like to acknowledge Fran Khoury who serves as my clinical assistant. She was responsible for ensuring that the clinical aspect of my practice continued smoothly, despite the time I needed to commit to this book.

Finally, John Insall, M.D. for his help and guidance throughout the years. He has been an inspiration to me in all phases of my professional life for his clinical expertise, his academic excellence, and his research efforts. Above all, I value his friendship.

Contributors

Kirk Aadalen, M.D.
Orthopaedic Resident
Department of Orthopaedic Surgery
Northwestern University Medical School;
Department of Pediatric Orthopaedic Surgery
Children's Memorial Hospital
Chicago, Illinois

Michael S. Bednar, M.D.
Associate Professor
Department of Orthopaedic Surgery and Rehabilitation
Stritch School of Medicine
Loyola University
Maywood, Illinois

Matthew Bernstein, M.D.
Orthopaedic Resident
Department of Orthopaedic Surgery
Northwestern University Medical School
Chicago, Illinois

Mark K. Bowen, M.D.
Associate Clinical Professor of Orthopaedic Surgery
Department of Orthopaedic Surgery
Northwestern University Medical School
Chicago, Illinois

Daniel D. Buss, M.D.
Associate Professor
Department of Orthopaedic Surgery
University of Minnesota
Minneapolis, Minnesota

Charles Carroll IV, M.D.
Assistant Professor of Clinical Orthopaedic Surgery
Department of Orthopaedic Surgery
Northwestern University Medical School
Chicago, Illinois

Franklin Chen, M.D.
Attending Hand Surgeon
Edison-Metuchen Orthopaedic Group
Edison, New Jersey

Scott D. Cordes, M.D.
Assistant Professor of Clinical Orthopaedic Surgery
Department of Orthopaedic Surgery
Northwestern University Medical School
Chicago, Illinois

Angelo DiFelice, M.D.
Fellow, Sports Medicine
Department of Orthopaedic Surgery
Northwestern University Medical School
Chicago, Illinois

Roger Dunteman, M.D.
Orthopaedic Resident
Department of Orthopaedic Surgery
Northwestern University Medical School;
Department of Pediatric Orthopaedic Surgery
Children's Memorial Hospital
Chicago, Illinois

Mark E. Easley, M.D.
Orthopaedic Fellow
Department of Orthopaedic Surgery
Beth Israel Medical Center
New York, New York

John J. Grayhack, M.D.
Assistant Professor
Department of Orthopaedic Surgery
Northwestern University Medical School
Chicago, Illinois

John R. Green III, M.D.
Assistant Professor
Department of Orthopaedic Surgery
LSU Medical Center
Shreveport, Louisiana

Brian J. Hartigan, M.D.
Clinical Instructor
Department of Orthopaedic Surgery
Northwestern University Medical School
Chicago, Illinois

Serena S. Hu, M.D.
Associate Professor
Department of Orthopaedic Surgery
University of California San Francisco
San Francisco, California

William C. Jacobsen, M.D.
Fellow, Sports Medicine
Minneapolis Sports Medicine Center
Minneapolis, Minnesota

David M. Kalainov, M.D.
Instructor of Clinical Orthopaedic Surgery
Department of Orthopaedic Surgery
Northwestern University Medical School
Chicago, Illinois

Armen S. Kelikian, M.D.
Associate Professor
Department of Orthopaedic Surgery
Northwestern University Medical School
Chicago, Illinois

Erik C. King, M.D.
Instructor
Department of Orthopaedic Surgery
Northwestern University Medical School
Chicago, Illinois

Steven Kodros, M.D.
Assistant Professor of Clinical Orthopaedic Surgery
Department of Orthopaedic Surgery
Northwestern University Medical School
Chicago, Illinois

Michael Kuczmanski, M.D.
Orthopaedic Resident
Department of Orthopaedic Surgery
Northwestern University Medical School;
Department of Pediatric Orthopaedic Surgery
Children's Memorial Hospital
Chicago, Illinois

Stephen G. Manifold, M.D.
Orthopaedic Fellow
Department of Orthopaedic Surgery
Beth Israel Medical Center
New York, New York

Bradley R. Merk, M.D.
Instructor of Orthopaedic Surgery
Department of Orthopaedic Surgery
Northwestern University Medical School
Chicago, Illinois

Srdjan Mirkovic, M.D.
Assistant Clinical Professor of Orthopaedic Surgery
Department of Orthopaedic Surgery
Northwestern University Medical School
Chicago, Illinois

Gordon W. Nuber, M.D.
Academic Professor of Clinical Orthopaedic Surgery
Department of Orthopaedic Surgery
Northwestern University Medical School
Chicago, Illinois

Douglas E. Padgett, M.D.
Assistant Professor of Orthopaedic Surgery
Hospital for Special Surgery
Cornell University Medical College
New York, New York

John F. Sarwark, M.D.
Associate Professor of Orthopaedics
Department of Orthopaedic Surgery
Northwestern University Medical School;
Interim Division Head
Department of Pediatric Orthopaedic Surgery
Children's Memorial Hospital
Chicago, Illinois

Giles R. Scuderi, M.D.
Assistant Clinical Professor of Orthopaedic Surgery
Department of Orthopaedic Surgery
Beth Israel Medical Center
New York, New York

Steven H. Stern, M.D.
Associate Professor of Clinical Orthopaedics
Department of Orthopaedic Surgery
Northwestern University Medical School
Chicago, Illinois

Section One

Shoulder and Arm

CHAPTER 1

Open Acromioplasty

Mark K. Bowen and Angelo DiFelice

Indications

1. Radiographically documented impingement that has failed nonsurgical management (rest, local modalities, nonsteroidal anti-inflammatory drugs (NSAIDs), physical therapy, and judicious subacromial cortisone injections)
2. Full-thickness rotator cuff tears—not repairable
3. Partial-thickness rotator cuff tears—less than 50% thickness of tendon

Contraindications

1. Neuropathic joint
2. Active soft tissue or glenohumeral infection
3. Failed prior surgical treatment with associated deltoid insufficiency
4. Degenerative glenohumeral arthritis (relative); consider combining acromioplasty with shoulder arthroplasty
5. Patient's overall medical condition (relative)
6. Patient unable to comply with postoperative rehabilitation (relative)

Preoperative Preparation

1. Physical examination should include assessment of acromioclavicular (AC) joint tenderness and/or pain with shoulder adduction.
2. Obtain radiographs

   a. Anteroposterior (AP) in plane of scapula ("true AP")
   b. AP shoulder (check distal clavicle for "spurs")
   c. Axillary view (check for os acromiale, glenohumeral arthritis)
   d. Supraspinatus outlet view (assess acromion shape [types I–III], spinoacromial angle)
   e. Twenty-five degree caudal tilt ("Rockwood view") (optional)

3. Consider magnetic resonance imaging (MRI): Helps evaluate extent ("full" versus "partial" thickness) of rotator cuff tears, and presence of muscle atrophy or tendon retraction; observe mass effect of acromion and AC joint on supraspinatus tendon (impingement).

Special Instruments, Position, and Anesthesia

1. Small sagittal or oscillating saw for bone resection
2. 1.6-mm drill bit for deltoid reattachment
3. Small, half-circle curved free Mayo needle, and #2 braided nonabsorbable suture
4. 5-mm round burr and broad flap rasp to "fine-tune" acromioplasty
5. Semisitting or beach chair position. The patient is moved as close to the side of the table as possible while still being stable. A beanbag-type McConnell head holder (McConnell Surgical Mfg., Greenville, TX) or AMSCO "captain's chair" is useful to secure

and stabilize the head in a safe neutral position. Care must be taken to pad all bony prominences.

6. The head may be secured gently with a padded strap or tape across a pad on the forehead. Care must be taken to avoid the strap or tape from sliding down over the eyes.

7. The procedure can be done with either general or interscalene block anesthesia.

Tips and Pearls

1. Prior to initiating surgery use a marking pen to outline prominent anatomic landmarks. Identification of the acromion, scapular spine, and clavicle is critical for accurate arthroscopic portal and skin incision placement.

2. Consider arthroscopic evaluation of the glenohumeral joint including the articular surfaces, glenohumeral ligaments, biceps tendon, and the undersurface of the rotator cuff for completeness. Threading an absorbable suture through a spinal needle placed through the torn area can mark partial-thickness tears.

3. Arthroscopic evaluation of the subacromial space may reveal near complete full-thickness rotator cuff tears in the setting of an apparent intact cuff on intra-articular examination.

What To Avoid

1. Make sure the patient is properly positioned on the operating room table. Avoid excessive cervical traction or brachial plexus traction. Ensure proper padding of all bony prominences to minimize risk of neuropraxias.

2. Avoid fracturing the acromion during either the acromioplasty or deltoid reattachment.

3. Avoid inadequate or insecure repair of the deltoid to the acromion.

Postoperative Care Issues

1. A sling is used for comfort.
2. Start the patient on pendulum-type passive exercises the day of surgery.

3. Physical therapy is begun approximately 2 weeks postoperatively. Initially, the patient starts performing passive and active assisted range-of-motion exercises. The patient must avoid active motions for 4 weeks to protect the deltoid repair. The patient begins strengthening exercises as tolerated.

Operative Technique

Approach

1. Position the patient on the operating room table as outlined above.

2. Prepare and drape the entire arm and shoulder girdle "free."

3. Carefully outline prominent anatomic landmarks: coracoid process, clavicle, AC joint, acromion, and scapular spine.

4. Draw the planned skin incision with a marker. The incision should extend 2 in from the lateral aspect of the anterior third of the acromion toward the lateral tip of the coracoid process acromion halfway between the anterolateral and posterolateral corners of the acromion. Place the skin incision in Langer's lines that parallel the lateral border of the acromion (**Fig. 1–1**).

5. If an excision of the distal clavicle is indicated, move the incision approximately 1 cm medial to the standard incision (**Fig. 1–1**).

6. Infiltrate the skin and subcutaneous tissue with 1:200,000 concentration of epinephrine.

7. Incise the skin and subcutaneous tissue down to the deltoid fascia. Develop the prefascial plane to expose the entire anterolateral corner of the acromion and the lateral aspect of the deltoid. If AC joint excision is planned, dissect further medially to expose the distal 2 cm of the clavicle.

8. Split the deltoid muscle in the raphe between the anterior and middle deltoid. Begin at the anterolateral corner and extend the dissection distally 2 to 3 cm. The direction of the split is approximately perpendicular to the skin incision. Consider placing a stay suture to avoid injuring the terminal branches of the axillary nerve (**Fig. 1–2A**).

9. Starting from the split, release the deltoid subperiosteally along the anterior acromion using

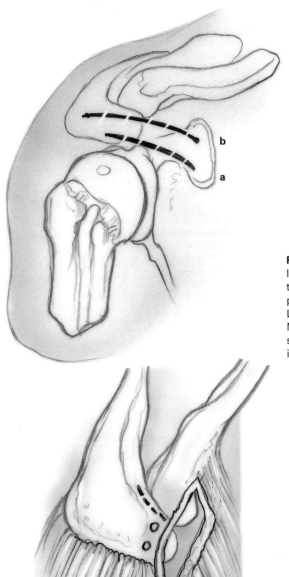

Figure 1–1 Skin incision. The incision should extend 4 cm from the lateral aspect of the anterior third of the acromion toward the lateral tip of the coracoid process halfway between the anterolateral and posterolateral corners of the acromion. Place the skin incision in Langer's lines that parallel the lateral border of the acromion **(a)**. Note that if excision of the distal clavicle is planned, the skin incision should be positioned approximately 1 cm medial to the standard incision **(b)**.

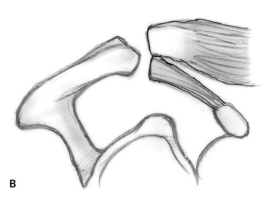

Figure 1–2 (A) Deltoid exposure. Split the deltoid muscle in the raphe between the anterior and middle deltoid. This incision should begin at the anterolateral corner and extend distally 2 to 3 cm. The direction of the split is approximately perpendicular to the skin incision. Consider placing a stay suture to avoid injuring the terminal branches of the axillary nerve. Starting from the split, you should release the deltoid subperiosteally along the anterior acromion using an electrocautery. Extend the incision along the clavicle when a distal clavicle excision is planned. **(B)** Lateral view of deltoid detachment. Completely detach the coracoacromial ligament, usually along with the deep deltoid fascia, from its attachment on the acromion.

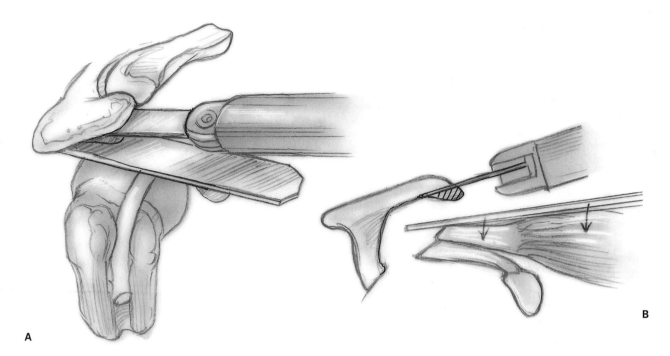

Figure 1–3 (A) Acriomioplasty. Perform the acromioplasty utilizing either a sagittal saw or sharp osteotome. This should create a flat or slightly angled-up acromion. Note the position of the retractor which serves to protect the rotator cuff. **(B)** Acromioplasty (lateral view). Lateral view of acromioplasty creating a type I acromion.

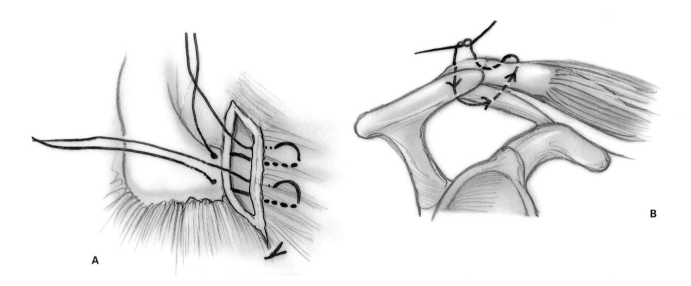

Figure 1–4 (A) Deltoid repair. The deltoid is repaired to the anterior acromion through two 1.6-mm drill holes in the acromion, at least 5 mm back from the anterior edge. Note that both the superficial and deep fascia are incorporated in the repair using #2 braided nonabsorbable sutures. **(B)** Deltoid repair (lateral view). Sutures are placed through drill holes in acromion and passed full thickness through the deltoid muscle.

electrocautery. Start several millimeters back from the anterior edge of the acromion (**Fig. 1–2A**). Bovie electrocautery is more effective than sharp dissection for this step.

10. Release the superficial and deep deltoid fascia. Tag these with heavy nonabsorbable suture, which aids retraction and deltoid repair. Carefully coagulate the acromial branch of the thoracoacromial artery, which is usually encountered near the anterolateral acromion between the superficial and deep deltoid.

11. Completely detach the coracoacromial ligament, usually along with the deep deltoid fascia, from its attachment on the acromion (**Fig. 1–2B**). Usually it is not necessary to dissect these out separately.

12. Extend the deltoid release past the AC joint. Expose the distal clavicle when distal clavicle excision is planned (**Fig. 1–2A**).

13. Release bursal adhesions with a blunt instrument or an index finger.

Acromioplasty

14. Protect the rotator cuff with a blunt retractor, such as a medium chandler. Perform the acromioplasty, utilizing either a sagittal saw or sharp osteotome (**Fig. 1–3**). The wedge of bone excised should be the full width of the acromion from the medial to the lateral.

  a. The goal of acromioplasty is to shape the acromion so that its undersurface is flat from anterior to posterior and medial to lateral. After surgery, the acromion's undersurface should have a smooth contour for optimal subacromial contact. There should be neither ridges or "sharp spikes of bone" nor anterior overhang of the acromion.

  b. The deep deltoid fascia attachment to the lateral acromion can be used as a landmark to judge the amount of acromion resected. After an acromioplasty, the acromion should be flush with the deep deltoid attachment to the lateral acromion.

15. Use a burr or file to smooth the undersurface of the acromion.

16. Identify the subacromial bursa and perform a complete subdeltoid bursectomy. Fully rotate the arm as this exposes the rotator cuff tendons.

Closure

17. Copiously irrigate the wound.

18. Carefully secure the deltoid to the anterior acromion. This is best achieved by making two 1.6-mm drill holes in the acromion, at least 5 mm back from the anterior edge (**Fig. 1–4**).

19. Repair the deltoid to the acromion. Incorporate both the superficial and deep fascia in the repair using #2 braided nonabsorbable sutures (**Fig. 1–4**).

20. Close the subcutaneous tissues and skin with a cosmetic subcuticular closure.

21. Apply a sterile dressing. Place the patient's arm in a sling.

Suggested Readings

Iannotti JP, Williams GR Jr. *Disorders of the Shoulder: Diagnosis and Management.* Philadelphia, PA: Lippincott Williams & Wilkins, 1999.

Rockwood CA, Matsen FA. *The Shoulder.* Philadelphia, PA: W.B. Saunders, 1998.

CHAPTER 2

Open Rotator Cuff Tendon Repair

Mark K. Bowen and Angelo DiFelice

Indications (Rotator Cuff Repair)

1. Patients with chronic shoulder pain or weakness with a documented rotator cuff tear that has failed nonsurgical management (rest, local modalities, NSAIDs, physical therapy, and judicious subacromial cortisone injections)
2. Acute, traumatic full-thickness rotator cuff tears
3. Partial-thickness rotator cuff tears greater than 50%

Indications for associated acromioclavicular (AC) joint resection

➢ AC joint tenderness on physical examination
➢ Radiographic changes of AC joint arthritis
➢ Exposure optimization of a retracted supraspinatus tendon in chronic or massive rotator cuff tears

Contraindications

1. Active soft tissue or glenohumeral infection
2. Neuropathic joint
3. Chronic axillary nerve injury
4. Failed prior surgical treatment with associated deltoid insufficiency (relative)
5. Degenerative arthritis (relative); consider combining rotator cuff repair with shoulder arthroplasty
6. Patient's overall medical condition (relative)
7. Parkinson's disease or other diseases that cause uncontrolled muscle activity (relative)
8. Patient unable to comply with postoperative rehabilitation

Preoperative Preparation

1. Physical examination to include assessment of AC joint tenderness and/or pain with shoulder adduction
2. Obtain radiographs

   a. Anteroposterior (AP) in plane of scapula (true AP)
   b. AP shoulder (check distal clavicle for "spurs")
   c. Axillary view (check for os acromiale, glenohumeral arthritis)
   d. Supraspinatus outlet view (assess acromion shape [types I–III], spinoacromial angle)
   e. 25 degree caudal tilt ("Rockwood view") (optional)

3. Consider magnetic resonance imaging (MRI): helps evaluate extent ("full" versus "partial" thickness) of rotator cuff tears, and presence of muscle atrophy or tendon retraction; observe mass effect of acromion and AC joint on supraspinatus tendon (impingement).

Special Instruments, Position, and Anesthesia

1. Small sagittal or oscillating saw for bone resection
2. 1.6-mm drill bit for deltoid reattachment
3. Small, half-circle curved free Mayo needle, and #2 braided nonabsorbable suture
4. 5-mm round burr and broad flap rasp to "fine-tune" acromioplasty

5. Semi-sitting or beach chair position. The patient is moved as close to the side of the table as possible while still being stable. A beanbag-type McConnell head holder (McConnell Surgical Mfg., Greenville, TX) or AMSCO "captain's chair" is useful to secure and stabilize the head in a safe neutral position. Care must be taken to pad all bony prominences.

6. The head may be secured gently with a padded strap or tape across a pad on the forehead. Care must be taken to avoid the strap or tape from sliding down over the eyes.

7. The procedure can be done with either general or interscalene block anesthesia.

Tips and Pearls

1. A thorough preoperative evaluation is critical to a successful rotator cuff repair. A complete physical examination, review of plain radiographs, and MRI provide meaningful information to plan surgery and counsel patients preoperatively. The size of tear and the degree of tendon retraction and muscle atrophy can suggest the degree of difficulty in attempting to repair the rotator cuff and the possible need for postoperative abduction brace immobilization.

2. Check passive range of motion preoperatively and under anesthesia. Gentle shoulder manipulation may be necessary to release capsular adhesions. If adhesive capsulitis is severe, consider a staged manipulation and subsequent rotator cuff repair to minimize post-surgical loss of motion.

3. Mobilization of the rotator cuff tendon along its superior and inferior surfaces and release of a contracted coracohumeral ligament is important to minimize undesirable tension on the tissue and repair.

4. Define the anterior and posterior aspects of the rotator cuff tear and advance and secure these areas first. This closes the tear and relieves tension on the repair at the tuberosity.

5. A secure deltoid repair to the acromion is as important as the rotator cuff repair in restoring shoulder strength and function.

What To Avoid

1. Make sure the patient is properly positioned on the operating room table. Avoid excessive cervical traction and brachial plexus traction. Ensure proper padding of all bony prominences to minimize risk of neuropraxias.

2. Avoid fracturing the acromion during either the acromioplasty or deltoid reattachment.

3. Do not mistake the flimsy bursal tissue for the rotator cuff tendon and use it in the cuff repair.

4. Avoid inadequate or insecure repair of the deltoid to the acromion.

Postoperative Care Issues

1. A sling or abduction pillow is used postoperatively to protect the rotator cuff repair. The choice of postoperative protection depends on the type of patient, the quality of the tendon tissue, the tension on the sutures, and the adequacy of the cuff and deltoid repair.

2. Three phases of rehabilitation—time in each stage depends on tendon quality and assessment of repair.

   a. *Phase 1.* Passive range of motion: includes pendulum saw, and tummy rub exercises
   b. *Phase 2.* Active-assisted range of motion exercises and gentle cuff isometrics
   c. *Phase 3.* Active range of motion and resistance exercises

Operative Technique

Approach

1. Position the patient on the operating room table as outlined above.

2. Prepare and drape the entire arm and shoulder girdle "free."

3. Carefully outline prominent anatomic landmarks: coracoid process, clavicle, AC joint, acromion and scapular spine.

4. Draw the planned skin incision with a marker. The incision should extend 2 in from the lateral aspect of the anterior third of the acromion toward the lateral tip of the coracoid process acromion halfway between the anterolateral and posterolateral corners of the acromion. Place the skin incision in Langer's lines that parallel the lateral border of the acromion (see Fig. 1–1).

5. If an excision of the distal clavicle is indicated, move the incision approximately 1 cm medial to the standard incision (see Fig. 1–1).

6. Infiltrate the skin and subcutaneous tissue with 1:200,000 concentration of epinephrine.

7. Incise the skin and subcutaneous tissue down to the deltoid fascia. Develop the prefascial plane to expose the entire anterolateral corner of the acromion and the lateral aspect of the deltoid. If AC joint excision is planned, dissect further medially to expose the distal 2 cm of the clavicle.

8. Split the deltoid muscle in the raphe between the anterior and middle deltoid. Begin at the anterolateral corner and extend the dissection distally 2 to 3 cm. The direction of the split is approximately perpendicular to the skin incision. Consider placing a stay suture to avoid injuring the terminal branches of the axillary nerve (see Fig. 1–2A).

9. Starting from the split, release the deltoid subperiosteally along the anterior acromion using an electrocautery. Start several millimeters back from the anterior edge of the acromion (see Fig. 1–2A). Bovie electrocautery is more effective than sharp dissection for this step.

10. Release the superficial and deep deltoid fascia. Tag these with heavy nonabsorbable suture, which aids retraction and deltoid repair. Carefully coagulate the acromial branch of the thoracoacromial artery that is usually encountered near the anterolateral acromion between the superficial and deep deltoid.

11. Completely detach the coracoacromial ligament, usually along with the deep deltoid fascia, from its attachment on the acromion (see Fig. 1–2B). Usually it is not necessary to dissect these out separately.

12. Extend the deltoid release past the AC joint. Expose the distal clavicle when distal clavicle excision is planned (see Fig. 1–2A).

13. Release bursal adhesions with a blunt instrument or an index finger.

Acromioplasty

14. Protect the rotator cuff with a blunt retractor, such as a medium chandler. Perform an acromioplasty utilizing either a sagittal saw or a sharp osteotome (see Fig. 1–3A). The wedge of bone excised should be the full width of the acromion from the medial to lateral.

   a. The goal of the acromioplasty is to shape the acromion so its undersurface is flat from anterior to posterior and medial to lateral. After surgery, the acromion's undersurface should have a smooth contour for optimal subacromial contact. There should be no ridges or sharp spikes of bone, nor should there be anterior overhang of the acromion.

   b. The deep deltoid fascia attachment to the lateral acromion can be used as a landmark to judge the amount of acromion resected. After an acromioplasty, the acromion should be flush with the deep deltoid attachment to the lateral acromion.

15. Use a burr or file to smooth the undersurface of the acromion.

Rotator cuff repair

16. Identify the subacromial bursa and perform a complete subdeltoid bursectomy. Fully rotating the arm exposes the rotator cuff tendons.

17. Assess the size of the rotator cuff tendon tear, the precise rotator cuff tendon anatomy, the shape of the tendon tear, the tendons involved, the degree of tendon retraction, the anterior and posterior extent of the tear, and the quality of the tendon available for repair.

18. Tag the torn edges of the rotator cuff with heavy nonabsorbable suture. Assess the need for mobilization of the tendon.

19. Several methods are useful in mobilizing the rotator cuff

   a. Release and excision of the subacromial and subdeltoid bursa

   b. Release of the coracohumeral ligament, which is a thick band of tissue between the coracoid

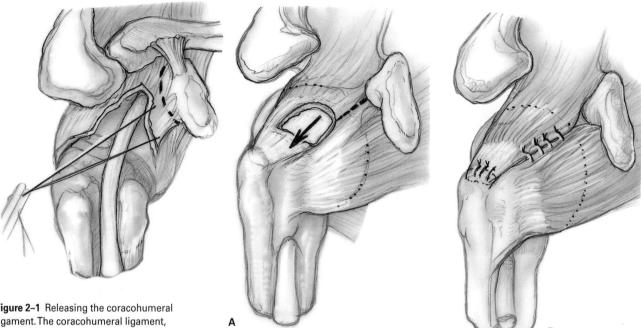

Figure 2–1 Releasing the coracohumeral ligament. The coracohumeral ligament, which is a thick band of tissue between the coracoid process and the supraspinatus tendon, can be released to mobilize the rotator cuff.

A

B

Figure 2–2 (A) Longitudinal releasing incisions. Longitudinal releasing incisions in the anterior tendon (in the rotator interval) or posterior tendon can help to advance the supraspinatus. **(B)** Closure of the interval. The interval is closed after the tendon is repaired to bone.

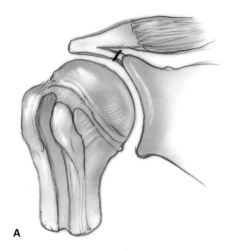

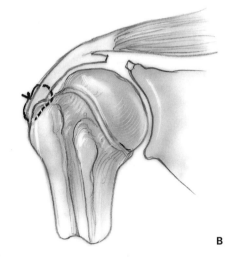

A

B

Figure 2–3 Releasing intra-articular adhesion. In large, chronic tears, consider intra-articular release of the adhesions between the capsule and the rotator cuff. If the tendon is retracted and tethered by the capsule at the glenoid, the capsule is incised. Use a blunt elevator to lift the muscle tendon tissue off the glenoid neck. Take care when dissecting superior and posterior to avoid injuring the suprascapular nerve as it passes through the spinoglenoid notch. **(B)** Intra-articular adhesion release. These steps demonstrate the mobilization, advancement, and repair of the rotator cuff tendon.

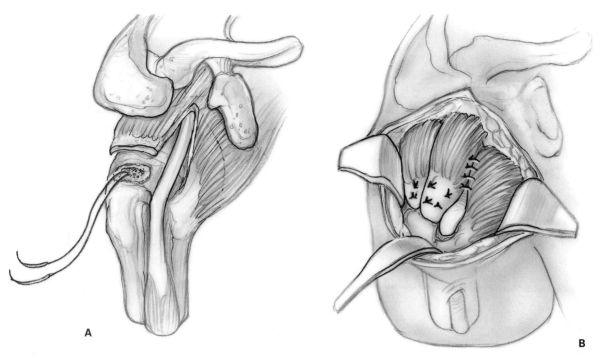

Figure 2–4 (A) Preparation of humeral bed. An area of bone between the articular surface of the humeral head and the greater tuberosity is prepared to serve as the bed for the rotator cuff repair. Use rongeurs, curettes, or a motorized burr to create a bleeding surface to optimize tendon healing. Take care not to create troughs or weaken the cortical bone. After preparation of the "bed" to receive the tendon has been completed, soft tissue anchors are placed approximately 1 cm apart in a staggered fashion. **(B)** Repairing the rotator cuff with suture anchors. The sutures are tied with tension minimized by holding the arm in abduction.

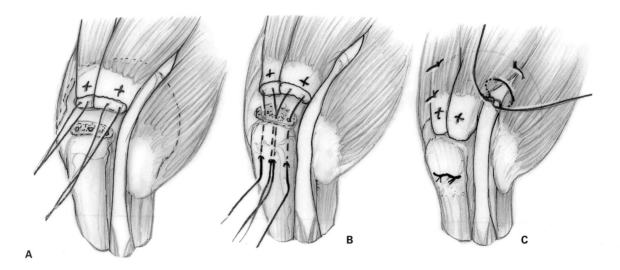

Figure 2–5 (A) Repairing the rotator cuff through bony tunnels. The sutures can be placed through the tendon and passed through bone tunnels from the tuberosity to the lateral cortex. **(B)** Repairing the rotator cuff through bony tunnels. Placement of sutures through bone tunnels with appropriate spacing in the greater tuberosity. **(C)** Repairing the rotator cuff through bony tunnels after final repair and closure of the rotator interval.

process and the insertion of the supraspinatus tendon (**Fig. 2–1**)

c. Longitudinal releasing incisions in the anterior tendon (in the rotator interval) or posterior tendon can help to advance the supraspinatus (**Fig. 2–2**).

d. In large, chronic tears, consider intra-articular release of the adhesions between the capsule and the rotator cuff (**Fig. 2–3**). After sharply releasing the capsule, use a blunt elevator to lift the muscle tendon tissue off the glenoid neck. Take care when dissecting superior and posterior to avoid injuring the suprascapular nerve as it passes through the spinoglenoid notch.

20. Minimally trim the torn tendon so fresh tendon is available for insertion to the bone.

21. Once the tendon has been adequately mobilized, prepare an area of bone between the articular surface of the humeral head and the greater tuberosity to serve as the bed for the rotator cuff repair (**Fig. 2–4A**). Use rongeurs, curettes, or a motorized burr to create a bleeding surface to optimize tendon healing. Take care not to create troughs or weaken the cortical bone.

22. Inspect the biceps tendon. Occasionally if the biceps tendon is completely torn, it can be used to augment deficient and larger rotator cuff tears. If the biceps tendon is significantly degenerated, consider tenodesing it at the bicipital groove.

23. After preparation of the "bed" to receive the tendon has been completed, place soft tissue anchors in the humeral head approximately 1 cm apart in a staggered fashion (**Fig. 2–4A**).

24. Pass nonabsorbable sutures through the tendon in a similar pattern to their placement in the tuberosity bone.

25. Tie the sutures with tension minimized by holding the arm in abduction (**Fig. 2–4B**). Alternatively, place sutures in the tendon and pass them through bone tunnel from the tuberosity to the lateral cortex (**Fig. 2–5A–C**).

26. Once the repair is secure, gently range the shoulder through an arc of motion. Assess the integrity of the repair and the safe postoperative range of motion. If the rotator interval was opened for exposure, close it with absorbable sutures.

27. In patients with a tear of the subscapularis tendon, replace the biceps tendon (if it is intact) in the bicipital groove and stabilize it by securing the cuff on either side of it. Alternatively, the biceps tendon can be tenodesed in the bicipital groove.

Closure

28. Copiously irrigate the wound.

29. Carefully secure the deltoid to the anterior acromion. This is best achieved by making two 1.6-mm drill holes in the acromion, at least 5 mm back from the anterior edge (**see Fig. 1–4**).

30. Repair the deltoid to the acromion. Incorporate both the superficial and deep fascia in the repair using #2 braided nonabsorbable sutures (**see Fig. 1–4**).

31. Close the subcutaneous tissues and skin with a cosmetic subcuticular closure.

32. Apply a sterile dressing. Place the arm in a sling.

Suggested Readings

Iannotti JP, Williams GR Jr. *Disorders of the Shoulder: Diagnosis and Management.* Philadelphia, PA: Lippincott Williams & Wilkins, 1999.

Rockwood CA, Matsen FA. *The Shoulder.* Philadelphia, PA: W.B. Saunders, 1998.

CHAPTER 3

Open Anterior Shoulder Stabilization

Daniel D. Buss and William C. Jacobsen

Indications

1. Recurrent anterior shoulder instability with pain that limits activities

Contraindications

1. Voluntary shoulder instability
2. History of psychiatric disease
3. Active infection
4. Multidirectional shoulder instability or generalized ligamentous laxity (relative)
5. Glenohumeral arthritis (relative)
6. Presence of a large Hill-Sachs lesion or glenoid deficiency may alter approach

Preoperative Preparation

1. Shoulder radiographs

   a. True anteroposterior (AP) view
   b. Axillary lateral view
   c. Consider an AP view with internal rotation of the humerus.
   d. Consider Stryker-notch view.
   e. Consider West Point modified axillary view.
   f. Consider scapular "Y" views.

2. Consider computed tomography (CT) arthrography, magnetic resonance imaging (MRI), or magnetic resonance (MR) arthrogram (if necessary).
3. Assess passive and active range of motion.

4. Document neurovascular examination.
5. Consider diagnostic arthroscopy (if examination under anesthesia [EUA] is not consistent with clinical diagnosis).
6. Appropriate medical and anesthesia preoperative evaluation.

Special Instruments, Position, and Anesthesia

1. Specialized shoulder retractors for soft tissues and humeral head
2. Suture anchors
3. Beach chair position with beanbag
4. If available, a McConnell arm holder is helpful (McConnell Surgical Mfg., Greenville, TX).
5. All pressure points should be well padded.
6. The procedure can be done with regional anesthesia (interscalene block) and/or general anesthesia.

Tips and Pearls

1. Intravenous antibiotics are administered prior to the skin incision.
2. A concealed anterior axillary skin incision is preferred. The arm is adducted across the body after sterile prepping and draping is completed. This helps define the natural axillary skin folds, which can then be marked with a sterile pen.
3. Limit arthroscopy time so that the soft tissues do not become too edematous.

4. EUA is performed to assess the direction and degree of shoulder instability and the results compared with the contralateral shoulder.

What To Avoid

1. Avoid incisions outside the natural skin lines.
2. If possible, avoid injury to the cephalic vein. Commonly, it is preserved and retracted laterally with the deltoid.
3. Attempt to avoid injury to the axillary and musculoskeletal nerves by protecting them at all times.
4. Avoid damaging the glenohumeral articular cartilage.
5. Avoid "overtightening" the shoulder during the capsular shift and/or repair of the subscapularis tendon.

Postoperative Care Issues

1. The neurovascular examination should be performed and documented. The examination may be affected by regional anesthesia in the immediate postoperative period.
2. Consider using an ice and compression device, which helps with swelling and pain control.
3. The shoulder is immobilized in a sling for up to 3 to 4 weeks for comfort only. The patient may use the elbow and hand normally for light activity.
4. Postoperative rehabilitation begins by working on achieving adequate range of shoulder motion, then progresses to strengthening of the shoulder muscles, and finally to a functional program to reestablish proprioception and muscular coordination.
5. Exercises commence with pendulum exercises, forward flexion in the plane of the scapula using pulleys and wands, and passive range-of-motion exercises including external rotation in the predetermined safe zone. The safe zone is determined by the surgeon at the time of surgical repair.
6. Active and active-assisted range-of-motion exercises are started at 4 to 6 weeks postoperatively to strengthen the deltoid, rotator cuff, and scapular muscles.
7. At 3 months postoperatively, therapy is directed at regaining full strength and endurance of the shoulder.

8. At 4 months postoperatively, functional exercises are added.
9. At 4 to 6 months postsurgery, it is possible for the patient to return to sports and to engage in full activity.

Operative Technique

Approach

1. Position the patient supine on the table. Place blankets or pillows under the patient's thighs. Flex the waist approximately 35 degrees, the knees approximately 40 degrees, and the back approximately 20 degrees.
2. With the head and neck in neutral position, contour the beanbag around the patient and deflate the bag.
3. Position the patient so the operative shoulder is pulled to the bed's edge to allow adequate access. Secure the patient to the bed.
4. Prepare and drape the limb in the hospital's standard sterile fashion.
5. Draw the bony landmarks, including the acromion, clavicle, spine of the scapula, and coracoid tip, on the skin.
6. Perform glenohumeral arthroscopy (optional—see Chapter 4 on shoulder arthroscopy).
7. Infiltrate the incision site with a dilute epinephrine solution.
8. Make a 5- to 8-cm incision. Start 2 cm below the coracoid tip and extend the incision down toward the anterior axillary line. Elevate skin flaps to aid retraction (**Fig. 3–1**).
9. Identify the deltopectoral interval and the cephalic vein, which is usually seen as a fat stripe between the deltoid and pectoralis major.
10. Expose and mobilize the cephalic vein. Commonly, dissection is performed on the vein's medial side, which allows the vein to be retracted laterally with the deltoid.
11. Open the deltopectoral interval. Carry the dissection 1 cm proximal to the coracoid tip. Stay lateral to the coracoid.
12. Undermine the deltoid and pectoralis to aid retraction. The upper portion of the pectoralis may have to be released to aid in retraction in well-muscled

individuals. Place a self-retaining retractor under the deltoid and pectoralis.

13. Open the clavipectoral fascia. Identify the lateral edge of the conjoined tendon.

14. Identify the subscapularis tendon, long head of the biceps tendon and lesser tuberosity. Internal and external rotation helps define the subscapularis tendon.

15. Palpate the axillary nerve by sliding your finger down the subscapularis tendon and internally rotate the arm when you reach the inferior border of the subscapularis. This is known as the "tug test."

16. Protect the axillary nerve with a retractor.

17. Identify the rotator interval. The superior edge of the subscapularis is at the rotator interval and the anterior humeral circumflex vessels ("three sisters") mark the inferior edge. Expose and cauterize these vessels.

18. With the arm externally rotated, divide the subscapularis tendon in its midportion. Typically this is at a point 1 to 1.5 cm medial to the lesser tuberosity. Carry the dissection down to but not through the shoulder capsule. The fibers of the tendon run transversely. The tendon can be divided completely or partially (**Fig. 3–2**).

19. Place stay sutures along the edge of the tendon (**Fig. 3–3**).

20. Define the plane between the subscapularis and capsule. Using a Cobb elevator, separate the muscle and capsule medially and tendon and capsule laterally.

21. Evaluate the rotator interval. It will need to be closed later if it is widened or electively opened.

Procedure

22. Perform an arthrotomy. This can be done either laterally (humeral) or medially (glenoid) (**Fig. 3–4**).

23. Carry the arthrotomy down to the humeral attachment. Use a periosteal elevator to elevate the capsule off the anterior glenoid.

24. For a lateral arthrotomy, elevate the capsule off the humerus inferiorly in a similar fashion. Do not incise the capsule too inferiorly, that is, through the axillary pouch. This will result in an ineffective shift of the inferior capsule.

25. If there is excessive inferior capsular redundancy, it may be necessary to make a "T" incision. This allows a superior shift of the inferior capsule. The "T" should be made between the inferior and middle glenohumeral ligaments.

26. The advantages of the lateral versus medial arthrotomy are described by Bigliani (1996).

27. Use a humeral head retractor to help visualize the glenoid.

28. Evaluate the labrum to determine if reattachment is needed.

29. Roughen the anterior glenoid neck with a curette. Consider "rose-pedaling" the area with a small osteotome.

30. Evaluate the joint for loose bodies, articular cartilage damage, and humeral head defects.

Labral reattachment

31. We prefer suture anchors for labral reattachment. This can also be accomplished with transosseous drill holes.

32. Place suture anchors along the glenoid rim at the 7, 9, and 11 o'clock position for the left shoulder and at the 1, 3, and 5 o'clock position for the right shoulder (**Fig. 3–5**).

33. If a Bankart lesion is present, pass both suture limbs of each anchor through the labrum and tie them down. If desired, these can be passed through the "shifted" capsule.

34. For a medial arthrotomy, shift the capsule superiorly as far as possible and medially 2 to 3 mm.

35. For the lateral arthrotomy, the capsule is shifted superiorly and laterally.

36. Use the stay sutures placed along the edges of the capsule to pull it in the desired direction.

37. Reattach the edges of the shifted capsule to the capsular edge not involved in the shift with a nonabsorbable suture on a noncutting needle.

38. For the "T" incision, the inferior capsule is shifted as described above. The superior limb is then brought inferiorly and medially for the medial arthrotomy and inferiorly and laterally for the lateral arthrotomy. These arthrotomies are reattached similarly.

39. Proper arm position is important to ensure that the capsular shift is effective and allows adequate shoulder function. Place the arm in approximately 20 degrees of external rotation and abduction and 10 degrees of forward flexion. For overhead athletes, consider positioning the arm with slightly greater external rotation and abduction.

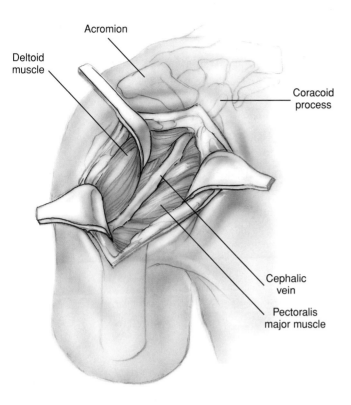

Figure 3–1 Skin incision and subcutaneous exposure.

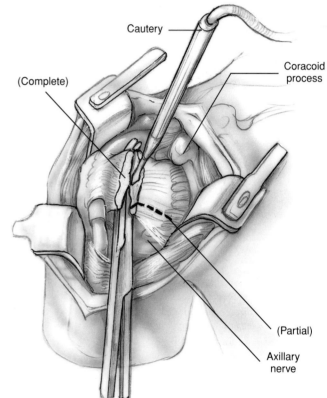

Figure 3–2 Deep exposure depicting a complete or a partial tenotomy of the subscapularis tendon.

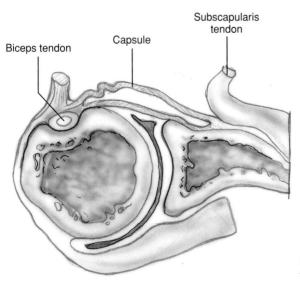

Figure 3–3 Axial view of the cut subscapularis tendon and underlying capsule.

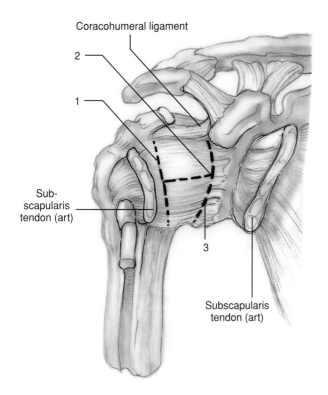

Coracohumeral ligament

2

1

Sub-
scapularis
tendon (art)

3

Subscapularis
tendon (art)

Figure 3–4 Capsular incisions. (1) "T" based off the humeral side (lateral shift). (2) "T" based off the glenoid side (medial shift). (3) Medial arthrotomy without a shift.

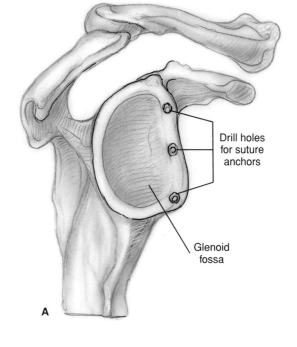

Drill holes
for suture
anchors

Glenoid
fossa

A

Figure 3–5 (A) Correct position for transosseous drill holes for a repair of a Bankart lesion. **(B)** Axial view of the correct position for intraosseous anchors.

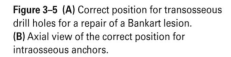
Anchor

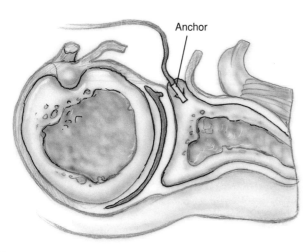

B

Closure

40. Thoroughly irrigate the wound with antibiotic irrigation.
41. Ensure adequate hemostasis has been achieved.
42. A drain is usually not necessary.
43. Remove all retractors. Repeat the "tug-test" to verify continuity and mobility of the axillary nerve.
44. If necessary, close the rotator interval.
45. Reapproximate the subscapularis tendon with the arm in slight external rotation to avoid loss of external rotation. Nonabsorbable suture is preferred.
46. If the pectoralis was released, reapproximate it with a single, nonabsorbable suture.
47. Close the deltopectoral interval with absorbable sutures. Protect the cephalic vein.
48. Close the subcutaneous tissue with absorbable suture.
49. Close the skin with staples or a running subcuticular stitch and steristrips.
50. Apply a sterile compressive dressing.
51. Place the arm in a sling device. Transfer the patient to the recovery room.

Suggested Readings

Bigliani, Louis U, eds. *The Unstable Shoulder*. Rosemont, IL: American Academy of Orthopaedic Surgery, 1996.

Craig, EV, ed. The shoulder. *Master Techniques in Orthopedic Surgery*. New York, NY: Raven, 1995.

Rowe CR, Patel D, Southmayd WW. The Bankart procedure. *J Bone Joint Surg* 1978;60A:1–16.

CHAPTER 4

Shoulder Arthroscopy

Daniel D. Buss and John R. Green III

Indications

1. Loose body
2. Foreign body
3. Labral tear
4. Impingement syndrome
5. Instability
6. Acromioclavicular arthritis
7. Infection
8. Diagnostic dilemma

Contraindications

1. Acute adjacent soft tissue injury resulting in risk of neurovascular compromise from fluid extravasation (relative)

Preoperative Preparation

1. Shoulder radiographs including true anteroposterior (Grashe), outlet or "Y," and axillary views; Stryker-notch view is also obtained for patients with instability symptoms.
2. Consider magnetic resonance imaging (MRI) to confirm diagnoses.
3. Document preoperative neurovascular examination of upper extremity.

Special Instruments, Position, and Anesthesia

1. Beach chair position on full-body beanbag.

   a. Keep head midline with neck in neutral or slightly flexed position.
   b. Protract the scapula, which exposes the medial border of the scapula. Drape the shoulder free from the medial border of the scapula posteriorly to the midline of the clavicle anteriorly (**Fig. 4–1**).

2. Alternatively, consider using the modified lateral decubitus position which aligns the glenoid surface horizontal. The arm is slightly forward flexed and abducted 50 degrees with 10 to 15 lb of longitudinal suspension applied from a traction tower.
3. All pressure points should be padded, particularly the peroneal nerve.
4. The procedure can be performed with general and/or scalene block anesthesia.
5. Routine arthroscopy equipment is required for diagnostic arthroscopy. Additional specialized instrumentation is necessary for each operative procedure. Open shoulder instrumentation should be available.

Tips and Pearls

1. Perform a physical examination under anesthesia to assess shoulder stability and range of motion.

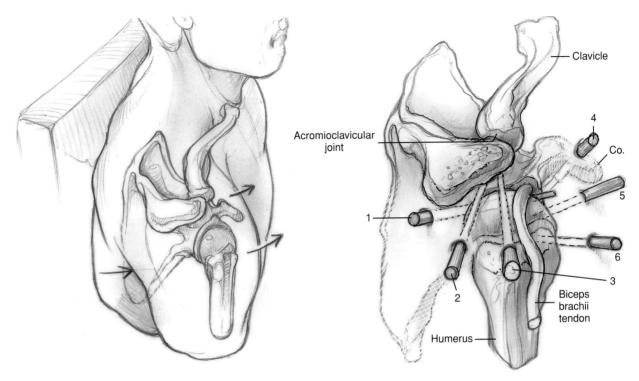

Figure 4–1 Patient position. Superior view of the shoulder in the beach chair position before draping. Note the exposure and scapular protraction.

Figure 4–2 Portals and vectors. Closeup superior view of shoulder demonstrating portal placement in relation to bony landmarks. 1—posterior portal, 2—lateral portal, 3—superolateral portal, 4—anterior superior portal, 5—anterior inferior portal, 6—5 o'clock portal.

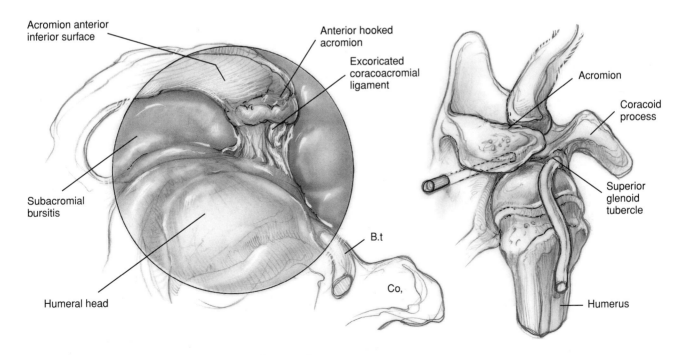

Figure 4–3 (A) Arthroscopic view of subacromial space demonstrating anterior hooked acromion, excoriated coracoacromial ligament, and subacromial bursitis.

21

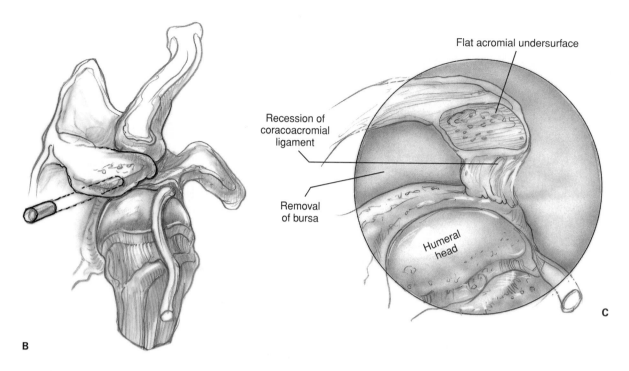

Flat acromial undersurface

Recession of coracoacromial ligament

Removal of bursa

Humeral head

B

C

Figure 4–3 *(Continued)* **(B)** Arthroscopic view of vector into subacromial space. **(C)** Arthroscopic view of subacromial space after decompression. Note the flattening of the undersurface of the acromion, recession of the coracoacromial ligament, and removal of the subacromial bursa.

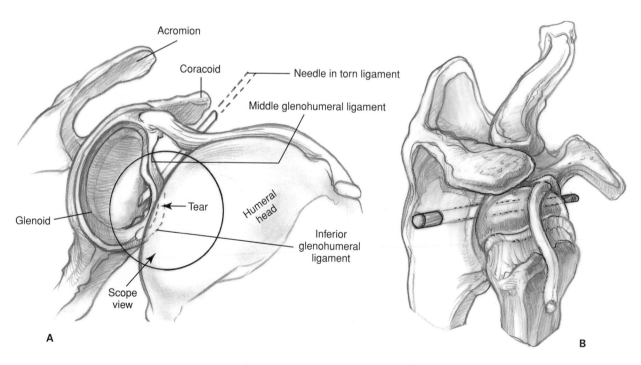

Acromion

Coracoid

Needle in torn ligament

Middle glenohumeral ligament

Tear

Humeral head

Glenoid

Inferior glenohumeral ligament

Scope view

A

B

Figure 4–4 **(A)** Arthroscopic view of Bankart lesion. **(B)** Arthroscopic view of vector into glenohumeral joint.

22

2. Drawing landmarks on the skin can help facilitate accurate portal placement.

3. Routine intravenous antibiotics should be administered prior to incision.

4. Confirm placement of the posterior portal with an 18-gauge 3½-in spinal needle. Distend the glenohumeral joint with 20 cc of 0.5% bupivicaine with epinephrine.

5. Infiltrate the portal sites with 0.5% bupivicaine with epinephrine.

6. Consider relative hypotensive anesthesia because this decreases intraoperative bleeding, thereby permitting lower fluid pressures which helps minimize fluid extravasation.

What To Avoid

1. Avoid chondral injury by using blunt obturators to enter the joint under careful control. Do not plunge!

2. Avoid inadvertent rotator cuff tendon tears during posterior portal placement by internal rotation of the humerus.

3. Minimize risk of neurovascular injury by placing the anterior portal lateral to the coracoid and keeping the humerus adducted when creating anterior portals.

Postoperative Care Issues

1. Use a sling with a 6-in elastic bandage wrapped around the body. The elastic bandage can be removed when the scalene block has worn off.

2. After arthroscopic shoulder decompression, the sling is removed after 2 days, and early active, active-assisted, and passive range-of-motion exercises are begun. In addition, isotonic rotator cuff strengthening and scapular stabilization exercises are also begun. The goal is full, active, pain-free range of motion 4 weeks after surgery.

3. After an arthroscopic Bankart repair, the sling is worn for 4 weeks. During this time, elbow range-of-motion exercises, squeezing a tennis ball for grip, co-contracture of the biceps and triceps, and pendulum exercises are instituted. At 4 weeks, isometric rotator cuff strengthening and active, active-assisted,

and passive range-of-motion exercises are begun. External rotation is limited to 20 degrees until 6 weeks after surgery. At 6 weeks, the patient begins isotonic strengthening exercises. Heavy lifting and throwing programs are deferred until 4 months after surgery.

Operative Technique

1. Position the patient supine on the table. Place blankets or pillows under the patient's thighs. Flex the waist approximately 35 degrees, the knees approximately 40 degrees, and the back approximately 40 degrees.

2. With the head and neck in neutral position, contour the beanbag around the patient and deflate the bag.

3. Position the patient so the operative shoulder is pulled to the bed's edge to allow adequate access. Secure the patient to the bed.

4. Prepare and drape the limb in the hospital's standard sterile fashion.

5. Draw the bony landmarks, including the acromion, clavicle, spine of the scapula, and coracoid tip, on the skin.

Diagnostic arthroscopy—posterior portal

6. Place the posterior portal in the "soft spot" between the infraspinatus, teres minor, and edge of deltoid. This is located 2 to 3 cm inferior and 1 to 2 cm medial to the posterolateral corner of the acromion. Localize the plane of the glenoid with an 18-gauge spinal needle. Enter the joint using a blunt obturator (Fig. 4–2).

7. Establish intra-articular orientation with the arthroscope looking straight inferior (the light cord facing straight up) by viewing the biceps tendon's insertion into the superior labrum and the plane of the glenoid. The inflow is through the arthroscope sheath.

8. Insert the arthroscope deeper into the shoulder to visualize the subscapularis tendon.

9. Rotate the arthroscope medially to view the subscapularis recess.

10. Rotate the arthroscope laterally to follow the subscapularis tendon. Visualize the undersurface of the biceps tendon, the superior glenohumeral ligament

crossing between the subscapularis tendon and the long head of the biceps tendon, and the transverse ligament securing the biceps tendon in the bicipital groove.

11. Retract the arthroscope and examine the anterior labrum. Externally rotate the humerus to accentuate and visualize the middle glenohumeral ligament.

12. "Drive through" the joint into the axillary recess by inserting the arthroscope deeper while rotating it to look inferiorly. Inspect the anterior band of the inferior glenohumeral ligament. The arthroscope's tip should be anterior to the articular surface to minimize the risk of abrasion.

13. Rotate the arthroscope to look superior. Raise the camera to view the inferior labrum and the humeral insertion of the anterior band of the inferior glenohumeral ligament.

14. Follow the labrum posteriorly, externally rotate the humerus to improve visualization.

15. Continue following the labrum superiorly. Examine the superior glenohumeral recess with the humerus abducted 20 to 30 degrees.

16. Follow the superior surface of the biceps tendon laterally. Forward flex the patient's arm slightly and begin abducting and externally rotating the humerus. Examine the supraspinatus tendon's insertion on to the greater tuberosity.

17. Visualize the insertion of the entire rotator cuff from greater tuberosity to axillary recess by slowly internally rotating the humerus and withdrawing the arthroscope. The bare area on the posterolateral humeral head is seen adjacent to the posterior cuff insertion. Minimize the risk of iatrogenic articular cartilage injury by using gentle pressure to keep the tip of the arthroscope off the chondral surface.

18. External rotation assists in viewing the articular surface of the posterior humeral head. A Hill-Sachs lesion is found on the superior posterolateral humeral head. Inspect the remaining humeral surface by internally rotating the arm.

Diagnostic arthroscopy—anterior portal

➤ An anterior portal is indicated to visualize posterior shoulder pathology. It provides the best view of the middle glenohumeral ligament and anterior labrum. Optimal position for the anterior portal depends upon the procedure being performed. A more superior position is desirable for stabilizing a superior labral tear or debriding a partial thickness rotator cuff tear, while a more inferior position is beneficial for performing an anterior capsulolabral repair, and a more medial position is advantageous for excising the distal clavicle excision (**Fig. 4–2**).

19. Evaluate the area between the subscapularis tendon and the supraspinatus tendon (rotator interval). Under direct vision insert an 18-gauge 3½-in spinal needle into this triangle passing the needle tip below the biceps tendon. The external entry point is generally midway between the coracoid and the anterior acromion. If an anterior portal is indicated, insert a cannula with a blunt obturator at the same angle as the spinal needle. If there is no indication for an anterior portal, use this needle to probe the superior labral attachment (**Fig. 4–2**). Alternatively, an anterior portal may also be made from inside-out. Drive the arthroscope anteriorly against the capsule in the triangle formed by the humeral head, glenoid, and biceps tendon. Remove the arthroscope from its sheath and insert a Wissinger rod or switching stick through the cannula so it can be palpated under the skin. Incise the tented skin with a scalpel. Pass a cannula over the rod into the joint (**Fig. 4–2**).

Diagnostic arthroscopy—subacromial space

20. Approach the subacromial space using the same skin incision as the posterior portal for the glenohumeral arthroscopy. With a blunt obturator in place, withdraw the arthroscopic sheath from the glenohumeral joint. Direct it superiorly in the subcutaneous tissue along the undersurface of the acromion until it rests against the coracoacromial ligament. Err on the side of scraping superiorly against the inferior acromion rather than inferiorly against the rotator cuff. Withdraw the cannula 1 cm, insert the arthroscope, and turn on the inflow through the arthroscopic sheath.

21. Initial visualization can sometimes be difficult in the presence of subacromial bursa pathology. In this situation, pass a switching stick through the arthroscopic cannula and out the anterior portal. Pass a second cannula over the rod anteriorly into the subacromial space. This cannula passes just

medial to the coracoacromial ligament. Insert a motorized shaver through the anterior cannula to clear away tissue and improve visualization in the subacromial space.

22. Diagnostic arthroscopy of the subacromial space includes assessment of the subacromial bursa, coracoacromial ligament, acromion, and outer surface of the rotator cuff. If indicated, dissect medially through a small fibrofatty layer to expose the undersurface of the acromioclavicular joint and the distal clavicle.

Arthroscopic subacromial decompression

➤ Always perform a diagnostic arthroscopy of the glenohumeral joint to rule out intra-articular causes of shoulder pain.

➤ Typical subacromial arthroscopic findings in impingement syndrome include bursal thickening, inflammation, or fibrosis, coracoacromial ligament thickening or excoriation, and subacromial spurring (**Fig. 4–3A**).

a. Place the arthroscope in the posterior portal and the inflow so it runs through an anterior portal (**Fig. 4–3B**).

b. Use a needle localization technique under direct vision to create a lateral portal. Start the needle approximately 2 cm distal to the lateral border of the acromion in the sagittal plane of the posterior aspect of the acromioclavicular joint (**Fig. 4–2**).

c. Work through a lateral portal. Alternate use of the electrocautery and motorized shaver to remove bursal tissue.

d. Cut across the soft tissue on the anterior half of the undersurface of the acromion in a cross-hatch fashion with the electrocautery. Remove the soft tissue with the motorized shaver.

e. Incise the coracoacromial ligament with the electrocautery from lateral to medial at its attachment to the anterior acromion. Minimize bleeding by staying close to bone. After the ligament is completely released from its acromial attachment, it will recess approximately 3 to 4 mm.

f. Perform an acromioplasty with a 6.0 oval burr. Resect bone starting from the lateral portal to remove the acromial hook in the sagittal plane.

Continue the resection to the level of the anterior aspect of the acromioclavicular joint.

g. Pass the burr over a switching stick to the posterior portal while viewing from the lateral portal. Flatten the inferior surface of the acromion with the burr. Minimize bone resection to the amount required to remove the anterior hook and flatten the undersurface to preserve the deltoid attachment.

h. With the patient's arm in 120 degrees of forward flexion, assess the adequacy of the decompression with a probe. If a question remains regarding the extent of the decompression, enlarge the lateral portal to facilitate introduction of a finger to manually palpate the acromion.

Arthroscopic anterior stabilization

➤ Always perform a diagnostic arthroscopy of the glenohumeral joint to rule out intra-articular causes of shoulder pain.

➤ The typical lesion in anterior instability is a detached anterior-inferior glenohumeral ligament with or without a detached labrum (Bankart lesion). You should evaluate the subscapularis and capsuloligamentous tissue for intrasubstance injury. If the anterior capsule is either absent or markedly attenuated, or a significant bone fragment has avulsed from the inferior glenoid (bony Bankart lesion), perform an alternative procedure (**Fig. 4–4A**).

➤ The goal of repair is to advance capsular tissue superiorly and medially, generally 3 to 4 mm. Doing so recreates a capsulolabral rim of tissue that is securely fixed as close as possible to the articular surface of the glenoid. The amount of imbrication depends upon the distance from the glenoid fixation point that the tissue is pierced by a suture or tack (up to 2 to 3 cm in extremely lax capsules). This can be accomplished by a variety of techniques including absorbable tacks or suture anchors, and generally proceeds from inferior (most difficult) to superior. Three points of fixation are routine with the exact number being determined by the extent and pattern of the lesion, and assessment of repair security.

➤ Consider rotator interval plication for shoulders with significant inferior laxity with the arm adducted (positive sulcus sign) during the initial examination under anesthesia.

   a. Use a needle localization technique (outside-in) under direct vision to create a superolateral portal. Insert the needle through the lateral edge of the rotator interval adjacent to the biceps tendon. Use this portal to view glenoid preparation, pass sutures, and place superior fixation (Fig. 4–4B).
   b. Place an anterior inferior portal at the inferior edge of the rotator interval using either an outside-in or inside-out technique. This portal should enter the skin just lateral to the coracoid and penetrate the joint just above the subscapularis tendon. Alternatively, create a more inferior portal from inside-out at the 5 o'clock position. Penetrate the subscapularis tendon as lateral as possible just superior to the anterior band of the inferior glenohumeral ligament. Keep the arm adducted during placement of all anterior portals to minimize danger to the musculocutaneous nerve. The cannulae should be large enough (8 mm) to accommodate instruments and threaded to prevent dislodgment.
   c. Prepare the glenoid neck with an arthroscopic elevator. Rasp this region down to bleeding bone. If sclerotic bone is encountered, use a small round motorized burr. Remove soft tissue debris with a motorized shaver.

Suture anchor technique

➤ The exact procedure for implanting specific suture anchors should be checked with the manufacturer's suggested technique manual. Insertion of some suture anchors requires predrilling.

➤ There are a variety of arthroscopic knots, which when well tied, provide secure fixation. Because they are all technically demanding to tie, you should practice them in the laboratory prior to surgery. Generally, knots are best seated by pushing past the knot with the knot pusher. Commonly, three alternating post, reversed half-hitches are placed to reinforce arthroscopic slipknots.

   a. Place the arthroscope in the more superior anterior portal. Place anchors through the more inferior cannula.

   b. Place the first suture anchor along the glenoid neck adjacent to the articular surface. Generally, the position of this anchor is as close as possible to the 6 o'clock position.
   c. Move the arthroscope to the posterior portal. Take both ends of the suture out the more superior anterior portal. Tag them with a hemostat.
   d. Assess anchor fixation by firmly pulling on both ends of the suture.
   e. Commonly, place additional anchors near the 2 and 4 o'clock positions. Adjust these positions as needed based on the location of the pathology.
   f. After each anchor is inserted, pull the sutures out the more superior anterior portal. Tag them with a hemostat. Assess anchor fixation by firmly pulling on both ends of the suture.
   g. Starting inferiorly, pull one suture limb into the inferior cannula with a crochet hook. Then pass it though the tissue under the labrum, inferior and lateral to the anchor, using a suture hook or suture punch. The amount of tissue imbricated depends upon the degree of soft tissue laxity present.
   h. Pass the other suture limb in a similar manner to create a horizontal mattress stitch. Alternatively, directly pull the suture out through the inferior cannula and tie it to form a simple stitch.
   i. Pass the knot pusher down one of the suture limbs to ensure no twists are present. Tie an arthroscopic knot outside the cannula. Seat it with a knot pusher.
   j. Test the knot's security with a probe. Cut the suture ends to prevent entanglement with other sutures.
   k. If needed, pass additional sutures through the capsulolabral tissue. Tie, test, and cut these in a similar fashion.

Absorbable tack technique

➤ The sequence of tack placement is also from inferior to superior.

   a. Position the arthroscope in the more superior anterior portal. Use the inferior portal as a working portal.
   b. Spear the capsulolabral tissue with a guide pin that protrudes 2 to 3 mm from the drill. The

distance from where the tissue is speared to where it is fixed determines the amount of soft tissue imbricated in the repair.

c. Advance the tissue superiorly and to the glenoid margin.

d. Insert the drill to the appropriate depth. Remove it leaving the guide wire in place.

e. Advance the absorbable tack over the wire. Seat it in position. Remove the guide wire.

f. Assess the security of the suture fixation by applying gentle pressure with a probe.

g. Visualize the tack from the anterior inferior portal. Recheck the tack's position and plan the appropriate insertion site for the next tack.

h. Place additional tacks superiorly. Commonly, these are near the 4 and 2 o'clock positions.

Capsular tightening

➤ Because a certain amount of capsular stretch injury occurs with a Bankart lesion, and patients have variable degrees of capsular laxity, capsulolabral repair even with tissue advancement may not completely stabilize the shoulder. Consider rotator interval plication for shoulders with significant inferior laxity with the arm adducted (positive sulcus sign) during the initial examination under anesthesia. Imbrication of the rotator interval is best performed prior to anterior capsulolabral repair so that the arm can be held in external rotation during the repair.

➤ Thermal capsulorrhaphy, although still a relatively new procedure with no long-term outcome studies, can be a helpful adjunct to arthroscopic anterior reconstruction by selective tissue shrinkage. It is best performed after capsulolabral repair and rotator interval plication are completed.

Arthroscopic rotator interval plication

➤ This procedure is best performed prior to arthroscopic Bankart repair.

a. Place the arthroscope in the posterior portal. Suturing is performed through the superolateral portal.

b. Place a suture with a suture hook angled at 45 degrees. Insert it between the superior glenohumeral ligament and the superior aspect of the middle glenohumeral ligament just lateral to

the glenoid. Pass the suture with the arm externally rotated.

c. Tie an arthroscopic knot and cut the suture ends.

d. Place a second, more lateral, suture in a similar fashion.

Thermal capsulorrhaphy

➤ This procedure is best performed after arthroscopic rotator interval and Bankart repair, when a persistent "drive-through sign" is present.

a. Vary the portals used depending on the pattern of persistent laxity. Commonly, the arthroscope is in the posterior portal and the thermal probe in the superolateral portal.

b. Treat lax areas of capsule, including the repaired tissue, by slowly passing the thermal probe over the tissue a single time with light pressure, as if painting.

Suggested Readings

Caspari RB, Thal R. A technique for arthroscopic subacromial decompression. *Arthroscopy* 1992;8(1):23–30.

Davidson PA, Tibone JE. Anterior-inferior (5 o'clock) portal for shoulder arthroscopy. *Arthroscopy* 1995;11(5):519–525.

Ellman H, Harris E, Kay SP. Early degenerative joint disease simulating impingement syndrome: arthroscopic findings. *Arthroscopy* 1992;8(4):482–487.

Gross RM, Fitzgibbons TC. Shoulder arthroscopy: a modified approach. *Arthroscopy* 1985;1(3):156–159.

Laurencin CT, Deutsch A, O'Brien SJ, et al. The superolateral portal for arthroscopy of the shoulder. *Arthroscopy* 1994;10(3):255–258.

Morrison DS, Schaefer RK, Friedman RL. The relationship between subacromial space pressure, blood pressure, and visual clarity during arthroscopic subacromial decompression. *Arthroscopy* 1995;11(5):557–560.

Skyhar MJ, Altchek DW, Warren RF, et al. Shoulder arthroscopy in the beach-chair position. *Arthroscopy* 1988;4(4):256–259.

Torpey BM, Ikeda K, Wang M, et al. The deltoid muscle origin: histologic characteristics and effects of subacromial decompression. *Am J Sports Med* 1998;26(3):379–383.

Warner JJ, Kann S, Maddox LM. The "arthroscopic impingement test". *Arthroscopy* 1994;10(2):224–230.

Wolf EM. Anterior portals in shoulder arthroscopy. *Arthroscopy* 1989;5(3):201–208.

CHAPTER 5

Proximal Humerus Fracture

Open Reduction and Internal Fixation

Angelo DiFelice and Gordon W. Nuber

Indications

1. Proximal humerus fracture with displacement of fracture fragments greater than 1 cm or 45 degrees of fracture angulation as described by Neer (1970)
2. Unstable fracture reductions
3. Irreducible fracture dislocation
4. Displaced tuberosity fracture
5. Three- or four-part fracture in younger patients
6. Open fracture
7. Fracture with an associated vascular injury

Contraindications

1. Poor bone quality (relative)
2. Patients with a guarded overall medical condition and poor rehabilitation potential (relative)
3. Marked deltoid dysfunction (relative)

Preoperative Preparation

1. Shoulder radiographs (trauma series) to include an AP shoulder view, an AP scapular view (Grashey view), and an axillary view
2. If needed, CT scan to define articular surface defects or assess reduction of the glenohumeral joint
3. Document status of preoperative neurovascular examination.

Special Instruments, Position, and Anesthesia

1. The patient is placed in the semi-sitting position (30 degrees upright).
2. All pressure points should be padded.
3. The procedure can be done with general or interscalene block anesthesia.
4. Trauma fixation sets should be available. These should include small and large fragment sets, as well as modified Enders rods.
5. Fluoroscopy should be available.

Tips and Pearls

1. Be sure to drape the entire shoulder girdle and arm free.
2. Check that the fracture can be adequately evaluated with the fluoroscopy prior to prepping the patient. If needed, adjust the patient accordingly.
3. Administer intravenous antibiotics prior to beginning the operation.

What To Avoid

1. Avoid excessive stripping of fracture fragments.
2. Avoid making shallow holes for the heavy suture or wire in the humeral shaft and tuberosities.

Postoperative Care Issues

1. A suction-type drain can be used and normally discontinued the morning after surgery.
2. A compressive dressing should be placed at the end of surgery and is normally changed approximately 48 hours after the procedure.
3. Assessment of the patient's distal neurovascular examination should be made the evening of surgery.
4. Early motion should be employed based on the stability of the fixation construct and the quality of the patient's bone.
5. Initiate three phases of rehabilitation based on 4- to 6-week intervals:

   a. *Phase 1.* Patient is allowed to come out of the brace and begin pendulum exercises, and saw and tummy rub exercises
   b. *Phase 2.* Patient works with a therapist to begin active-assistive exercises and more aggressive passive range-of-motion exercises
   c. *Phase 3.* Once radiographic evidence of healing is noted, resistive and stretching exercises for the rotator cuff muscles are instituted

Operative Technique

Approach

1. Place the patient in the semi-sitting position (30 degrees upright) on the operating room table.
2. Place a small bump under the operative scapula to help access the entire shoulder girdle.
3. Make a standard deltopectoral incision. Open the deltopectoral interval and mobilize the cephalic vein laterally.
4. Retract the deltoid muscle laterally. If needed, partially release the deltoid at its insertion.
5. If additional exposure is required, release the coracoacromial ligament proximally and partially release the pectoralis major tendon distally. The pectoralis tendon should be repaired at the time of wound closure with heavy nonabsorbable suture.
6. Identify the long head of the biceps. This structure helps outline the fracture pattern and serves as a guide to fracture reduction (**Fig. 5–1**).

Reduction and fixation

7. Mobilize the fracture fragments. Take care to preserve bone fragment vascularity by avoiding extensive soft tissue dissection.
8. Place stay sutures in the fracture fragments. Inspect the humeral head for impaction or malposition.
9. Consider using a Cobb elevator to reduce the humeral head into the glenoid and to clear the fracture site of hematoma.
10. Reduce the fracture fragments. If needed, provisionally hold them in place with 0.062 K-wires.
11. After the humeral head is reduced, make two drill holes through the anterior aspect of the humeral shaft on each side of the bicipital groove (**Fig. 5–2A**).
12. Drill a 2-mm hole through the greater tuberosity and lesser tuberosity (**Fig. 5–2B**).
13. Use a 14-gauge angiocath as a guide for either an 18-gauge wire or a #5 braided nonabsorbable suture. Place the wire or suture through a hole in the anterior aspect of the humeral shaft (**Fig. 5–3**).
14. Use a 14-gauge angiocath as a guide for passing the previously positioned 18-gauge wire or #5 braided nonabsorbable suture through the rotator cuff tendon, greater tuberosity, subscapularis, and lesser tuberosity.
15. Ensure that the humeral head is reduced on the shaft and the tuberosities are anatomically reduced. Using the biceps and bicipital groove as landmarks, fix the suture or wire in a figure eight fashion.
16. After tensioning of the suture is complete, place a second wire or suture in a similar tension band technique, thereby securing the tuberosities to the humeral shaft (**Fig. 5–4**).
17. Ensure that the wires or sutures cross the fracture site. This allows them to apply compression and helps achieve a stable construct that moves as a unit (**Fig. 5–5**).

Closure

18. Loosely approximate the deltopectoral interval with an absorbable suture.
19. Close the subcutaneous tissue in layers over a suction drainage.
20. Close the skin using a subcuticular skin closure. Apply steristrips.

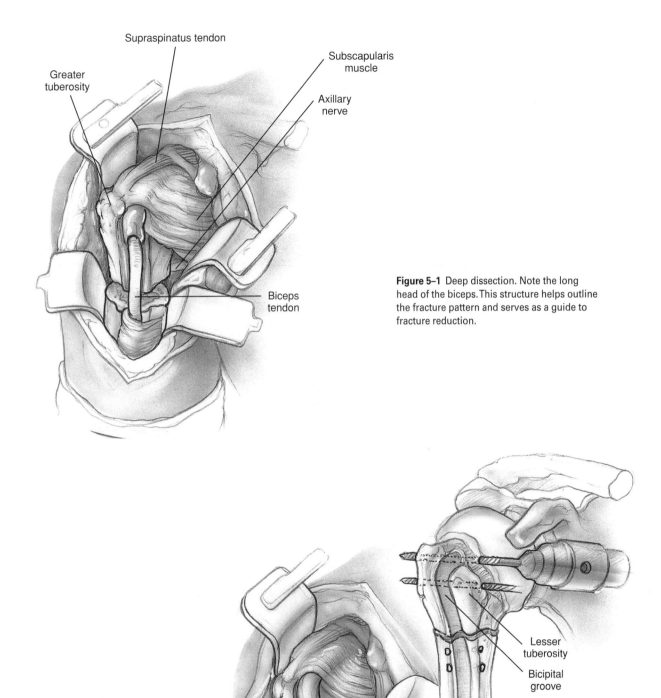

Figure 5–1 Deep dissection. Note the long head of the biceps. This structure helps outline the fracture pattern and serves as a guide to fracture reduction.

Figure 5–2 (A) Humeral drill holes. Two drill holes are made through the anterior aspect of the humeral shaft. They are positioned on each side of the bicipital groove. **(B)** Proximal drill holes. Two drill holes are made through the greater tuberosity and lesser tuberosity.

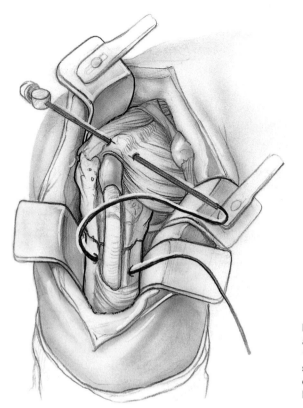

Figure 5–3 Wire or suture passage. A 14-gauge angiocath is used as a guide for either an 18-gauge wire or a #5 braided nonabsorbable suture. The wire or suture is passed through one of the holes in the anterior aspect of the humeral shaft.

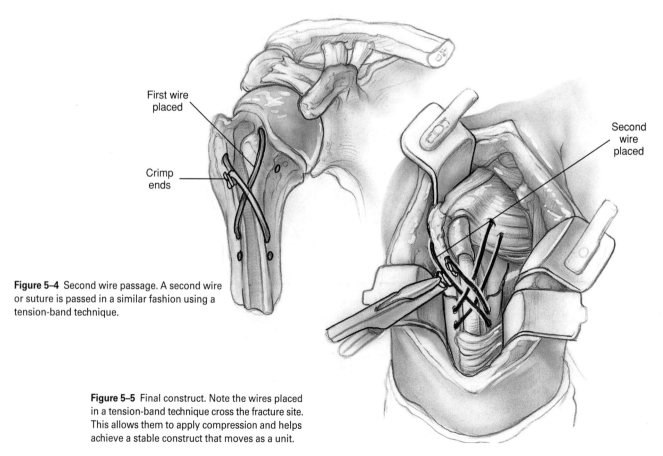

First wire placed

Crimp ends

Second wire placed

Figure 5–4 Second wire passage. A second wire or suture is passed in a similar fashion using a tension-band technique.

Figure 5–5 Final construct. Note the wires placed in a tension-band technique cross the fracture site. This allows them to apply compression and helps achieve a stable construct that moves as a unit.

Suggested Readings

Neer CS. Displaced proximal humerus fractures. I. Classification and evaluation. *J Bone Joint Surg* 1970;52A(6):1077–1089.

The shoulder. In: Hoppenfeld S, deBoer P, eds. *Surgical Exposures in Orthopaedics: The Anatomic Approach.* 2nd ed. Philadelphia, PA: J.B. Lippincott, 1994:5–13.

CHAPTER 6

Proximal Humerus Fracture

Hemiarthroplasty

Mark K. Bowen and Angelo DiFelice

Indications

1. Four-part proximal humerus fractures and fracture dislocations of the proximal humerus
2. Humeral head splitting fractures
3. Displaced anatomic humeral neck fractures that cannot be adequately reduced or fixed
4. Chronic shoulder dislocations with impaction fractures involving greater than 40% of the humeral head's articular surface
5. Selected three-part proximal humerus fractures in older patients with osteoporotic bone

Contraindications

1. Soft tissue infection
2. Chronic osteomyelitis
3. Paralysis of the rotator cuff muscles
4. Deltoid muscle paralysis (relative)

Preoperative Preparation

1. Perform a complete history. Attempt to determine the cause of the fracture. Obtain pertinent medical history including history of seizures or syncope. Consider metastatic disease.
2. Document the preoperative neurovascular status of the limb, especially the axillary nerve.
3. Obtain radiographs (shoulder trauma series)
   a. Anteroposterior (AP) in plane of scapula ("true AP")
   b. Transscapular lateral
   c. Axillary view
   d. AP and lateral of the unaffected shoulder to assist with templating
4. Templates of the prosthesis to be implanted
5. If needed, obtain computed tomography (CT) scan to assess degree of fracture displacement or to evaluate the humeral head's articular surface in head splitting fractures or chronic dislocations.

Special Instruments, Position, and Anesthesia

1. Patient is placed in a modified beach chair position with head up 20 to 30 degrees. Position patient so the involved shoulder extends over the edge of the table to allow free humeral extension and rotation **(Fig. 6–1)**. The head should be stabilized in a neutral position to avoid traction on the brachial plexus. The McConnell head holder (McConnell Surgical Mfg., Greenville, TX) facilitates stable positioning of the patient.
2. Routine orthopaedic surgical instruments. Implant specific instruments for prosthesis: humeral preparation, head sizing, trials, etc.
3. Small drill bits for greater tuberosity reattachment
4. Curved Mayo needles; #2 and #5 braided nonabsorbable suture

Tips and Pearls

1. Intravenous antibiotics should be given prior to the beginning of the operation.
2. The patient must be positioned with the arm able to hang free over the table's side so that it can be easily hyperextended and internally and externally rotated.
3. Restoring the proper length of the humerus is critical to proper function: if the prosthesis is left proud stiffness will result; if the prosthesis is inserted too deep loss of soft tissue tension may cause instability.
4. Restoring proper humeral retroversion is critical to optimizing shoulder function and stability.
5. Achieving secure fixation of the greater and lesser tuberosities to each other, as well as the prosthesis and humeral shaft is the important final step in performing a successful shoulder reconstruction.

What To Avoid

1. Avoid excessive operating room traffic.
2. Avoid excessive or aggressive reaming or broaching of the humeral canal to minimize the risk of intraoperative humeral fracture.
3. Avoid dissection beyond the medial border of the coracoid to minimize the risk of injuring the neurovascular structures.
4. Avoid implanting the humeral component in anteversion.
5. Avoid deep or proud placement of the humeral component that may significantly change glenohumeral mechanics or lead to shoulder instability.

Postoperative Care Issues

1. Passive motion is usually begun on the first postoperative day under the supervision of a therapist. The range of motion is limited by the stability of the intraoperative tuberosity fixation. The patient usually performs pendulum, saw, and tummy rub exercises for approximately 4 weeks.
2. After 4 weeks, the patient generally begins active assisted range-of-motion exercises to improve the shoulder's range of motion.

3. After radiographic evidence of tuberosity union, active range-of-motion exercises may be added to the rehabilitation program.
4. Usually by 10 to 12 weeks, the patient is able to begin resistance-type exercises and a more aggressive stretching program.

Operative Technique

Approach

1. Position the patient on the operating room table as outlined above.
2. Prepare and drape the entire shoulder girdle. Isolate an operative field that extends to the midclavicle anteriorly, below the axilla inferiorly, and to the middle of the scapular spine posteriorly.
3. Make a long deltopectoral incision. Begin the incision just below the clavicle and extend it over the lateral aspect of the coracoid to the deltoid insertion on the humeral shaft (Fig. 6–2).
4. Identify the cephalic vein. Retract it laterally with the deltoid muscle.
5. To aid exposure, partially elevate the insertion of the deltoid and partially release the pectoralis major tendon one-half of its length. Tag the pectoralis tendon to facilitate its repair during closure.
6. To further facilitate exposure, resect the coracoacromial ligament for humeral shaft preparation and implant placement.

Fracture exposure

7. Place retractors underneath the deltoid muscle and underneath the lateral borders of the coracoid muscles to assist in exposing the fracture.
8. Evacuate the hematoma. Debride bone and soft tissue debris.
9. Identify by palpation the musculocutaneous and axillary nerves. Carefully retract and protect these structures at all times.
10. Identify the long head of the biceps tendon distally and followed proximally to its insertion on the glenoid. The biceps tendon is a key landmark to identify fracture fragments and aids in assessing soft tissue tension during prosthesis insertion. The biceps tendon identifies the interval between the lesser and greater tuberosities.

11. Expose and mobilize the fracture fragments. Fractures usually involve the bicipital groove. Commonly, the humeral head is a free-floating fragment.

12. Open the rotator interval to help with prosthesis insertion and with securing the tuberosities to the prosthesis.

13. Free the greater and lesser tuberosities. Tag them at the bone-tendon junction with #2 or #5 braided nonabsorbable suture.

14. Gently retract the tuberosities and remove the humeral head fragment. Try to maintain the bony integrity of the tuberosities and the shaft, which will be needed during prosthesis fixation.

15. Compare the removed humeral head fragment with humeral head trials to determine optimal prosthetic size and curvature.

16. Inspect the glenoid for degenerative changes, loose fragments or fractures.

17. Assess the acromion and the rotator cuff tendon. If indicated, perform an acromioplasty or tendon repair.

Humeral component insertion (cement fixation)

➤ Commonly, proximal humeral fractures occur in osteoporotic bone, so care must be taken when extending or rotating the arm.

➤ If a nondisplaced fracture of the proximal shaft occurs, place a cerclage wire or heavy suture prior to humeral shaft preparation. Generally, the cerclage fixation and a cemented prosthesis will provide a stable construct for the fracture.

➤ Normally, there is not sufficient or adequate bone available for press-fit fixation, so the humeral canal should be prepared for cement insertion.

18. Remove blood and bone fragments from the humeral canal.

19. Carefully prepare the medullary canal with rasps and reamers per the specific implant protocol. Determine desired humeral stem size.

20. To restore proper humeral length, place the appropriate trial and desired head size into the canal. With the arm in the plane of the body and the elbow flexed 90 degrees, pull gently on the extremity exerting longitudinal traction, and slide the prosthesis proximally so that the head seats well in the glenoid.

Measure the distance from the collar of the prosthesis to the fractured shaft of the humerus (**Fig. 6–3**).

21. During insertion of the humeral prosthesis, retroversion must be maintained to restore the anatomic alignment of the proximal humerus and to prevent instability of the glenohumeral joint. The goal is approximately 25 to 40 degrees of retroversion. The most reliable landmark is the bicipital groove. The lateral fin of the prosthesis should be just posterior to the bicipital groove. Palpating the distal humeral epicondyles, and confirming that the angle of the prosthesis is 25 to 40 degrees posterior to a line through the epicondyles can also test retroversion.

22. Create a notch at the location of the humeral component's fin to serve as a landmark to be used later during cementing (**Fig. 6–4**).

23. Prior to prosthesis implantation, drill three to four 1.6-mm holes in the area of the greater tuberosity and two to three in the area of the lesser tuberosity for sutures to hold both tuberosities.

24. Use a suture passer to pass #2 or #5 braided nonabsorbable sutures through each hole. Label each suture with a hemostat (**Fig. 6–5**).

25. Irrigate the canal with pulsatile, antibiotic solution. Dry the canal. If desired, a small cement restrictor can be placed at this time. Use a syringe to inject the cement.

26. Cement the proper-sized humeral component into place. Take care not to overpressurize the cement since the cement can be extruded through the medullary canal into the soft tissues.

27. Attempt to optimize proper prosthesis placement. Analysis of tension on the biceps tendon, if still intact, can aid in determining the most appropriate depth of component insertion. The height of the prosthesis should be slightly above the level of the greater tuberosity. Determine final head size and perform a trial reduction prior to final implant selection.

Closure

28. After the cement has cured and the prosthesis is stable, secure the tuberosities. Secure both tuberosities to the prosthesis, proximal humeral shaft, and each other using the heavy sutures placed earlier (**Fig. 6–5**). If needed, place bone graft from the humeral head under the tuberosities.

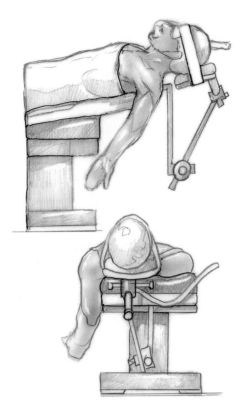

Figure 6–1 Position of the patient. The patient is placed in a modified beach chair position with the head up 20 to 30 degrees. The involved shoulder extends over the edge of the table to allow free humeral extension and rotation. The head should be stabilized in a neutral position to avoid traction on the brachial plexus. The McConnell head holder facilitates stable positioning of the patient.

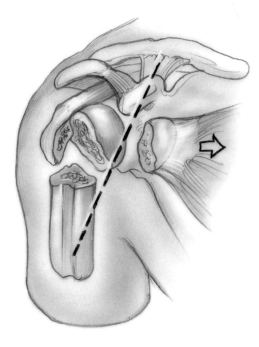

Figure 6–2 Deltopectoral skin incision. The incision begins just below the clavicle and extends over the lateral aspect of the coracoid to the deltoid insertion on the humeral shaft.

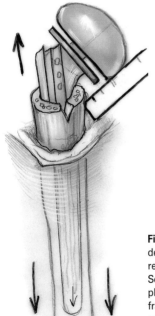

Figure 6–3 Placement of the prosthesis. The appropriate trial and desired head size is placed into the humeral canal. During trial reduction, the head should be well seated within the glenoid. Soft tissue tension can be used to assess the depth of prosthesis placement. The distance from the collar of the prosthesis to the fractured shaft of the humerus is measured to help restore proper soft tissue tension.

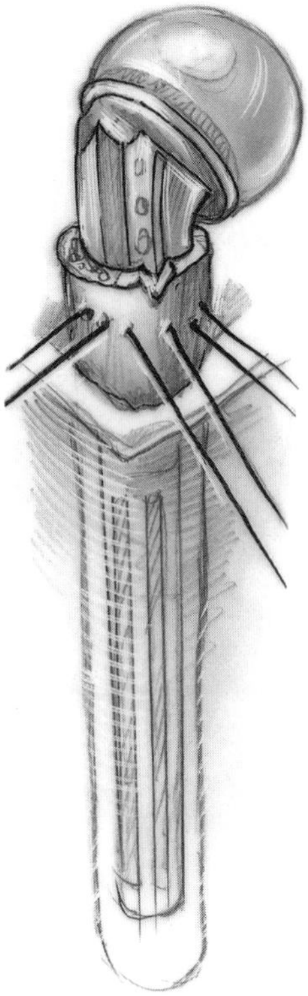

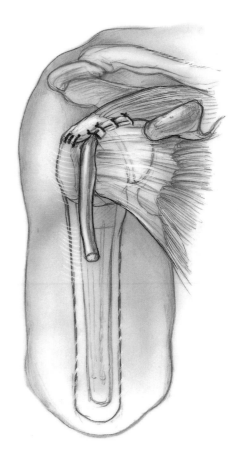

Figure 6–4 Trial reduction. A notch is created at the location of the humeral component's fin to serve as a landmark for rotation to be used later during cementing. Nonabsorbable #2 or #5 braided sutures are passed through holes drilled in the greater and lesser tuberosity.

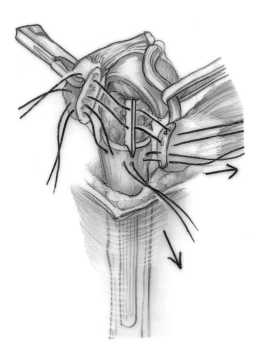

Figure 6–5 Tuberosity repair. Tuberosity repair is accomplished using the preplaced sutures. After the cement has polymerized, the sutures are passed through the prosthesis and tuberosities and tied.

Figure 6–6 Rotator interval repair. The biceps tendon is replaced in the bicipital groove and the lateral aspect of the rotator interval is repaired with #1 braided absorbable suture.

29. Replace the biceps tendon in the bicipital groove. Repair the rotator interval with #1 braided absorbable suture **(Fig. 6–6)**.
30. Gently internally and externally rotate the arm to test the stability of the tuberosity repair.
31. Loosely close the deltopectoral interval. Close the subcutaneous tissues in layers using absorbable sutures over a suction drain.

Suggested Readings

Iannotti JP, Williams GR Jr. *Disorders of the Shoulder: Diagnosis and Management.* Philadelphia, PA: Lippincott Williams & Wilkins, 1999.

Rockwood CA, Matsen FA. *The Shoulder.* Philadelphia, PA: W.B. Saunders, 1998.

CHAPTER 7

Humeral Shaft Fracture

Open Reduction and Internal Fixation

Bradley R. Merk

Indications

1. Humeral shaft fracture which failed nonoperative treatment ("acceptable" nonoperative treatment requires maintenance of fracture reduction with less than 20 degrees of sagittal and 30 degrees of coronal angulation and less than 5 cm of shortening)
2. Open humeral shaft fracture
3. Humeral shaft fracture associated with a vascular injury
4. Humeral shaft fracture in a polytrauma patient
5. Humeral shaft fracture associated with a floating elbow
6. Bilateral humeral fractures
7. Segmental humeral shaft fracture
8. Humeral shaft fracture associated with an ipsilateral brachial plexus injury
9. Humeral shaft fracture associated with pelvic or lower extremity injuries necessitating crutch ambulation
10. Pathologic humeral shaft fracture (intramedullary device generally preferred)
11. Humeral shaft fracture associated with a secondary radial nerve palsy (controversial)
12. Nonunion or malunion after a humeral shaft fracture

Contraindications

1. Acceptable fracture alignment in a closed isolated injury

2. Gustillo grade IIIB or IIIC open fracture with extensive wound contamination (external fixation generally preferred)

Preoperative Preparation

1. Careful documentation of the admitting neurovascular status (especially the radial nerve); the neurovascular status should be reevaluated and again documented after fracture reduction.
2. Careful assessment of soft tissue injuries (obvious or occult); administer appropriate antibiotics and tetanus prophylaxis in the event of an open fracture
3. Appropriate examination of the spine, pelvis, and other limbs to rule out associated injury
4. Radiographs to include AP and lateral views of the shoulder, humerus, and elbow
5. Displaced or angulated fractures should be reduced and provisionally splinted with a coaptation splint or a hanging arm cast prior to surgical stabilization.
6. Postreduction AP and lateral views of the humerus should be obtained to evaluate the postreduction fracture alignment.
7. The fracture should be classified by descriptive terminology (i.e., location, fracture pattern, soft tissue injury, and bone quality) or with the AO/OTA classification scheme.
8. Preoperative templating and planning should be undertaken to facilitate fracture reduction and stabilization as outlined by the AO group.

Special Instruments, Position, and Anesthesia

1. Supine position on the operating room table for the anterolateral approach
2. Prone position for the posterior approach
3. The patient's condition and preference dictate anesthetic choice.
4. Basic orthopedic surgical tray
5. Large fragment plate and screw set (preferred implant is the broad 4.5-mm DC plate although the 4.5-mm LC-DC plate may be required in smaller patients)

Tips and Pearls

1. In a patient with polytrauma, supine positioning is often preferred and may dictate an anterolateral approach.
2. The anterolateral approach is the classic extensile exposure and may be used to expose the entire humerus from the shoulder to the elbow.
3. However, for distal third fractures, a posterior approach affords better exposure and a flat surface for plate application.
4. The radial nerve should be identified and protected in all approaches to the humeral shaft (**Fig. 7–1**).
5. As with all fracture surgery, meticulous handling of the fracture fragments with minimal soft tissue stripping will facilitate union.
6. Indirect reduction techniques and bridge plating using the femoral distractor or articulated tensioning device are useful in the management of segmental comminuted fractures.
7. If possible, interfragmentary screw fixation is used to enhance fixation rigidity.
8. Plates should be selected to allow for a minimum of six, but preferably eight, cortices proximal and distal to the fracture site.

What To Avoid

1. Avoid "guessing" the location of the radial nerve.
2. Avoid circumferential stripping of the periosteum during the surgical approach.
3. Avoid extensive soft tissue stripping of comminuted fracture fragments because the blood supply to these fragments arises via these soft tissue attachments.
4. Avoid injury to the radial nerve at the level of the spiral groove when drilling holes for anterior plating.
5. Avoid inadvertent pressure on the radial nerve from Hohman, Chandler, or other retractors.

Postoperative Care Issues

1. Postoperatively, a posterior mold splint is applied for comfort. It can be removed after several days.
2. The postoperative neurovascular status should be assessed and documented in the recovery room.
3. Ice and elevation are useful in limiting postoperative pain and edema.
4. Suction drainage may be discontinued on the first postoperative day.
5. If fracture fixation is stable, passive and active-assisted shoulder and elbow range-of-motion exercises can begin after splint removal.

Operative Technique

Anterolateral approach (Figs. 7–2 and 7–3)

1. Place the patient supine on the operating room table with the limb resting on a hand table.
2. Prepare and drape the limb from the hand to the shoulder in the hospital's usual sterile fashion.
3. If possible, use a sterile tourniquet cuff to enhance operative exposure.
4. Make an incision along the line from the coracoid process to the deltopectoral interval to the lateral border of the biceps muscle belly to the elbow. The incision's exact placement and length are dictated by the fracture pattern.
5. Incise the deep fascia of the arm in line with the skin incision.
6. Retract the biceps muscle medially. Avoid injury to the lateral antebrachial cutaneous nerve as it emerges from the distal interval between the biceps and brachialis.
7. Identify the radial nerve distally in the interval between the brachialis and brachioradialis near the elbow.

8. Dissect the radial nerve proximally until it pierces the lateral intermuscular septum. Protect it with vessel loops.

9. Incise the lateral border of the brachialis down to bone. Perform subperiosteal dissection as needed for fracture exposure.

10. Perform proximal dissection as needed by dissecting in the internervous plane between the deltoid and pectoralis major.

11. Protect the cephalic vein which lies in this interval.

12. Longitudinally incise the periosteum just lateral to the pectoralis major insertion at the lateral lip of the bicipital groove. Carry the dissection distally.

13. Complete the exposure with subperiosteal dissection as needed.

14. If a very proximal exposure is required, the anterior humeral circumflex vessels will be encountered crossing the surgical field. These vessels often require ligation.

Posterior approach (Fig. 7–4)

1. Place the patient prone on the operating room table with appropriate padding and eye protection. Abduct the arm 90 degrees. Allow the hand to hang free over a table attachment.

2. Prepare and drape the limb from the hand to the shoulder in the hospital's usual sterile fashion.

3. If possible, use a sterile tourniquet cuff to enhance operative exposure.

4. Make a midline posterior incision.

5. Incise the arm's deep fascia in line with the skin incision.

6. Bluntly develop the interval between the long and lateral triceps head proximal to the tendon confluence.

7. Sharply split the triceps tendon in the midline to the level of the bluntly developed interval.

8. Identify the radial nerve in the middle third of the humeral shaft as it crosses obliquely from medial to lateral above the medial triceps muscle origin in the spiral groove of the humerus.

9. Carefully dissect the radial nerve and the accompanying profunda brachial artery. Protect them with vessel loops.

10. Make a midline incision through the medial head of the triceps and periosteum.

11. Complete the exposure with subperiosteal dissection as needed.

Fracture fixation

1. After appropriate exposure is achieved, evacuate the fracture hematoma.

   a. For spiral or oblique fractures, perform a reduction and maintain it with a pointed reduction clamp. Place an interfragmentary lag screw using standard technique at 90 degrees to the fracture line in a location that does not interfere with plate application.

   b. Since transverse fractures are not amenable to lag screw fixation, consider Kirschner wire stabilization after reduction to facilitate plate application, or fixing the plate to one of the fragments and then reducing the other to the plate.

   c. Comminuted fractures may require indirect reduction techniques using the femoral distractor under fluoroscopic control and a bridge-plating technique to avoid devascularization of the fracture site.

2. Select a 4.5-mm broad DC plate or LC-DC plate that allows for a minimum of 6 cortices of fixation on either side of the fracture.

3. Consider slightly prebending the plate at the fracture level to facilitate fracture compression.

4. Use a Verbrugge clamp to stabilize the plate on the cortical surface.

5. Place 4.5-mm cortical screws in compression mode adjacent to the fracture site.

6. If possible, place interfragmentary screws through the plate.

7. Place the remainder of the screws in routine fashion.

Closure

8. Copiously irrigate the wound.

9. Perform a layered closure over a medium hemovac suction drain.

10. Apply a posterior mold splint over a bulky sterile dressing.

11. Transfer the patient to the recovery room.

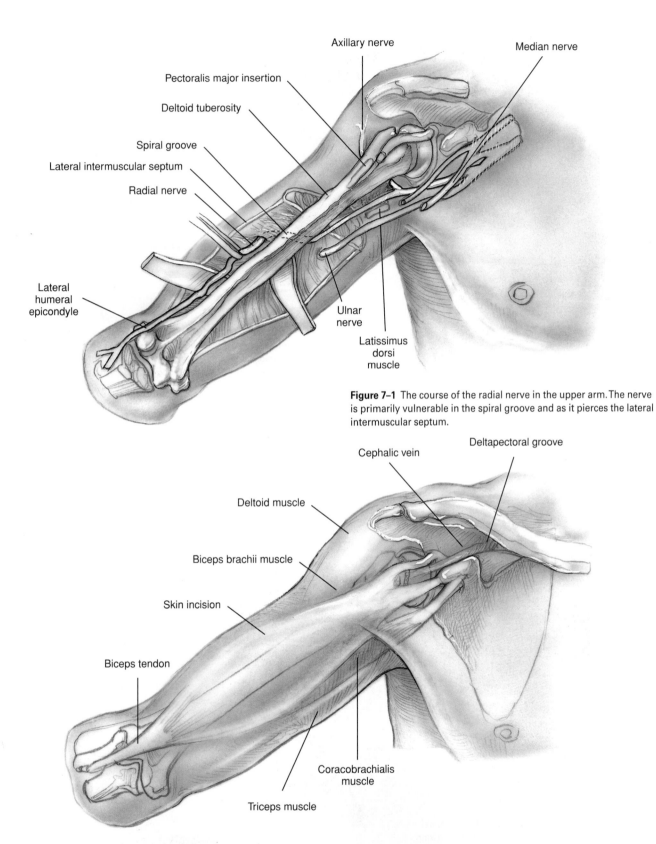

Figure 7–1 The course of the radial nerve in the upper arm. The nerve is primarily vulnerable in the spiral groove and as it pierces the lateral intermuscular septum.

Figure 7–2 Topographic anatomy of the anterolateral approach to the humerus. The incision can be made at any point along the line connecting the coracoid process and the lateral aspect of the biceps brachii to the elbow.

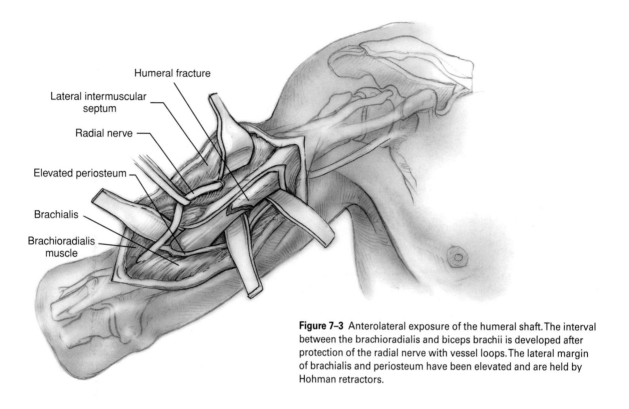

Humeral fracture

Lateral intermuscular
septum

Radial nerve

Elevated periosteum

Brachialis

Brachioradialis
muscle

Figure 7–3 Anterolateral exposure of the humeral shaft. The interval between the brachioradialis and biceps brachii is developed after protection of the radial nerve with vessel loops. The lateral margin of brachialis and periosteum have been elevated and are held by Hohman retractors.

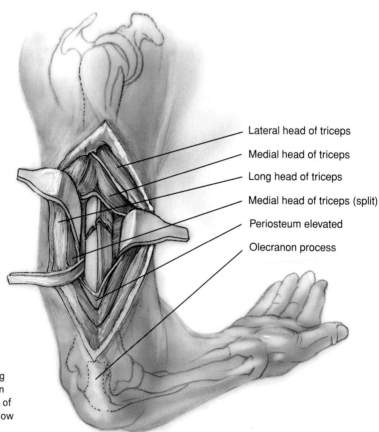

Lateral head of triceps

Medial head of triceps

Long head of triceps

Medial head of triceps (split)

Periosteum elevated

Olecranon process

Figure 7–4 Posterior exposure of the humeral shaft. The interval between the lateral and long triceps head has been developed. Visualization of the radial nerve allows for the safe division of the medial (deep) head of triceps brachii to allow exposure of the posterior humeral shaft.

Suggested Readings

Allgower M, ed. *Manual of Internal Fixation.* 3rd ed. New York, NY: Springer Verlag, 1995.

Chapman MW, ed. *Operative Orthopaedics.* 2nd ed. Philadelphia, PA: J.B. Lippincott, 1994.

Hoppenfeld S, deBoer MA. *Surgical Exposures in Orthopaedics: The Anatomic Approach.* 2nd ed. Philadelphia, PA: J.B. Lippincott, 1994.

Section Two

Elbow and Forearm

CHAPTER 8

Radial Head Fracture

Brian J. Hartigan

Indications

1. Displacement greater than 2 mm or angulation of the neck
2. Large fragment (more than marginal lip or greater than 25% articular surface)
3. Elbow motion or forearm rotation mechanically blocked
4. Associated injury to interosseous ligament/distal radioulnar joint, elbow collateral ligaments or coronoid process

Contraindications

1. Severe comminution precluding rigid internal fixation; consider excision or excision and prosthetic replacement when associated with injury to interosseous ligament/distal radioulnar joint, collateral ligament, or coronoid process
2. Low demand patient (relative); consider excision
3. Open fracture with contaminated wound

Preoperative Preparation

1. Evaluation

   a. Document complete neurovascular examination, especially posterior interosseous nerve.
   b. Assess medial collateral ligament—tenderness and valgus stress test at 30 degrees flexion.
   c. Assess interosseous ligament/distal radioulnar joint—tenderness along forearm and wrist.
   d. Assess for mechanical block; consider sterile intra-articular injection of local anesthetic to allow evaluation of range of motion.

2. Adequate radiographs

   a. AP and lateral of the elbow
   b. Neutral PA view of the wrist with contralateral comparison view to assess for longitudinal stability
   c. Consider CT scan with axial, sagittal and coronal cuts to assess fragment size, comminution, and degree of displacement.

3. Prepare patient for possible need for excision if reduction and internal fixation technically impossible.

Special Instruments, Position, and Anesthesia

1. Patient supine on operating table with affected arm positioned over the chest
2. Tourniquet placed high up on arm
3. Can be done with general or regional anesthetic
4. Instrumentation

   a. Kirschner wires
   b. Mini-fragment internal fixation set with reconstruction plates
   c. Herbert mini-screw set

Tips and Pearls

1. Place tourniquet as high on the arm as is possible to ensure adequate exposure available. If the arm is short or obese, consider using sterile tourniquet.
2. Administer IV antibiotics prior to tourniquet inflation.
3. Hold arm in position by clamping stockinette over hand to drapes using nonpenetrating clamp.
4. Place hardware on the radial head/neck within the "safe zone": 110 degree arc on the lateral side of the radial head extending 65 degrees anteriorly and 45 degrees posteriorly from the midpoint of the radial head with the arm in neutral rotation (**Fig. 8–1**).
5. Check for impingement of hardware in the proximal radioulnar joint prior to closure by visualizing the radial head while pronating and supinating the forearm at various positions of elbow flexion/extension.
6. Repair lateral capsule complex carefully to avoid instability.

What To Avoid

1. Avoid injury to posterior interosseous nerve.

   a. Keep forearm pronated in order to move nerve out of operative field (**Fig. 8–2**).
   b. Avoid placing retractors such as Hohman or Chandler around the radial neck; instead use right angle retractors.
   c. When extending the exposure distally for neck fixation, identify the posterior interosseous nerve.

2. Avoid placing hardware that will impinge on the proximal radioulnar joint by placing it in the safe zone or counter-sinking.
3. Avoid definitive use of Kirschner wires, as they do not provide stable fixation.
4. Avoid passive motion exercises postoperatively.

Postoperative Care Issues

1. Remove drain (if used) on the first postoperative day.
2. Splint arm in 90 degrees flexion and neutral rotation.

3. Remove splint after 5 to 10 days. Use sling for comfort. Begin active and active-assisted motion exercises with emphasis on achieving extension.
4. *Do not* use passive motion exercises.
5. If not progressing with regard to extension, consider use of dynamic splinting program.

Operative Technique

Approach

1. Prepare and drape the arm in the hospital's standard sterile fashion ensuring adequate exposure available.
2. Exsanguinate the arm and inflate the tourniquet.
3. Make a lateral incision beginning proximally at the lateral epicondyle and extending distally over the radial head and neck (**Fig. 8–3**). Dissect down through the subcutaneous fat while attempting to preserve cutaneous nerves.
4. Identify the interval between the anconeus (posterior) and the extensor carpi ulnaris (anterior). Divide the fascia at this interval and carefully separate the two muscles. Proximally, continue to expose the capsule to at least the lateral epicondyle.
5. With the forearm fully pronated to keep the posterior interosseous nerve away from the operative field (**Fig. 8–2**), incise the capsule beginning at the lateral epicondyle and extend distally (**Fig. 8–4**). Proximally, elevate the capsule off of the anterior aspect of the lateral epicondyle. Avoid posterior dissection so as not to injure the lateral collateral ligament complex. Distally, the annular ligament may need to be divided and elevated in order to gain access to the neck.
6. If further exposure of the neck is necessary, identify the posterior margin of the supinator (look for oblique fiber direction). With the forearm in full pronation, divide the supinator at its posterior margin. Identify the posterior interosseous nerve to avoid injury.

Procedure

7. Debride fracture hematoma in order to visualize the fracture pattern.
8. Reduce the fracture fragments to reconstruct the radial head. Provisional fixation with small Kirschner wires may be possible, although often difficult due to the small size of the fragments.

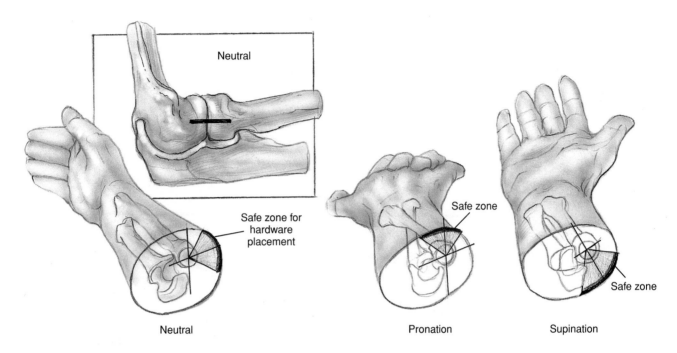

Neutral

Safe zone for hardware placement

Neutral

Safe zone

Pronation

Safe zone

Supination

Figure 8–1 Safe zone. Place hardware on the radial head/neck within the "safe zone": 110 degree arc on the lateral side of the radial head extending 65 degrees anteriorly and 45 degrees posteriorly from the midpoint of the radial head with the arm in neutral rotation.

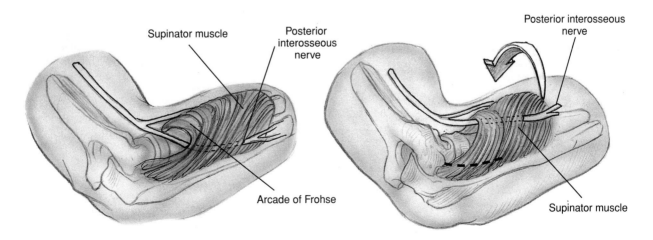

Supinator muscle

Posterior interosseous nerve

Arcade of Frohse

Posterior interosseous nerve

Supinator muscle

Figure 8–2 Posterior interosseous nerve. Note how pronating the forearm moves the posterior interosseous nerve away from the operative field.

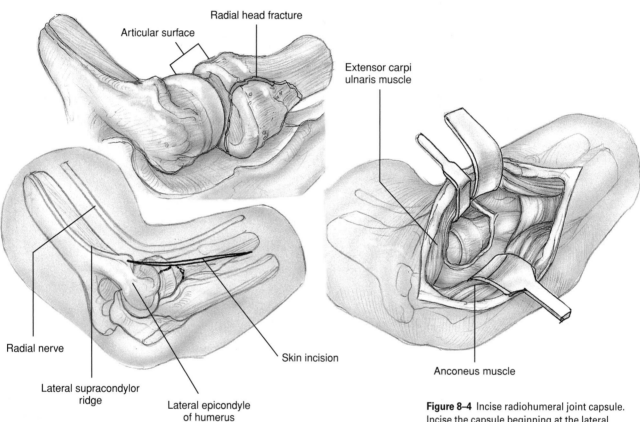

Radial head fracture

Articular surface

Extensor carpi
ulnaris muscle

Radial nerve

Skin incision

Lateral supracondylor
ridge

Lateral epicondyle
of humerus

Anconeus muscle

Figure 8–3 Skin incision. Make a lateral incision beginning proximally at the lateral epicondyle and extending distally over the radial head and neck. Dissect down through the subcutaneous fat while attempting to preserve cutaneous nerves.

Figure 8–4 Incise radiohumeral joint capsule. Incise the capsule beginning at the lateral epicondyle and extend distally. Proximally, elevate the capsule off of the anterior aspect of the lateral epicondyle. Avoid posterior dissection so as not to injure the lateral collateral ligament complex. Distally, the annular ligament may need to be divided and elevated in order to gain access to the neck.

9. Fill defects with cancellous bone graft.
10. Fixation—obtain rigid internal fixation.

   a. Radial head fracture alone: choices for fixation include minifragment screws (1.5 to 2.7 mm) placed in the safe zone (**Fig. 8–1**). If unable to place in the safe zone, consider counter-sinking a minifragment screw or using a small Herbert screw that can be placed below the articular surface. Avoid overdrilling of the proximal cortex for lag technique which could result in comminution of fragment. Therefore, consider placement of the screw without overdrilling by manually compressing the fracture during insertion or using a self-compressing Herbert screw.

   b. Radial head and neck fracture: reconstruct the radial head as above and use 2.0-, 2.4-, or 2.7-mm contoured T-, L-, or Y-plate or condylar plate for fixation to proximal radius.

   c. Radial neck fracture alone: use contoured 2.0-, 2.4-, or 2.7-mm T-, L-, or Y-plate or condylar plate for fixation to proximal radius.
   Note: If unable to obtain rigid fixation, consider excision and possible prosthetic replacement.

11. Assess reduction and check for hardware impingement by pronating and supinating the forearm in various positions of flexion and extension. Modify hardware placement if impingement occurs at the proximal radioulnar joint.
12. Assess valgus stability and consider repair of medial collateral complex if unstable.

Closure

13. Irrigate the wound.
14. Release the tourniquet and obtain hemostasis. Consider using a drain if unable to obtain acceptable hemostasis.
15. Repair the lateral capsular complex primarily in interrupted fashion with absorbable sutures. Consider reattaching the capsule to the lateral epicondyle with suture anchors.
16. Close subcutaneous tissue in interrupted, inverted fashion with absorbable sutures.
17. Close skin with staples, nylon or prolene.
18. Dress in sterile fashion and place in bulky dressing with splint arm in 90 degrees flexion and neutral rotation.

Suggested Readings

The elbow. In: Hoppenfeld S, deBoer P, eds. *Surgical Exposures in Orthopaedics: The Anatomic Approach.* 2nd ed. Philadelphia, PA: J.B. Lippincott, 1994, pp. 103–109.

Hotchkiss RN. Fractures and dislocations of the elbow. In: Rockwood CA, Green DP, Bucholz RW, Heckman JD, eds. *Rockwood and Green's Fractures in Adults.* 4th ed. Philadelphia, PA: Lippincott-Raven, 1996, pp. 929–1024.

Hotchkiss RN. Fractures of the radial head. In: Norris TR, ed. *Orthopaedic Knowledge Update: Shoulder and Elbow.* Rosemont, IL: American Academy of Orthopaedic Surgeons, 1997, pp. 387–395.

Hotchkiss RN. Displaced fractures of the radial head: internal fixation or excision? *J Am Acad Orthop Surg* 1997;5:1–10.

Morrey BF. Surgical exposures of the elbow. In: Morrey BF, ed. *The Elbow and Its Disorders.* 2nd ed. Philadelphia, PA: W.B. Saunders, 1993, pp. 139–165.

Morrey BF. Radial head fracture. In: Morrey BF, ed. *The Elbow and Its Disorders.* 2nd ed. Philadelphia, PA: W.B. Saunders, 1993, pp. 383–404.

CHAPTER 9

Olecranon Fracture

Brian J. Hartigan

Indications

1. Any displaced olecranon fracture

   a. Tension band fixation

      i. Transverse fracture without comminution or joint instability
      ii. Large avulsion fracture

   b. Interfragmentary and/or plate fixation

      i. Comminuted fracture
      ii. Oblique fracture with or without comminution
      iii. Small avulsion fracture in high demand patient

   c. Excision of Fragment and Advancement of Triceps

      i. Extensively comminuted fracture
      ii. Small avulsion fracture in low demand patient (consider nonoperative treatment)

Contraindications

1. Open fracture with contaminated wound
2. Inadequate soft tissue coverage
3. Avoid excision and triceps advancement when associated with disruption of coronoid or anterior soft tissues, dislocation of radial head and/or ulna, or comminution of distal aspect (consider plate fixation).

Preoperative Preparation

1. Document complete neurovascular examination, especially ulnar nerve function.
2. Obtain adequate radiographs including AP and true lateral of elbow.
3. Splint arm at 90 degrees flexion and neutral rotation and ice/elevate arm until surgery.
4. Determine tentative plan for fixation and ensure instrumentation options available.

Special Instruments, Position, and Anesthesia

1. Patient supine on operating table with affected arm positioned over the chest, possibly on sterile Mayo stand (**Fig. 9–1A**)
2. Tourniquet placed high on the arm
3. Can be done with general or regional anesthetic
4. Instrumentation

   a. Bone reduction clamps
   b. Kirschner wires
   c. Stainless steel wire
   d. 3.5-mm AO recon plate and small fragment set

Tips and Pearls

1. Test for active elbow extension before determining a fracture to be nondisplaced.

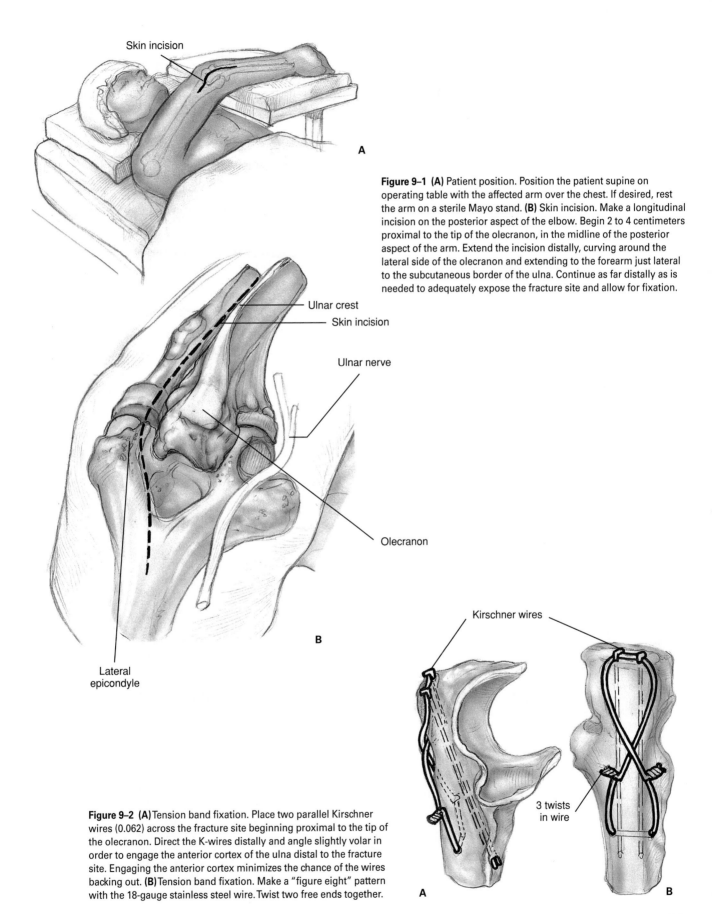

Skin incision

A

Figure 9–1 (A) Patient position. Position the patient supine on operating table with the affected arm over the chest. If desired, rest the arm on a sterile Mayo stand. **(B)** Skin incision. Make a longitudinal incision on the posterior aspect of the elbow. Begin 2 to 4 centimeters proximal to the tip of the olecranon, in the midline of the posterior aspect of the arm. Extend the incision distally, curving around the lateral side of the olecranon and extending to the forearm just lateral to the subcutaneous border of the ulna. Continue as far distally as is needed to adequately expose the fracture site and allow for fixation.

Ulnar crest
Skin incision
Ulnar nerve
Olecranon

B

Lateral epicondyle

Kirschner wires

3 twists in wire

Figure 9–2 (A) Tension band fixation. Place two parallel Kirschner wires (0.062) across the fracture site beginning proximal to the tip of the olecranon. Direct the K-wires distally and angle slightly volar in order to engage the anterior cortex of the ulna distal to the fracture site. Engaging the anterior cortex minimizes the chance of the wires backing out. **(B)** Tension band fixation. Make a "figure eight" pattern with the 18-gauge stainless steel wire. Twist two free ends together.

A

B

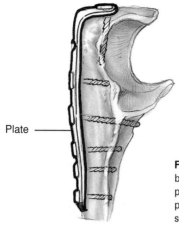

Plate —

Figure 9–3 Plate fixation. If a plate is used for fixation, contour it to the bony anatomy. Proximally, use cancellous screws with unicortical purchase including a screw placed longitudinally in the ulna beginning proximal to the olecranon tip. Distal to the olecranon fossa, cortical screws with bicortical purchase can be used.

Lateral view

Correct

Incorrect

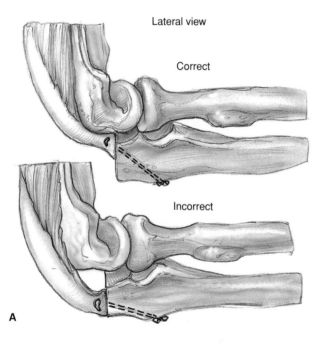

A

Figure 9–4 (A) Triceps advancement. Create three small parallel drill holes in the ulna beginning adjacent to the articular surface and exiting on the posterior surface of the ulna. **(B)** Triceps advancement. Pass the sutures through the drill holes such that the center hole has two sutures (one from each Kessler stitch) and the side holes have one suture each. Ensure that triceps is opposed to bone and tie the sutures over the bone.

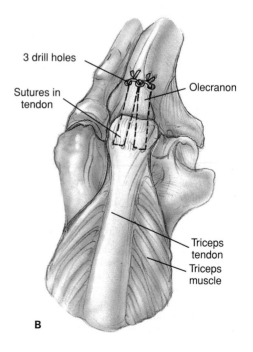

3 drill holes

Sutures in tendon

Olecranon

Triceps tendon

Triceps muscle

B

2. Consider the need for a bone graft preoperatively to allow for preoperative discussion with the patient and appropriate exposure during draping.

3. Place tourniquet as high on the arm as is possible to ensure adequate exposure available. If the arm is short or obese, consider using a sterile tourniquet.

4. Administer IV antibiotics prior to tourniquet inflation.

5. Protect ulnar nerve during procedure by avoiding medial dissection.

6. Use fluoroscopy during hardware placement to avoid intra-articular placement.

7. For tension band fixation, penetrate anterior cortex of ulna with Kirschner wires to minimize chance of wires backing out (**Fig. 9–2A**).

8. For plate fixation use template to aid in contouring plate.

9. If fragment is excised and triceps advanced, attach triceps adjacent to the remaining articular surface (**Fig. 9–4A**).

10. Assess fixation and "safe"/stable range of motion prior to closure by moving elbow through range of motion.

What To Avoid

1. Avoid elevating skin flaps during the exposure.
2. Avoid medial dissection.
3. Avoid penetration of articular surface with hardware.
4. Avoid over-compression of fracture site, causing impingement of trochlea.
5. Avoid prominent hardware, especially Kirschner wires used for tension band fixation.

Postoperative Care Issues

1. Splint arm in 90 degrees flexion.
2. Remove splint after 7 to 10 days. Begin active and active-assisted motion if wound is healed satisfactorily. Avoid full flexion for first 3 to 6 weeks depending on the quality of fixation.
3. Begin strengthening exercises after the fracture is healed or after 8 weeks following excision of fragment.
4. *Do not* use passive motion exercises.

Operative Technique

Approach

1. Prepare and drape the arm in the hospital's standard sterile fashion ensuring adequate exposure available.

2. Exsanguinate the arm and inflate the tourniquet.

3. Make a longitudinal incision on the posterior aspect of the elbow. Begin 2 to 4 cm proximal to the tip of the olecranon, in the midline of the posterior aspect of the arm. Extend the incision distally, curving around the lateral side of the olecranon and extending to the forearm just lateral to the subcutaneous border of the ulna. Continue as far distally as is needed to adequately expose the fracture site and allow for fixation (**Fig. 9–1B**).

4. Divide the deep fascia in line with the incision between the aconeus/extensor carpi ulnaris and flexor carpi ulnaris.

5. Identify the subcutaneous border of the ulna and divide the periosteum longitudinally. Dissect medially and laterally in the subperiosteal plane to adequately expose the fracture site.

   a. If tension band fixation is to be used, the triceps insertion does not need to be divided unless it interferes with exposure of the fracture site.

   b. If plate fixation is to be used, the ulna needs to be exposed both proximally and distally to allow for application of a plate. Proximally, the insertion of the triceps may need to be divided longitudinally to contour the plate over the tip of the olecranon.

Procedure

6. Reduce the fracture by extending the elbow and using manual manipulation of the fragments. Obtain temporary stabilization of the fragments with bone reduction clamps. A small drill hole in distal fragment can be made to secure reduction clamp with the other end of clamp proximal to olecranon tip.

7. Elevate any areas of articular depression. If necessary, use cancellous bone graft to support the articular reconstruction and fill subcortical defects.

8. Fixation techniques.

Tension band fixation (Figs. 9–2A and 2B)

a. Place two parallel Kirschner wires (0.062) across the fracture site, beginning proximal to the tip of the olecranon. Direct the K-wires distally and angle slightly volar in order to engage the anterior cortex of the ulna distal to the fracture site. Once the anterior cortex is engaged, back the K-wires out 2 to 3 mm (**Fig. 9–2A**).

b. Drill a transverse hole (2 mm) through the ulna to pass 18-gauge stainless steel wire. The hole should be 2.5 to 3 cm distal to the fracture site or roughly the same distance from the fracture as the distance from the olecranon tip to the fracture.

c. Pass an 18-gauge angiocath through the tricep aponeurosis adjacent to the bone and just proximal to the protruding K-wires. Use the plastic canula of the angiocath as a guide to pass a length of 18-gauge stainless steel wire. Remove the angiocath.

d. Cross one free end of the 18-gauge stainless steel wire over the posterior surface of the olecranon leaving enough slack to allow for a loop to be twisted for tensioning.

e. Continue to pass the 18-gauge stainless steel wire through the transverse hole in the olecranon distal to the fracture and back to the other free end of the wire in order to complete the "figure eight." Twist two free ends together (**Fig. 9–2B**).

f. Grasp both of the twists in the wire with heavy needle-drivers and twist uniformly to tension the wire. While twisting, pull away from the bone to prevent kinking. Do not allow wire to twist on itself.

g. Obtain intraoperative radiograph or fluoroscopic image to assess reduction.

h. Move elbow through a range of motion to ensure fixation is secure.

i. Cut the two twisted segments leaving 3 to 4 complete twists. Turn the wire toward the bone and impact.

j. Bend the two K-wires 90 degrees and cut. Twist cut end to point proximally over the stainless steel wire. Impact K-wires through small cuts made in the tricep aponeurosis.

Plate fixation (Fig. 9–3)

a. Expose enough ulna in order to apply 3.5-mm AO recon plate. If the fracture is proximal, this may require dividing the triceps aponeurosis so that the plate can extend proximal to the olecranon tip.

b. Contour a 3.5-mm recon plate to fit along posterolateral cortex of ulna and over olecranon tip if necessary.

c. If fracture is oblique, place 3.5-mm interfragmentary lag screw(s) across fracture.

d. Place the contoured plate on the ulna and temporarily secure with clamp.

e. Fix the plate to the ulna. Proximally, use cancellous screws with unicortical purchase including a screw placed longitudinally in the ulna beginning proximal to the olecranon tip. Distal to the olecranon fossa, cortical screws with bicortical purchase can be used.

f. Move elbow through a range of motion to ensure fixation is secure and hardware does not enter joint.

g. Obtain intra-operative radiograph to ensure adequate reduction and placement of hardware. Ensure that no screws penetrate articular surface.

Excision of fragment and advancement of triceps (Figs. 9–4A and 4B)

a. Excise the proximal fragment of bone from the triceps aponeurosis leaving as much soft tissue as possible.

b. Using a grasping stitch, (i.e., Kessler, Bunnel, or locking loop) place two heavy nonabsorbable sutures (#2, #1, 0) side-by-side in the triceps tendon.

c. Smooth the proximal end of the remaining ulna.

d. Create three, small parallel drill holes in the ulna beginning adjacent to the articular surface and exiting on the posterior surface of the ulna.

e. Pass the sutures through the drill holes so that the center hole has two sutures (one from each Kessler stitch) and the side holes have one suture each.

f. Ensure that triceps is opposed to bone and tie the sutures over the bone. Move elbow through a range of motion to ensure repair is secure.

g. Repair rents in the medial and lateral aspects of the triceps aponeurosis using nonabsorbable suture.

Closure

9. Irrigate the wound.

10. Repair the triceps aponeurosis in an interrupted fashion using absorbable sutures.

11. Close the fascia in interrupted fashion using absorbable sutures.
12. Close the subcutaneous tissue in interrupted, inverted fashion using absorbable sutures.
13. Close the skin using nylon or prolene.
14. Dress the wound in a sterile fashion and splint the arm in 90 degrees flexion.

Suggested Readings

The elbow. In: Hoppenfeld S, deBoer P, eds. *Surgical Exposures in Orthopaedics: The Anatomic Approach*. 2nd ed. Philadelphia, PA: J.B. Lippincott, 1994, pp. 84–89.

Cabanela ME, Morrey BF. Fractures of the proximal ulna and olecranon. In: Morrey BF, ed. *The Elbow and Its Disorders*. 2nd ed. Philadelphia, PA: W.B. Saunders, 1993, pp. 405–428.

Cooper JL, D'Ambrosia RD. Fractures and fracture-dislocations about the elbow. In: Chapman MW, ed. *Operative Orthopaedics*. 2nd ed. Philadelphia, PA: J.B. Lippincott, 1993, pp. 439–456.

Hotchkiss RN. Fractures and dislocations of the elbow. In: Rockwood CA, Green DP, Bucholz RW, Heckman JD, eds. *Rockwood and Green's Fractures in Adults*. 4th ed. Philadelphia, PA: Lippincott-Raven, 1996, pp. 929–1024.

Morrey BF. Surgical exposures of the elbow. In: Morrey BF, ed. *The Elbow and Its Disorders*. 2nd ed. Philadelphia, PA: W.B. Saunders, 1993, pp. 139–165.

O'Driscoll SW. Olecranon and coronoid fractures. In: Norris TR, ed. *Orthopaedic Knowledge Update: Shoulder and Elbow*. Rosemont, IL: American Academy of Orthopaedic Surgeons, 1997, pp. 405–413.

CHAPTER 10

Distal Humeral Fractures

Brian J. Hartigan

Indications

1. Intra-articular fracture
2. Unstable nonarticular fracture
3. Associated vascular injury requiring repair

Contraindications

1. Open fracture with contaminated wound
2. Inadequate soft tissue coverage
3. High-operative risk (relative)
4. Severe osteoporosis or comminution (relative)

Preoperative Preparation

1. Evaluate patient for other injuries.
2. Assess for open wounds.
3. Document complete neurologic and vascular examination.

   a. If vascular compromise, perform closed reduction and reassess. If continued vascular compromise, plan for operative exploration and vascular repair/bypass in addition to skeletal stabilization.

4. Obtain adequate radiographs.

   a. AP and lateral of elbow
   b. Consider AP and lateral with longitudinal traction.
   c. Consider radiographs of contralateral extremity for preoperative planning purposes.
   d. Consider CT scan, especially for intra-articular comminuted fractures.

5. Splint elbow at 90 degrees flexion and ice/elevate until definitive operative fixation.
6. Understand normal elbow anatomy (**Fig. 10–1**).

   a. Lateral column diverges approximately 20 degrees from sagittal axis and projects 30 to 40 degrees anteriorly, ending at the capitellar articular surface (**Fig. 10–1D**).
   b. Medial column diverges approximately 45 degrees from sagittal axis and projects 10 to 20 degrees anteriorly, ending proximal to the trochlea (**Fig. 10–1C**).
   c. Olecranon fossa and coronoid fossa lie between lateral and medial columns and proximal to the trochlea.
   d. Trochlea internally rotated 3 to 8 degrees and has valgus inclination of 94 to 98 degrees (**Figs. 10–1A and 1B**).
   e. Diameter of trochlear sulcus is much smaller than that of the medial trochlear ridge and the lateral condyle.

7. Create operative plan for exposure, reduction and fixation.
8. Consider the need for bone graft.

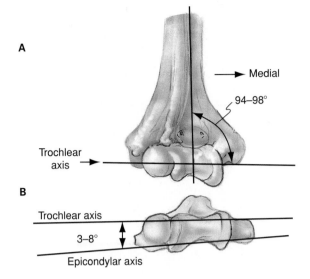

A

Medial

94–98°

Trochlear
axis

B

Trochlear axis

3–8°

Epicondylar axis

Figure 10–1 (A) Normal elbow anatomy. Trochlea has valgus inclination of 94 to 98 degrees. **(B)** Normal elbow anatomy. Trochlea internally rotated 3 to 8 degrees. **(C)** Normal elbow anatomy. Medial column projects 10 to 20 degrees anteriorly, ending proximal to the trochlea. **(D)** Normal elbow anatomy. Lateral column projects 30 to 40 degrees anteriorly, ending at the capitellar articular surface

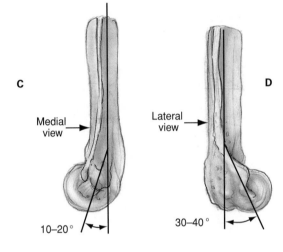

C

Medial
view

10–20°

D

Lateral
view

30–40°

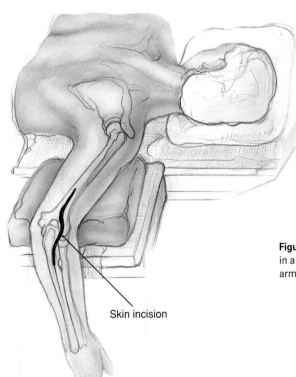

Skin incision

Figure 10–2 Patient position. The patient is placed in a prone position with the arm on a short armboard and the elbow flexed.

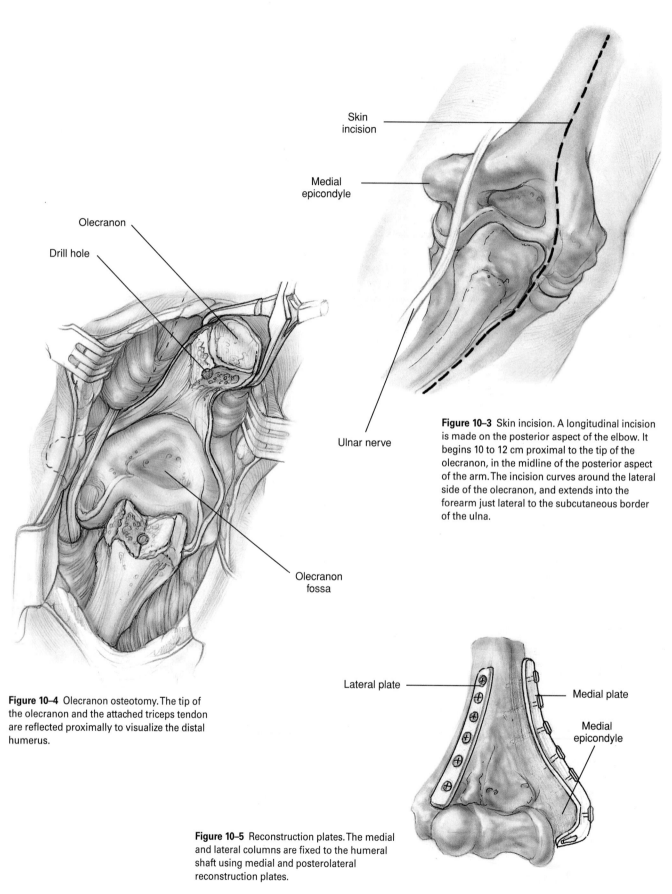

Olecranon

Drill hole

Olecranon
fossa

Skin
incision

Medial
epicondyle

Ulnar nerve

Figure 10–3 Skin incision. A longitudinal incision
is made on the posterior aspect of the elbow. It
begins 10 to 12 cm proximal to the tip of the
olecranon, in the midline of the posterior aspect
of the arm. The incision curves around the lateral
side of the olecranon, and extends into the
forearm just lateral to the subcutaneous border
of the ulna.

Figure 10–4 Olecranon osteotomy. The tip of
the olecranon and the attached triceps tendon
are reflected proximally to visualize the distal
humerus.

Lateral plate

Medial plate

Medial
epicondyle

Figure 10–5 Reconstruction plates. The medial
and lateral columns are fixed to the humeral
shaft using medial and posterolateral
reconstruction plates.

Special Instruments, Position, and Anesthesia

1. Patient is positioned in a prone position with the arm on a short armboard and the elbow flexed or in a lateral decubitus position with the involved arm draped over a bolster (**Fig. 10–2**).
2. If bone graft may be needed, drape out a portion of the iliac crest.
3. General anesthesia
4. Sterile tourniquet placed high on the arm
5. Instrumentation
   a. Small fragment set
   b. 3.5-mm reconstruction plates
   c. 3.5-mm pelvic long screw set
   d. Reduction clamps
   e. 6.5-mm screw set
   f. Herbert screw set and/or mini fragment set for articular fractures

Tips and Pearls

1. Look for other injuries since fracture is usually the result of high-energy trauma.
2. Identify the ulnar nerve and protect it throughout the procedure.
3. Transpose the ulnar nerve if hardware is placed medially to prevent irritation from the hardware.
4. Perform the olecranon osteotomy in the area of the olecranon that is normally devoid of articular cartilage.
5. Drill and tap olecranon prior to performing the osteotomy.
6. When performing the olecranon osteotomy, remember that the semilunar notch is "V-shaped" with the central area being the thickest. Use an osteotome inserted obliquely to complete the osteotomy in order to protect the trochlea.
7. Distally, use cannulated screws and intraoperative fluoroscopy to optimize screw placement. Avoid multiple drill holes.
8. Screws through the trochlea must be centered accurately because the diameter at the center of the trochlea is less than at the edges (**Fig. 10–1**).
9. Use an oscillating drill and drill sleeves to protect neurovascular structures.

10. Attempt to preserve or repair the medial and lateral collateral ligaments.

What To Avoid

1. Avoid injury to the radial nerve by identifying the nerve if proximal exposure is necessary.
2. Avoid narrowing the trochlea with lag fixation in cases with articular comminution.
3. Avoid placement of intra-articular hardware or hardware placed in the olecranon fossa or coronoid fossa.
4. Avoid prominent hardware when fixing olecranon osteotomy.

Postoperative Care Issues

1. Splint arm in 90 degrees flexion.
2. Drain is removed on postoperative day #1.
3. Remove splint after 5 to 7 days. Begin active and active-assisted motion if wound is healed satisfactorily. Place arm in a sling during the day and in a removable splint at night. Emphasize elbow extension with therapy program.
4. Avoid strengthening exercises until fracture has healed (approximately 8 to 12 weeks).

Operative Technique

Approach

1. Prepare and drape the arm in the hospital's standard sterile fashion ensuring adequate exposure available.
2. Place a sterile tourniquet on the upper arm as high as possible.
3. Exsanguinate the arm and inflate the tourniquet.
4. Make a longitudinal incision on the posterior aspect of the elbow. Begin 10 to 12 cm proximal to the tip of the olecranon, in the midline of the posterior aspect of the arm. Extend the incision distally, curving around the lateral side of the olecranon, and extending to the forearm just lateral to the subcutaneous border of the ulna (**Fig. 10–3**).
5. Divide the deep fascia in line with the incision.

6. Elevate the subcutaneous tissues medially to identify the ulnar nerve within the cubital tunnel. Release the fascia over the nerve and transpose the nerve anteriorly out of the tunnel using a vascular loop. Leave loop around the nerve for identification at all times during the procedure.

7. Olecranon osteotomy **(Fig. 10–4)**

   a. Use a 3.2-mm drill to make a longitudinal drill hole in the ulna. Begin proximal to the olecranon tip, starting through the triceps aponeurosis.

   b. Tap the hole with the 6.5-mm tap (for the 6.5-mm cancellous screw). Ensure that the hole is long enough for the threads of the screw to pass the osteotomy site.

   c. Measure the depth of the hole to determine screw length.

   d. Dissect the soft tissues off of the posterior aspect of the olecranon, leaving the triceps attachment intact. Identify the medial and lateral borders of the olecranon down to the articular surface.

   e. Identify the site for the osteotomy—about 2 cm distal to the olecranon tip. If possible visualize the joint and position the osteotomy to enter the joint where the semilunar notch is devoid of cartilage.

   f. While protecting the articular cartilage on the trochlea with a freer, create a chevron osteotomy with the apex pointing distally. Begin the osteotomy using an oscillating saw with a thin blade and complete the osteotomy with a sharp, thin osteotome.

8. Reflect the tip of the olecranon and the attached triceps tendon proximally to visualize the distal humerus **(Fig. 10–4)**. If proximal exposure is necessary, identify and protect the radial nerve, and reflect the triceps further proximally.

9. Medial and lateral subperiosteal dissection is used as needed for adequate exposure.

Procedure

10. Assess the fracture and modify the preoperative plan accordingly.

11. Reduce and internally fix the fracture. Although the intra-articular and/or intercondylar components are normally fixed before the supracondylar component, the entire construct for fixation must be considered at this stage because screws for intra-articular fixation can be placed through the plate used for supracondylar fixation, adding to the strength of the construct.

12. Intra-articular/Intercondylar fixation

   a. Reduce the fracture under direct visualization and obtain provisional fixation with Kirschner wires (0.045–0.062) or guide pins for the cannulated screws.

   b. If there is no intra-articular comminution, fixation is obtained with a 3.5-mm or 4.5-mm lag screw placed in a medial-to-lateral or lateral-to-medial direction.

   c. If intra-articular comminution is present, avoid lag screw fixation, as this will narrow the trochlea. Use bone graft to fill the defect and place screws without lag fixation. Tricortical bone graft from the iliac crest can be used to fill large defects in the articular surface.

   d. Small articular fragments can be fixed by either counter-sinking a mini-fragment screw or using a Herbert screw placed beneath the articular surface.

13. The supracondylar portion is then addressed by reconstructing the medial and lateral columns and fixing them to the humeral shaft using medial and posterolateral plates.

   a. Contour two 3.5-mm reconstruction plates **(Fig. 10–5)**.

      i. Medial aspect of the medial column—can extend either medially or posteriorly around the medial epicondyle if distal fixation is necessary.

      ii. Posterior aspect of the lateral column—can extend distally to the posterior border of the capitellum. Distal screws are aimed proximally to avoid the anterior aspect of the capitellum.

   b. Fix the plates to the bone.

14. Move elbow through a complete range of motion to evaluate stability and ensure that hardware will not impinge on joint motion.

15. Obtain intraoperative radiographs to assess the reduction of the fracture and placement of hardware.

16. Reduce the olecranon osteotomy and hold with a bone clamp. Place a 6.5-mm cancellous screw (length determined prior to osteotomy) through a washer to secure the osteotomy.

17. Move the elbow through a complete range of motion to evaluate stability of the osteotomy. If unstable, consider use of figure eight wire.

18. Obtain intraoperative radiographs to assess the reduction of the fracture/osteotomy and placement of hardware.

Closure

19. Repair rents along medial and lateral triceps using absorbable suture in an interrupted fashion.

20. Transpose the ulnar nerve anterior to the medial epicondyle and create a fascial sling to prevent posterior displacement.

21. Close the deep fascia in interrupted fashion using absorbable sutures.

22. Place the drain superficial to deep fascia and exit proximal to wound.

23. Close the subcutaneous tissue in interrupted, inverted fashion using absorbable sutures.

24. Close the skin using nylon or prolene.

25. Dress the wound in a sterile fashion and splint the arm in 90 degrees flexion.

Suggested Readings

The elbow. In: Hoppenfeld S, deBoer P, eds. *Surgical Exposures in Orthopaedics: The Anatomic Approach*. 2nd ed. Philadelphia, PA: J.B. Lippincott, 1994, pp. 84–89.

Asprinio D, Helfet DL. Fractures of the distal humerus. In: Levine AM, ed. *Orthopaedic Knowledge Update: Trauma*. Rosemont, IL: American Academy of Orthopaedic Surgeons, 1996, pp. 35–46.

Hotchkiss RN. Fractures and dislocations of the elbow. In: Rockwood CA, Green DP, Bucholz RW, Heckman JD, eds. *Rockwood and Green's Fractures in Adults*. 4th ed. Philadelphia, PA: Lippincott-Raven, 1996, pp. 929–1024.

Webb LX. Distal humerus fractures in adults. *J Am Acad Orthop Surg* 1996;4:336–344.

Weber BG. Fractures of the distal humerus. In: Chapman MW, ed. *Operative Orthopaedics*. 2nd ed. Philadelphia, PA: J.B. Lippincott, 1993, pp. 439–456.

CHAPTER 11

Forearm Diaphyseal Fractures
Radius and Ulna

David M. Kalainov and Charles Carroll IV

Indications

1. Radial shaft fracture with angulation greater than 10 degrees, malrotation, or disturbance of the normal radial bow
2. Ulnar shaft fracture with angulation greater than 10 degrees, malrotation, displacement greater than 50%, or shortening with distal radio-ulnar joint incongruency
3. Both-bones forearm fracture
4. Monteggia fracture
5. Galeazzi fracture
6. Open fracture
7. Segmental or comminuted fracture (relative)
8. Concomitant soft-tissue injury requiring frequent wound care (e.g., burn)
9. Compartment syndrome

Contraindications

1. Nondisplaced radial shaft fracture
2. Minimally displaced ulnar shaft fracture ("nightstick" fracture)
3. Severe coexisting medical illness
4. Childhood injury (relative). In general, a greater degree of initial displacement can be accepted in children given their potential for remodeling during growth and high incidence of satisfactory functional outcomes with nonoperative treatment.

Preoperative Preparation

1. Standard AP and lateral radiographs of the injured forearm, elbow, and wrist
2. Comparative views of the contralateral forearm and wrist may be helpful.
3. Determine the radiographic characteristics of the fracture.

   a. One or both bones
   b. Shaft location—proximal, middle, or distal third
   c. Pattern of injury—transverse, oblique, spiral, comminuted, segmental, bone loss
   d. Degree and direction of displacement

4. Document the neurovascular status and evaluate the extremity for associated trauma (e.g., radial head dislocation, distal radio-ulnar joint instability).
5. Assess for elevated forearm compartment pressures.
6. Plan the surgical approach: anterior, posterior, ulnar.
7. Discuss with the patient the common potential complications associated with operative treatment of forearm fractures.

Special Instruments, Position, and Anesthesia

1. Supine position with a hand table extension
2. Regional or general anesthesia

3. Pneumatic arm tourniquet set at 250 mm Hg
4. If autogenous bone grafting is anticipated, prepare the anterior iliac crest.
5. Standard or minifluoroscopy unit
6. Consider low-power loop magnification (2.5×).
7. Basic hand tray and routine orthopaedic instruments (tissue scissors, retractors, fracture reduction clamps, dental probe, periosteal elevator, Freer elevator, currettes, osteotomes, mallet)
8. Internal fixation set with 3.5-mm screws and plates (dynamic compression plates, angled plates, T-plates); smaller 2.7-mm plates are useful for proximal radial and distal ulnar shaft fractures.
9. Availability of an external fixation device

Tips and Pearls

1. Administer intravenous antibiotics prior to tourniquet inflation. Avoid use of a tourniquet with extremely traumatized soft tissues or in the setting of a compartment syndrome.
2. Select the appropriate surgical exposure.

   a. Anterior approach (Henry)—preferred for fractures involving the distal third of the radial diaphysis (or any radial shaft fracture associated with elevated compartment pressures).
   b. Posterior approach (Thompson)—preferred for fractures involving the proximal and middle thirds of the radial diaphysis.
   c. Ulnar approach—applicable to all ulnar shaft fractures; additional incisions may be required for volar and dorsal fasciotomies.

3. Stabilize the fracture with a 3.5-mm dynamic compression plate(s).

   a. Allow for six to eight cortices of screw purchase both above and below the fracture line.
   b. Consider lag screw fixation either through the plate or separate from the plate for increased strength.
   c. A segmental radial or ulnar shaft fracture may necessitate two plates if the length of one plate is insufficient to bridge the fracture. Position the plates 90 degrees apart.

   d. When addressing a both bones injury, obtain provisional plate fixation with clamps to assess forearm rotation. If there is loss of normal supination or pronation, adjust the reduction before securing the plates with screws.

4. Bone graft areas of extensive comminution and bone loss.
5. Confirm reduction and stability of the distal radio-ulnar and proximal radio-capitellar joints after plate fixation. Be prepared to address residual problems at these sites.
6. Consider intramedullary nailing as an alternative method of stabilizing segmental forearm fractures in adults. This technique is particularly useful when addressing unstable diaphyseal fractures in children.
7. Apply an external fixator if early internal fixation is deemed inappropriate (e.g., significant soft-tissue destruction, wound contamination, polytrauma). Conversion to plate fixation at a later date is recommended.

What To Avoid

1. Do not expose the proximal third of the radius without protecting the posterior interosseous nerve.
2. Avoid injury to the dorsal cutaneous branch of the ulnar nerve when exposing the ulnar shaft distally. The nerve branches approximately 6 cm proximal to the ulnar head.
3. Avoid injury to the lateral antebrachial cutaneous and dorsoradial sensory nerves when approaching the radius anteriorly. The lateral antebrachial cutaneous nerve emerges from between the biceps tendon and brachialis proximally and courses down the volar-radial side of the forearm subcutaneously. The dorsoradial sensory nerve lies under cover of the brachioradialis in the proximal two thirds of the forearm and penetrates the fascial interval between the brachioradialis and extensor carpi radialis longus tendons distally.
4. Refrain from overzealous retraction of neurovascular structures.
5. Avoid excessive soft-tissue dissection, particularly with comminuted fractures.

6. Avoid stripping the interosseous membrane between the radius and ulna.

7. Do not close forearm fascia and avoid reapproximating wound edges under undue tension.

Postoperative Care Issues

1. Apply a well-padded gauze dressing and support the wrist and forearm in a volar plaster splint. A long-arm splint is indicated for fractures requiring stabilization of the radial head or distal radio-ulnar joint.

2. If a drain was placed, remove it on the first postoperative day.

3. Change the dressing 3 to 5 days after surgery and arrange for fabrication of a removable short-arm splint. If the ulnar styloid or distal radio-ulnar joint were addressed surgically, consider immobilizing the wrist and forearm in supination for 4 to 6 weeks.

4. Encourage finger and shoulder motion immediately after surgery.

5. Elbow, forearm, and wrist motion exercises are initiated 3 to 5 days postoperatively.

6. Remove skin sutures at 10 to 14 days.

7. Caution the patient against lifting heavy objects until bone union is evident on plain radiographs (approximately 4 months after surgery).

8. Plates and screws are not routinely extracted. Cortical remodeling under the implant is necessary to prevent subsequent fracture and may take up to 2 years following surgery.

Operative Technique

Anterior approach (Henry)

Preferred for distal third radial shaft fractures and for all radial shaft fractures associated with elevated compartment pressures.

1. With the involved extremity resting over a hand table, supinate the forearm and expose the volar surface.

2. Make a longitudinal incision along a line projecting from a point one fingerbreadth medial to the tip of the radial styloid to a point lateral to the biceps tendon. The length of the skin incision will depend upon the pattern and location of the fracture (**Fig. 11–1A**).

Distal third

a. Incise the antebrachial fascia in line with the skin incision. Retract the flexor carpi radialis medially along with the contents of the carpal canal. Retract the radial artery and brachioradialis laterally.

b. Release the insertion of the pronator quadratus from the radial shaft, preserving the origin of the volar radio-carpal ligaments. Elevate the muscle subperiosteally and retract medially to expose the fracture site. Proximal extension of the fracture or plate will necessitate partial detachment of the flexor pollicis longus muscle origin (**Fig. 11–1B**).

Proximal and middle thirds

a. Incise the antebrachial fascia in line with the skin incision. Develop the interval between the brachioradialis and pronator teres muscles proximally. In the middle third of the forearm, the interval lies between the brachioradialis and flexor carpi radialis muscles.

b. Retract the pronator teres, biceps tendon, and radial artery medially and the brachioradialis laterally. Ligate small arterial branches supplying the brachioradialis to mobilize the radial artery.

c. Release the supinator muscle from its radial insertion. Elevate the muscle subperiosteally and retract the fibers laterally, protecting the posterior interosseous nerve which courses through its substance (**Fig. 11–1C**).

d. For full exposure of the middle third of the diaphysis, pronate the forearm and release the attachments of the pronator teres and flexor digitorum superficialis from the radial shaft. Elevate both muscles subperiosteally and sweep medially with the radial artery.

3. Stabilize the fracture anteriorly with an appropriately sized 3.5-mm dynamic compression plate. An angled plate or T-plate is useful for distal third fractures at the metaphyseal-diaphyseal junction.

4. In the presence of a suspected compartment syndrome, perform a complete volar fasciotomy through a full-length incision. The release should

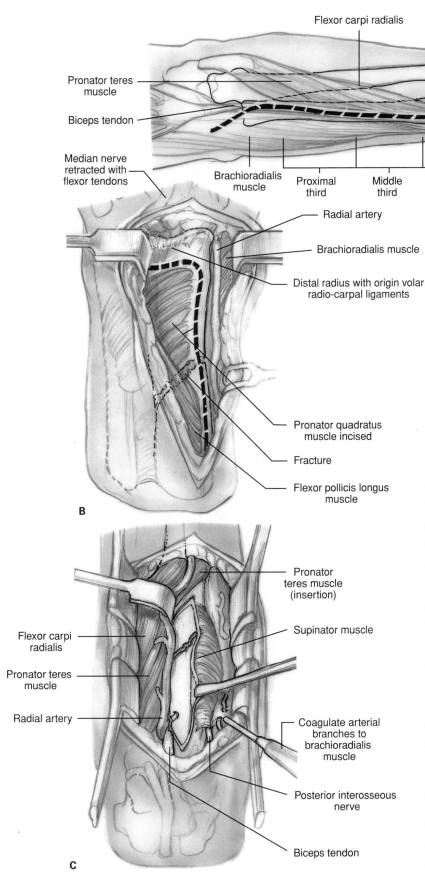

Flexor carpi radialis   Skin incision

Pronator teres muscle

Biceps tendon

Median nerve retracted with flexor tendons

Brachioradialis muscle

Proximal third

Middle third

Distal third

A

Radial artery

Brachioradialis muscle

Distal radius with origin volar radio-carpal ligaments

Pronator quadratus muscle incised

Fracture

Flexor pollicis longus muscle

B

Flexor carpi radialis

Pronator teres muscle

Radial artery

Pronator teres muscle (insertion)

Supinator muscle

Coagulate arterial branches to brachioradialis muscle

Posterior interosseous nerve

Biceps tendon

C

Figure 11–1 (A) Anterior approach. A longitudinal incision is made along a line projecting from a point one fingerbreadth medial to the tip of the radial styloid to a point lateral to the biceps tendon. The length of the incision will depend upon the pattern and location of the fracture. The antebrachial fascia is incised in-line with the skin incision. **(B)** Anterior approach (distal third). The forearm is supinated and the flexor carpi radialis is retracted medially with the contents of the carpal canal. The radial artery and brachioradialis are retracted laterally. The insertion of the pronator quadratus is released from the radius, preserving the origin of the volar radio-carpal ligaments. The muscle is elevated subperiosteally and retracted medially. More proximal exposure will necessitate partial detachment of the flexor pollicis longus muscle. **(C)** Anterior approach (proximal and middle thirds). Proximally, the pronator teres, biceps tendon, and radial artery are retracted medially and the brachioradialis laterally. With the forearm supinated, the origin of the supinator muscle is released and the muscle is elevated subperiosteally in a lateral direction. The posterior interosseous nerve is protected within the muscle fibers. For exposure of the mid-shaft, the forearm is pronated and the radial attachments of the pronator teres and flexor digitorum superficialis are released. Both muscles are elevated subperiosteally and retracted medially (not depicted).

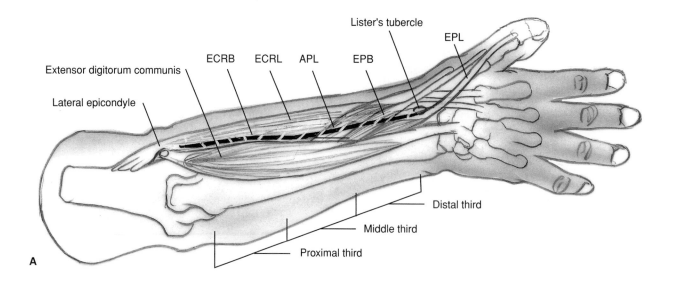

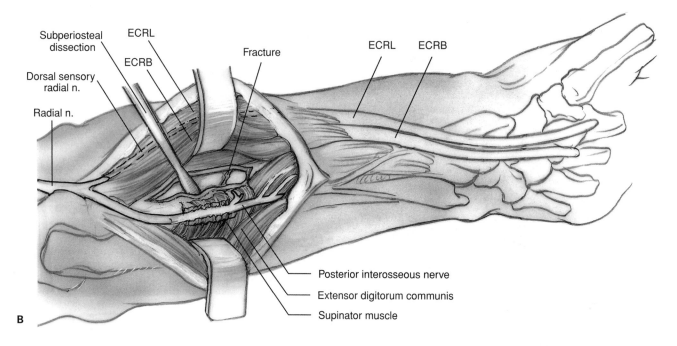

Figure 11–2 (A) Posterior approach. A longitudinal incision is made along a line projecting from the lateral epicondyle of the humerus to Lister's tubercle distally. The length of the incision will depend upon the pattern and location of the fracture. The antebrachial fascia is opened in line with the skin incision. **(B)** Posterior approach (proximal and middle thirds). Proximally, the interval between the extensor carpi radialis brevis (ECRB) and extensor digitorum communis muscles is developed. The posterior interosseous nerve is identified and carefully dissected from distal to proximal through the supinator muscle fibers. The supinator is then released from the radial shaft anteriorly and gently retracted laterally. Exposure of the mid-shaft necessitates elevation and retraction of the outcropping muscles (APL, EPB) distally. (APL = abductor pollicis longus; ECRB = extensor carpi radialis brevis; ECRL = extensor carpi radialis longus; EPL = extensor pollicis longus; EPB = extensor pollicis brevis.)

be carried distally into the palm to decompress the median nerve. Injury to the palmar cutaneous branch of the median nerve can be avoided by making a separate incision over the carpal canal. If pressures remain elevated in the dorsal and mobile wad compartments, make an additional incision over the extensor muscles to release the dorsal antebrachial fascia.

Posterior approach (Thompson)

Preferred for proximal and middle third radial shaft fractures.

1. With the injured extremity resting over a hand table, pronate the forearm and expose the dorsal surface.
2. Make a longitudinal incision along a line projecting from the lateral epicondyle of the humerus to Lister's tubercle distally. The length of the incision will depend upon the pattern and location of the fracture (**Fig. 11–2A**).
3. Incise the forearm fascia in-line with the skin incision.

Proximal and middle thirds

a. Develop the interval between the extensor carpi radialis brevis and extensor digitorum communis muscles. Distally, the outcropping muscles (abductor pollicis longus and extensor pollicis brevis) cross the forearm obliquely and will obscure the interval.
b. Identify the supinator muscle and posterior interosseous nerve proximally. Carefully dissect the nerve from distal to proximal through the supinator muscle fibers, preserving all visible nerve branches.
c. With the nerve protected, supinate the forearm and release the supinator from the anterior aspect of the radius. Expose the fracture site by subperiosteally elevating the muscle laterally (**Fig. 11–2B**).
d. If the fracture or planned fixation extends into the middle third of the radius, separate the fascia along the proximal margin of the outcropping muscles. Elevate these muscles as a unit from the radial shaft and retract distally.
e. Stabilize the fracture with a 3.5-mm dynamic compression plate placed across the dorsoradial bone surface.

Distal third

An anterior approach is preferred for fracture reduction and stabilization of distal third radial shaft fractures. If dorsal exposure is necessary, develop the interval between the extensor pollicis longus and extensor carpi radialis brevis tendons, distal to the outcropping muscles.

Ulnar approach

Appropriate for all ulnar shaft fractures.

1. With the injured extremity supported over a hand table, flex the elbow. Alternatively, the arm may be placed across the patient's chest.
2. Make a longitudinal incision slightly dorsal or volar to the palpable subcutaneous border of the ulna. The incision should be centered over the fracture site.
3. Sharply incise the fascia between the extensor carpi ulnaris and flexor carpi ulnaris muscles. Proximally, the interval lies between the anconeus and flexor carpi ulnaris muscles (**Fig. 11–3A**).
4. Deepen the incision through periosteum and elevate muscles subperiosteally to expose the fracture site. The ulna is covered dorsally by the anconeus, extensor carpi ulnaris, extensor pollicis longus, and extensor indicis muscles. The volar surface of the ulna is covered primarily by the flexor digitorum profundus proximally and the pronator quadratus distally.
5. In the region of the olecranon, identify and protect the ulnar nerve before elevating the flexor carpi ulnaris muscle.
6. Position the implant on either the dorsal or palmar surface of the ulna. Careful placement will avert problems associated with prominent hardware beneath the skin surface (**Fig. 11–3B**).

Closure

1. Deflate the tourniquet and apply pressure.
2. Irrigate the wound(s) and coagulate small bleeding vessels with bipolar cautery. Place a drain if necessary.
3. Reattach the supinator, pronator teres, and pronator quadratus muscles to periosteum with absorbable sutures if possible.
4. Loosely reapproximate subcutaneous tissues, leaving forearm fascia open.
5. Close the skin incision(s) with either interrupted nonabsorbable sutures or a running subcuticular stitch.

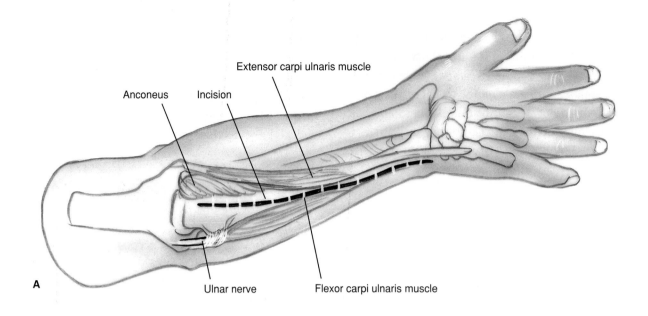

Anconeus Incision Extensor carpi ulnaris muscle

Ulnar nerve Flexor carpi ulnaris muscle

A

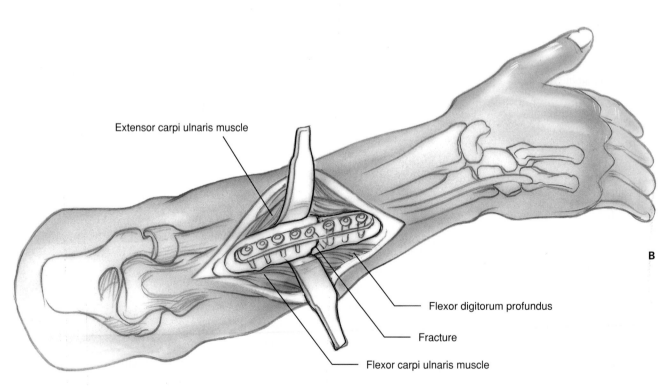

Extensor carpi ulnaris muscle

Flexor digitorum profundus

Fracture

Flexor carpi ulnaris muscle

B

Figure 11–3 (A) Ulnar approach. A longitudinal incision is made parallel to the subcutaneous border of the ulna. The length of the incision will depend upon the pattern and location of the fracture. The fascia between the extensor carpi ulnaris and flexor carpi ulnaris muscles is incised and the interval is developed. Proximally, the interval lies between the anconeus and flexor carpi ulnaris muscles. **(B)** Stabilization of a midshaft ulnar fracture with a dorsal 3.5-mm dynamic compression plate.

6. Apply a well-padded dressing and volar wrist splint. A long-arm splint is indicated for fractures requiring stabilization of the radial head or distal radio-ulnar joint. Support the extremity in a sling.

7. If there is undue tension on the repair, leave the wounds open and temporarily secure the skin edges with sterile elastic bands. A delayed primary wound closure or split-thickness skin graft procedure is performed 2 to 3 days later.

8. Injuries necessitating a compartmental release are similarly treated by delayed primary wound closure and/or split thickness skin grafting.

9. Significant contamination and soft-tissue destruction may also necessitate a delay in wound closure. Soft-tissue coverage requiring microvascular free tissue transfer is ideally performed within 1 week of injury. Bone grafting should be delayed until the time of definitive soft-tissue reconstruction.

Suggested Readings

Botte MJ, Cohen MS, Levernia CJ, et al. The dorsal branch of the ulnar nerve: an anatomic study. *J Hand Surg* 1990;15A:603–607.

Chapman, MW, Gordon JE, Zissimos AG. Compression plate fixation of acute fractures of the diaphysis of the radius and ulna. *J Bone Joint Surg* 1989;71A:159–169.

Godina M. Early microsurgical reconstruction of complex trauma of the extremities. *Plast Reconstr Surg* 1986;78:285–292.

Hanel DP. Volar plate fixation of distal radius fractures. *Atlas Hand Clin* 1997;2:1–24.

Hoppenfeld S, deBoer P. The forearm. In: Hoppenfeld S, deBoer P, eds. *Surgical Exposures in Orthopaedics: The Anatomic Approach.* 2nd ed. Philadelphia, PA: J.B. Lippincott, 1994, pp. 117–146.

Hotchkiss RN. Displaced fractures of the radial head: internal fixation or excision? *J Am Acad Orthop Surg* 1997;5:1–10.

Jupiter JB, Kellam JF. Diaphyseal fractures of the forearm. In: Browner BD, Jupiter JB, Levine AM, Trafton PG, eds. *Skeletal Trauma.* 2nd ed. Philadelphia, PA: W.B. Saunders, 1998, pp. 1421–1454.

Luhmann SJ, Gordon JE, Schoenecker PL. Intramedullary fixation of unstable both-bone forearm fractures in children. *J Pediatr Orthop* 1998;18:451–456.

Noonan KJ, Price CT. Forearm and distal radius fractures in children. *J Am Acad Orthop Surg* 1998;6:146–156.

Rowland SA. Fasciotomy: the treatment of compartment syndrome. In: Green DP, Hotchkiss RN, Pederson WC, eds. *Green's Operative Hand Surgery.* 4th ed. Philadelphia, PA: Churchill Livingstone, 1999, pp. 689–710.

CHAPTER 12

Forearm Fasciotomy

Michael S. Bednar

Indications

1. Increased forearm compartment pressure, either:

   a. Greater than 30 mm Hg *or*
   b. Greater than 20 mm Hg below diastolic blood pressure

2. Limb ischemia for greater than 6 h
3. Following open reduction and internal fixation of radius and ulna fractures in severe crush injury
4. Electrocution injury

Contraindications

None

Preoperative Preparation

Document status of preoperative neurovascular examination.

Special Instruments, Position, and Anesthesia

1. The patient is positioned supine on the operating table. The arm is positioned on an arm board.
2. An upper arm tourniquet is applied with cast padding.
3. The procedure may be done with general or regional anesthesia (not a Bier block).

4. Routine small-joint orthopaedic surgical instruments are required.

Tips and Pearls

1. Attempt to release the forearm compartments within 6 h from when increased compartment pressures begin.
2. The structures that need to be released are the lacertus fibrosis, the mobile wad (fascia of the brachioradialis, extensor carpi radialis longus, and extensor carpi radialis brevis), the palmar fascia, and the transverse carpal ligament. Therefore the skin incision must extend from the elbow to mid palm.
3. The median nerve exits from the muscle of the flexor digitorum superficialis in the distal 6 to 8 cm of the forearm. The skin incision should be ulnar at this distal location to provide soft tissue coverage for the nerve.
4. The epimysium of the individual muscles should be released in addition to the forearm fascia.

What To Avoid

1. Avoid leaving the median nerve exposed at the end of the procedure.
2. Avoid injury of the cutaneous nerves during the approach.
3. Avoid closing the skin. If possible, the skin should be left open or partially closed with rubber bands or vessel loops and staples.

Postoperative Care Issues

1. The extremity should be elevated so that it is above the level of the heart.
2. Active and passive range of motion of the fingers is encouraged as soon as the patient is comfortable.
3. Plan to return the patient to the operating room 48 to 72 h after the initial operation for a "second look" procedure. Consider possible debridement and skin closure (delayed primary or split-thickness skin graft).

Operative Technique

1. Place the patient supine on the operating room table. Extend the arm on an arm board. Place an upper arm tourniquet over cast padding on the proximal limb.
2. Prepare and drape the limb in the usual sterile fashion.

Anterior compartment release

3. Begin the incision at the cubital tunnel 1 to 2 cm anterior to the medial epicondyle. Extend the incision going radial toward the muscle of the brachioradialis. At the junction of the proximal and middle thirds to the forearm, swing the incision distally and ulnarly to lie just radial to the extensor carpi ulnaris tendon at the distal quarter of the forearm. Continue the incision distally to the flexor crease of the wrist. Extend the incision radially in the wrist crease to the location of the usual carpal tunnel release incision. This is found by drawing a line from the third web space. Distally, carry the incision 3 to 4 cm into the palm **(Fig. 12–1)**.
4. Identify and protect branches of the medial antebrachial cutaneous nerve near the medial epicondyle. This incision, which stays ulnar to the palmaris longus, will protect the palmar cutaneous branch of the median nerve.
5. Release the fascia of the anterior compartment.
6. Identify and release the lacertus fibrosis, which comes from the biceps tendon and passes distally and ulnarly.
7. Distally identify the median nerve as it exits from the muscle of the flexor digitorum superficialis in the distal quarter of the forearm. Protect the nerve distally while releasing the transverse carpal ligament.
8. Release of the transverse carpal ligament usually decompresses the ulnar nerve at the wrist. If the ulnar neurovascular structures appear compressed or if the patient had significant ulnar symptoms before the fasciotomy, consider releasing Guyon's canal.

   a. Identify the ulnar nerve and artery in the forearm under the flexor carpi ulnaris. The artery is more radial and more easily recognized. The transverse carpal ligament forms the floor of Guyon's canal.
   b. Protect the neurovascular structures while the fascia is released. At the distal end of the canal, the ulnar artery goes radial to form the superficial transverse arch. Since this passes superficial to the sensory nerves, take care to protect it during release of both Guyon's canal and the carpal tunnel.

9. After the median and ulnar nerves are identified and protected, release the fascia of the individual muscles. Make sure to release the muscles of the deep palmar compartment (flexor digitorum profundus, flexor pollicis longus, and pronator quadratus) **(Fig. 12–2)**.

Posterior compartment release

➤ Commonly, release of the anterior compartment will decompress the posterior compartment.
➤ Consider measuring posterior compartment pressure intraoperatively. If uncertainty exists, the posterior compartment should be released.

10. The line of the incision is between the lateral epicondyle and Lister's tubercle. Begin the incision 1 to 2 cm distal to the lateral epicondyle. Extend it to the junction of the middle and distal thirds of the forearm **(Fig. 12–3)**.
11. Take care to avoid injuring the posterior cutaneous nerves. Release the fascia of the extensor digitorum comminus and the extensor carpi ulnaris **(Fig. 12–4)**.

Closure

12. Deflate the tourniquet. Check the vascular status of the muscle. In most instances after a primary fasciotomy, poorly perfused muscle should be

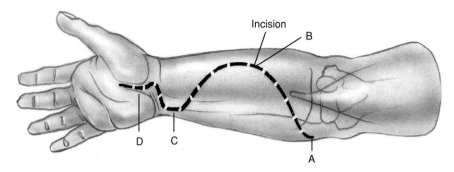

Figure 12–1 Incision for palmar forearm fasciotomy. The incision begins anterior to the medial epicondyle (A), goes distally and radially to open the mobile wad (B), then goes distally and ulnarly to form a flap to cover the median nerve proximal to the wrist (C). Finally, the incision crosses the carpal tunnel (D).

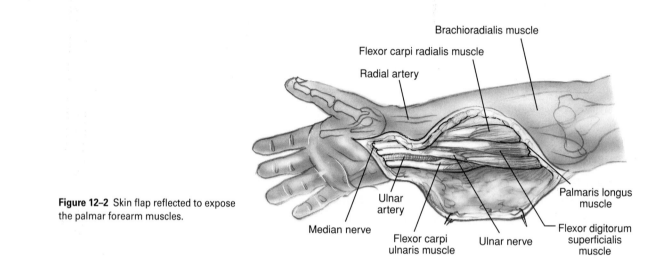

Figure 12–2 Skin flap reflected to expose the palmar forearm muscles.

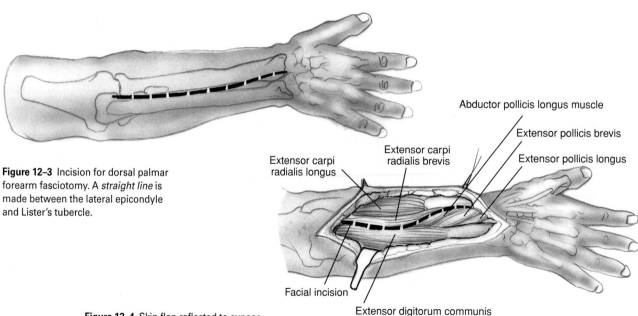

Figure 12–3 Incision for dorsal palmar forearm fasciotomy. A *straight line* is made between the lateral epicondyle and Lister's tubercle.

Figure 12–4 Skin flap reflected to expose the dorsal forearm muscles. The *dotted line* represents the fascial incision.

rechecked in 48 h before it is debrided. However, in the case of infection, debride all necrotic muscle at the original operation.

13. Do not close the fascia. Close the skin over the carpal tunnel primarily. Partially close the other wounds by using sterile vessel loops and staples. Tie the vessel loop in a knot and staple the knot to the proximal corner of the wound. Staple the vessel loop to the radial and ulnar wound borders approximately 2 cm distal to the corner. Crisscross the vessel loop over the wound and repeat the process.

14. Directly cover the wound with a nondesiccating dressing. Apply a bulky dressing followed with a sugartong plaster splint.

15. Transfer the patient to the recovery room with the arm elevated above the level of the heart.

Suggested Readings

Gelberman RH, Garfin SR, Hergenroeder PT, Mubarak SJ, Menon J. Compartment syndromes of the forearm: diagnosis and treatment. *Clin Orthop* 1981;161:252–261.

Rowland SA. Fasciotomy: the treatment of compartment syndrome. In: Green DP, Hotchkiss RN, Pederson WC, eds. *Green's Operative Hand Surgery*. 4th ed. New York, NY: Churchill Livingstone, 1999, pp. 689–710.

Section Three

Wrist and Hand

CHAPTER 13

Open Carpal Tunnel Release

Charles Carroll IV and David M. Kalainov

Indications

1. Persistent pain, numbness, or weakness in the median nerve distribution that is not due to cervical radiculitis, brachial plexopathy, pronator syndrome, or nerve laceration *and*
2. Positive findings on physical examination (Tinel, Phalen, carpal compression) *and*
3. Failure of nonoperative management (splinting, steroid injections)

Contraindications

1. Inconsistent clinical history and/or equivocal physical examination
2. Negative electrodiagnostic study (relative)
3. Psychological and socioeconomic issues that may preclude a good surgical outcome

Preoperative Preparation

1. Appropriate history and physical examination
2. AP and lateral wrist X-rays
3. Consider electrodiagnostic testing.

Special Instruments, Position, and Anesthesia

1. Position patient supine with the hand on a table extension.
2. Upper extremity padded tourniquet(s) set to 250-mm Hg
3. Hand instruments and low-power loupe magnification
4. Microscope if neurolysis is anticipated
5. Local or regional block with intravenous sedation

Tips and Pearls

1. Obtain hemostasis during exposure.
2. Identify the superficial palmar arch, Guyon's canal, and carpal tunnel before releasing the transverse carpal ligament.
3. Dissect beneath the transverse carpal ligament with a smooth curved clamp and divide the tissue sharply. Use curved blunt-tipped scissors to release proximal ligament/forearm fascia.
4. Dissect ulnar to the median nerve to minimize the risk of injury to the motor branch. The motor branch may vary in position beneath the ligament.

5. Be cognizant of the ulnar course of the common digital nerve to the long and ring fingers.

6. If the incision is carried proximally across the wrist creases, stay ulnar to the palmaris longus tendon to minimize the risk of injury to the palmar cutaneous branch of the median nerve. The incision should cross the wrist crease obliquely to minimize the risk of skin contracture.

7. Loosely reapproximate the skin edges.

What To Avoid

1. Avoid injury to visible palmar cutaneous nerve branches.

2. Avoid prolonged tourniquet time.

3. Avoid cutting any structures that have not been clearly identified.

4. Avoid injury to the ulnar nerve, median nerve (including motor branch), and palmar arch.

Postoperative Care Issues

1. Bulky dressing with fingers free; volar plaster splint optional

2. Commence immediate finger motion.

3. Dressing change at 3 to 5 days; removable wrist splint for comfort

4. Remove skin sutures 10 to 14 days after surgery.

5. Judicious use of hand therapy and return-to-work programs

6. Unrestricted activities at 2 to 3 months; full strength at 6 to 12 months

Operative Technique

Approach

1. Place the patient supine with the extremity resting over a hand table extension. Place a well-padded tourniquet(s) around the proximal arm.

2. Prepare and drape the extremity in the usual sterile fashion.

3. Secure the hand palm-up in a hand holding device.

4. The primary surgeon sits on the axillary side of the extremity.

5. Make a longitudinal incision approximately 3 to 4 cm in length. The incision should be positioned 0.5 cm ulnar to the thenar crease and in line with the third web space. For routine procedures, keep the incision distal to the wrist creases (**Fig. 13–1**).

6. Dissect through the subcutaneous fat by carefully spreading the tissue. Protect small palmar cutaneous nerve branches, which may transversely cross the proximal aspect of the incision.

7. Divide the palmar fascia sharply (**Fig. 13–2**).

Carpal tunnel release

8. Locate the distal end of the transverse carpal ligament where the tissue thins. Dissect into the interval between the superficial palmar arch and the distal transverse carpal ligament (**Fig. 13–3**).

9. Dissect beneath the transverse carpal ligament with a smooth curved clamp. Stay ulnar to the median nerve.

10. Sharply incise and divide the transverse carpal ligament. Avoid injury to crossing branches between the median and ulnar nerves (**Fig. 13–4**).

11. Under direct vision divide the volar forearm fascia with blunt-tipped scissors for a distance of 2 to 3 cm. The release should permit passage of one finger into the forearm.

12. Consider performing an external neurolysis if there are residual areas of focal compression.

Closure

13. Release the tourniquet.

14. Irrigate and cauterize small bleeders.

15. Anesthetize skin edges with 0.5% bupivacaine. Close the skin with 5-0 nylon sutures placed in an interrupted fashion.

16. Apply a loose bulky dressing that leaves the fingers free.

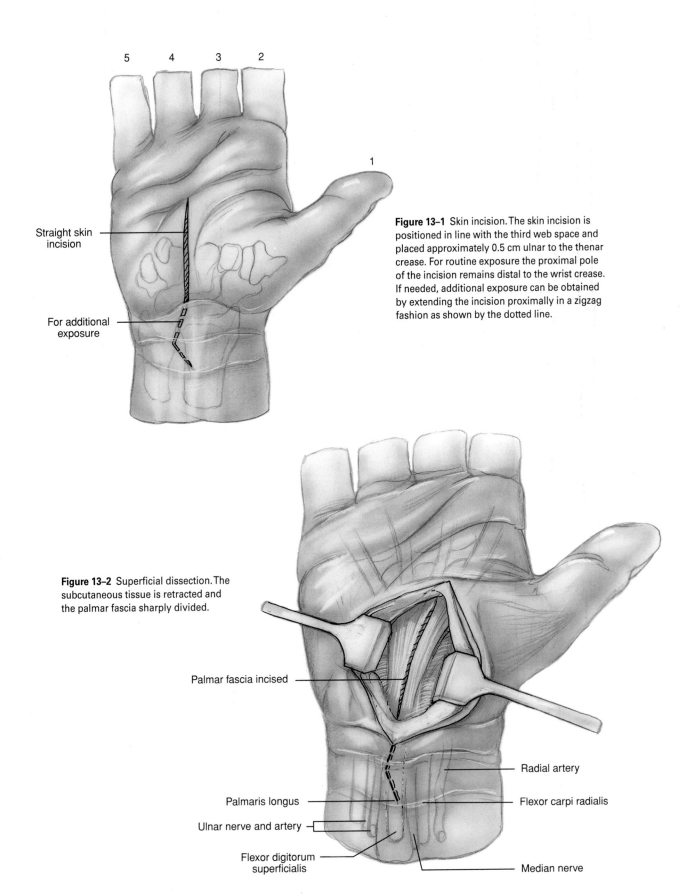

Figure 13–1 Skin incision. The skin incision is positioned in line with the third web space and placed approximately 0.5 cm ulnar to the thenar crease. For routine exposure the proximal pole of the incision remains distal to the wrist crease. If needed, additional exposure can be obtained by extending the incision proximally in a zigzag fashion as shown by the dotted line.

Straight skin incision

For additional exposure

5   4   3   2

1

Figure 13–2 Superficial dissection. The subcutaneous tissue is retracted and the palmar fascia sharply divided.

Palmar fascia incised

Palmaris longus

Ulnar nerve and artery

Flexor digitorum superficialis

Radial artery

Flexor carpi radialis

Median nerve

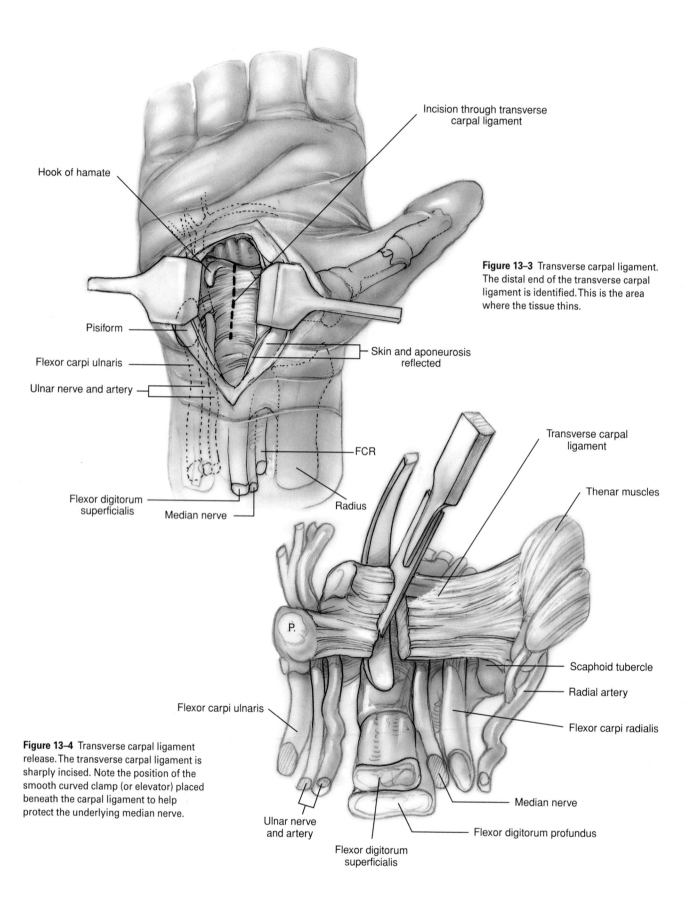

Hook of hamate

Incision through transverse
carpal ligament

Figure 13–3 Transverse carpal ligament.
The distal end of the transverse carpal
ligament is identified. This is the area
where the tissue thins.

Pisiform

Flexor carpi ulnaris

Ulnar nerve and artery

Skin and aponeurosis
reflected

FCR

Flexor digitorum
superficialis

Median nerve

Radius

Transverse carpal
ligament

Thenar muscles

Scaphoid tubercle

Radial artery

Flexor carpi radialis

Flexor carpi ulnaris

Figure 13–4 Transverse carpal ligament
release. The transverse carpal ligament is
sharply incised. Note the position of the
smooth curved clamp (or elevator) placed
beneath the carpal ligament to help
protect the underlying median nerve.

Median nerve

Flexor digitorum profundus

Ulnar nerve
and artery

Flexor digitorum
superficialis

Suggested Readings

Brown RA, Gelberman RH, Seiler JG III, et al. Carpal tunnel release. A prospective, randomized assessment of open and endoscopic methods. *J Bone Joint Surg Am* 1993;75A(9):1265–1275.

Phalen GS. The carpal-tunnel syndrome. Seventeen years' experience in diagnosis and treatment of six hundred fifty-four hands. *J Bone Joint Surg Am* 1966;48A(2):211–228.

Tomaino MM, Plakseychuk A. Identification and preservation of Palmar cutaneous nerves during open carpal tunnel release. *J Hand Surg [Br]* 1998;23(5): 607–608.

CHAPTER 14

Base of Thumb Metacarpal Fractures

Operative Repair

Matthew Bernstein, David M. Kalainov, and Charles Carroll IV

Indications

1. Inadequate closed reduction

    a. Epibasal fracture with greater than 30 degrees of angulation
    b. Intra-articular fracture with more than 1 to 2 mm of step-off
    c. Articular impaction
    d. Trapeziometacarpal joint subluxation/dislocation

2. Adequate closed reduction obtained but not maintained by cast immobilization.
3. Open fracture
4. Concomitant soft-tissue injury requiring frequent access to the wound (e.g., burn)

Contraindications

1. Nondisplaced fracture amenable to cast immobilization
2. Poor patient compliance or severe coexisting medical illness
3. Nonfunctional hand (relative)

Preoperative Preparation

1. Standard AP/lateral/oblique plain radiographs of the injured hand
2. True AP and lateral views of the thumb carpometacarpal joint
3. Comparative views of the contralateral thumb carpometacarpal joint
4. CT or tomograms if the extent of articular damage is difficult to assess with plain X-rays
5. Classify the fracture pattern.

    a. Extra-articular epibasal
    b. Intra-articular two-part (Bennett's fracture)
    c. Intra-articular three-part (Rolando's fracture)
    d. Intra-articular comminuted

6. Evaluate for concomitant injuries (e.g., tendon rupture, trapezial fracture, metacarpophalangeal joint instability).
7. Document the neurovascular status.
8. Plan the method of fixation: K-wires, interfragmentary screws, plate/screws, external fixation.
9. Discuss with the patient the common potential complications associated with operative treatment of thumb metacarpal fractures.

Special Instruments, Position, and Anesthesia

1. Supine position with a hand table extension
2. Upper extremity pneumatic tourniquet; include the forearm in the surgical field
3. Regional or general anesthesia
4. Low-power loop magnification (2.5X)
5. Basic hand tray and routine orthopedic instruments (e.g., tissue scissors, retractors, dental probe, sharp

pointed reduction clamp, periosteal elevator, Freer elevator, curettes, small osteotome, mallet)

6. Standard or mini-fluoroscopy unit

7. Powered wire driver and K-wires (0.028-, 0.035-, and 0.045-in)

8. Internal fixation set with 2-mm and 2.7-mm screws and plates (T-shaped and L-shaped); smaller screws for minute articular fragments (1 mm to 1.5 mm)

9. External fixation set if indicated (e.g., Mini External Fixator, Synthes, Paoli, PA)

Tips and Pearls

1. Intravenous antibiotics should be administered prior to tourniquet inflation.

2. Most unstable extra-articular (epibasal) and intraarticular two-part (Bennett's) fractures may be effectively treated by closed reduction and percutaneous pinning.

3. Displaced three-part fractures (Rolando's) can also be managed by closed reduction and percutaneous pinning. However, open reduction and screw/plate fixation will often permit a more accurate restoration of the joint surface and an earlier return to function. T-shaped and L-shaped plates are ideally suited for these fractures.

4. External fixation is helpful in situations of significant bone loss, comminution, soft-tissue injury, and/or infection. Dynamic skeletal traction through an oblique pin in the thumb metacarpal is an alternative to external fixation.

5. Bone grafting is necessary if the reduced articular surface requires metaphyseal support. An adequate amount of cancellous graft can usually be harvested from the distal radius through a small cortical window.

6. In rare instances of articular cartilage destruction involving both surfaces of the trapeziometacarpal joint, primary arthrodesis may be indicated.

What To Avoid

1. Avoid capturing the thumb flexor and extensor tendons in the fixation.

2. Review the anatomy of the dorsal radial sensory nerve branches. Avoid inadvertent injury with percutaneous pinning and open techniques.

3. Prevent unnecessary stripping of the periosteum and thenar muscles.

4. Refrain from releasing the anterior oblique ligament from the base of the first metacarpal. This ligament is an important stabilizer of the trapeziometacarpal joint and remains attached to the nondisplaced volar-ulnar beak fragment.

5. Avoid prominent hardware beneath the skin. This may impede tendon excursion and result in thumb stiffness, pain, and a cosmetic deformity.

6. The thread diameter of a screw should not exceed 30% of a fragment's surface width or length. If the screw is too large for the bone fragment, there is a risk of iatrogenic fracture.

7. Do not be overly aggressive in the elderly patient population. Pre-existing degenerative basilar joint arthritis may obviate any advantages from surgical intervention.

Postoperative Care Issues

1. Apply a light dressing and immobilize the thumb in a plaster spica splint.

2. Remove the dressing after 3 to 5 days and arrange for fabrication of a forearm-based thermal plastic splint. If the fixation is tenuous, apply a well-padded fiberglass thumb spica cast.

3. Leave the thumb interphalangeal joint free and encourage immediate motion of this joint and all fingers.

4. Remove skin sutures after 7 to 10 days.

5. Begin motion of the trapeziometacarpal joint after suture removal if internal fixation is secure and does not cross the joint.

6. Address superficial pin-tract infections, which may develop during the course of treatment, with oral antibiotics.

7. Remove pins and external fixation frames 4 to 6 weeks postoperatively if there is radiographic evidence of healing.

8. Initiate gentle pinch strengthening at 6 weeks and discontinue protective splinting 6 to 8 weeks postoperatively.

9. Consider removing buried implants after fracture union if the hardware is irritating and/or prominent.

Operative Technique

Closed reduction and percutaneous pinning

1. Epibasal fracture

   a. Apply longitudinal distraction and gentle pronation and extension forces to the thumb metacarpal with digital pressure across the fracture apex.
   b. Stabilize with two 0.045-in K-wires (Fig. 14–1A).

2. Bennett's fracture

   a. Apply longitudinal distraction and gentle pronation and extension forces to the thumb metacarpal with digital pressure against the dorsoradial margin of the trapeziometacarpal joint.
   b. Stabilize with two 0.045-in K-wires. Spearing the volar-ulnar fragment is not necessary (Fig. 14–1B).

3. Rolando's and comminuted fractures

   a. Apply longitudinal distraction to the thumb metacarpal.
   b. Manipulate the fracture fragments with a pointed reduction clamp and stabilize with two or more K-wires.
   c. Consider concomitant external fixation or dynamic pin traction for added stability.

Open reduction and internal fixation—radiovolar approach (Epibasal, Bennett's, Rolando's, comminuted)

1. Make a longitudinal incision over the subcutaneous border of the thumb metacarpal along the demarcation of the glabrous and nonglabrous skin. At the distal wrist crease, curve the incision ulnarly toward the radial edge of the flexor carpi radialis tendon (Fig. 14–2A).
2. Bluntly dissect through the subcutaneous tissues to expose the base of the first metacarpal, thenar muscles, and carpometacarpal joint capsule. Protect branches of the radial sensory nerve that course parallel to and/or cross the incision. Branches of the

lateral antebrachial cutaneous nerve, palmar cutaneous branch of the median nerve, and the superficial palmar branch of the radial artery may be encountered proximally.

3. Elevate the thenar muscles (abductor pollicis brevis and opponens pollicis) subperiosteally from the volar base of the first metacarpal and dissect the fibers off the carpometacarpal joint capsule. Avoid releasing the bony insertion of the abductor pollicis longus tendon from the base of the metacarpal (Fig. 14–2B).
4. Open the carpometacarpal joint capsule transversely for a limited distance, preserving capsular attachments between the trapezium and nondisplaced metacarpal fracture fragment(s). Pay particular attention to the capsular thickening medially which represents the anterior oblique ligament. Clean and irrigate the fracture site (Fig. 14–2C).
5. Develop the interval between the abductor pollicis longus and extensor pollicis brevis tendons to serve as a portal for hardware placement.
6. Apply appropriate reduction forces to the thumb metacarpal and manipulate the fragments into position with a dental pick, Freer elevator, K-wire, and/or pointed reduction clamp.
7. Elevate areas of articular cartilage impaction and bone graft subchondral defects.
8. Obtain provisional fixation with K-wires.
9. Confirm the reduction under direct visualization and with the image intensifier.
10. Achieve final stabilization with K-wires, interfragmentary screws, and/or a plate (Figs. 14–3A and 3B).

External fixation

1. Place one or two pins across the intact diaphysis of the first metacarpal through a small incision. The pins should be positioned in the mid-lateral plane to avoid tethering the thenar muscles and thumb extensor tendons.
2. Place one or two additional pins into the trapezium, distal radius, or second metacarpal.
3. Assemble clamps and connecting bars onto the pins, reduce the fracture, and tighten the construct.
4. If significant articular displacement remains, consider open reduction and supplemental K-wire fixation. Subchondral defects should be bone grafted (Fig. 14–4).

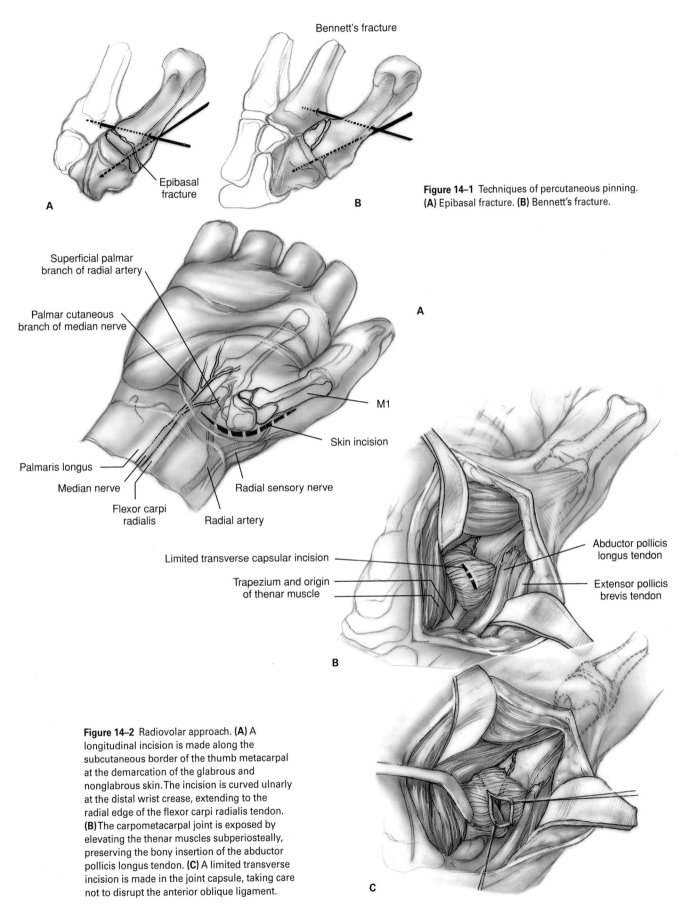

Bennett's fracture

Epibasal
fracture

A

B

Figure 14–1 Techniques of percutaneous pinning.
(A) Epibasal fracture. **(B)** Bennett's fracture.

A

Superficial palmar
branch of radial artery

Palmar cutaneous
branch of median nerve

M1

Skin incision

Palmaris longus

Median nerve

Radial sensory nerve

Flexor carpi
radialis

Radial artery

Limited transverse capsular incision

Abductor pollicis
longus tendon

Trapezium and origin
of thenar muscle

Extensor pollicis
brevis tendon

B

Figure 14–2 Radiovolar approach. **(A)** A
longitudinal incision is made along the
subcutaneous border of the thumb metacarpal
at the demarcation of the glabrous and
nonglabrous skin. The incision is curved ulnarly
at the distal wrist crease, extending to the
radial edge of the flexor carpi radialis tendon.
(B) The carpometacarpal joint is exposed by
elevating the thenar muscles subperiosteally,
preserving the bony insertion of the abductor
pollicis longus tendon. **(C)** A limited transverse
incision is made in the joint capsule, taking care
not to disrupt the anterior oblique ligament.

C

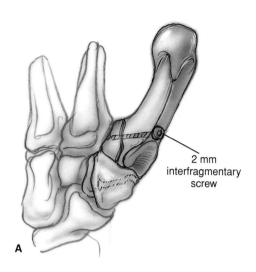

2 mm
interfragmentary
screw

A

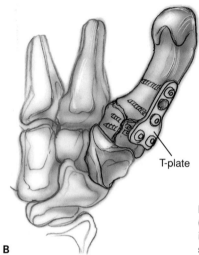

T-plate

B

Figure 14–3 Methods of internal fixation.
(A) Bennett's fracture stabilized with a 2-mm
interfragmentary screw. **(B)** Rolando's fracture
stabilized with a 2.7-mm T- plate.

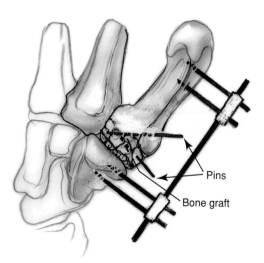

Pins

Bone graft

External fixation

Figure 14–4 Comminuted intra-articular fracture
treated by a combination of K-wires, external
fixation, and bone grafting.

Closure

1. Close the carpometacarpal joint capsule with 4-0 reabsorbable sutures.
2. Reapproximate periosteum over retained implants and reattach the thenar muscles to periosteum with additional 4-0 reabsorbable sutures.
3. After repairing the deep structures, release the tourniquet and apply pressure to the wound.
4. Copiously irrigate the wound and coagulate small bleeding vessels with bipolar cautery.
5. Reapproximate the skin edges with either superficial sutures or a subcuticular closure.
6. Cut the pins external to the skin surface and bend or cap the ends.
7. Apply a light dressing and thumb spica splint.
8. Support the arm in a temporary sling in the setting of regional anesthesia.

Suggested Readings

Buchler U, McCollam SM, Oppikofer C. Comminuted fractures of the basilar joint of the thumb; combined treatment by external fixation, limited internal fixation, and bone grafting. *J Hand Surg* 1991;16A:556–560.

DeBartolo TF. Screw fixation of Bennett's fracture. In: Blair WF, ed. *Techniques in Hand Surgery*. Baltimore, MD: Williams & Wilkins, 1996, pp. 265–273.

Foster RJ, Hastings H II. Treatment of Bennett, Rolando, and vertical intraarticular trapezial fractures. *Clin Orthop* 1987;214:121–129.

Gelberman RH, Vance RM, Zakaib GS. Fractures at the base of the thumb: treatment with oblique traction. *J Bone Joint Surg* 1979;61A:260–262.

Jupiter JB, Axelrod TS, Belsky MR. Fractures and dislocations of the hand. In: Browner BD, Jupiter JB, Levine AM, Trafton PG, eds. *Skeletal Trauma*. 2nd ed. Vol. 2. Philadelphia, PA: W.B. Saunders, 1998, pp. 1269–1282.

Leibovic SJ. Treatment of Bennett's and Rolando's fractures. *Tech Hand Upper Extrem Surg* 1998;2:36–46.

Proubasta IR. Rolando's fracture of the first metacarpal; treatment by external fixation. *J Bone Joint Surg* 1992; 74B:416–417.

Stern PJ. Fractures of the metacarpals and phalanges. In: Green DP, Hotchkiss RN, Pederson WC, eds. *Green's Operative Hand Surgery*. 4th ed. Vol. 1. Philadelphia, PA: Churchill Livingstone, 1999, pp. 758–764.

Wagner CJ. Method of treatment of Bennett's fracture dislocation. *Am J Surg* 1950;80:230–231.

CHAPTER 15

Distal Radius Fractures

Open Reduction and Internal Fixation

Franklin Chen and David M. Kalainov

Indications

1. Fractures that cannot be adequately reduced by closed means
2. Displaced dorsal and volar shear fractures (i.e., dorsal Barton's and volar Barton's fractures)
3. Fractures involving the lunate fossa with separation of the dorsal and palmar components
4. In combination with external fixation for radiocarpal fracture-dislocations and complex, high-energy fractures with greater than 2 mm of articular displacement

Contraindications

1. Stable nondisplaced fractures
2. Fractures amenable to treatment by closed means
3. Severe coexisting medical illness or patient non-compliance
4. Active local infection
5. Significant soft-tissue or bone loss

Preoperative Preparation

1. AP/lateral/oblique plain radiographs; comparative views of the contralateral wrist may be helpful.
2. Determine the fracture pattern: extra-articular, intra-articular, articular gap/step-off, direction of displacement, amount of displacement, comminution, ulnar styloid involvement.
3. The classification scheme used to describe the fracture is less important than a general understanding of the fracture pattern.
4. Consider CT scanning if the complexity of the fracture is not clearly evident on plain radiographs. CT has been shown to be more reliable than plain radiography in quantifying articular surface incongruencies.
5. Evaluate the entire extremity for associated injuries (e.g., scaphoid fracture, scapholunate dissociation, distal radioulnar joint instability, compartment syndrome).
6. Document the neurovascular status; median nerve symptoms are not uncommon. Worsening signs and symptoms of median nerve compression should be addressed by carpal tunnel release.

Special Instruments, Position, and Anesthesia

1. Supine position with a hand table extension
2. Upper extremity pneumatic tourniquet
3. Basic hand tray and routine orthopedic instruments
4. Standard or mini-fluoroscopy unit
5. Familiarize yourself with the available plating system. Plates and screws ranging in size from 2 to 3.5 mm are recommended.
6. Intra-operative traction is sometimes necessary and can be achieved with temporary external fixation or finger-trap traction.

7. The procedure is performed under regional or general anesthesia.

Tips and Pearls

1. A clear understanding of the fracture pattern is critical for planning the surgical approach and method of fracture stabilization.
2. Autogenous bone grafting may be necessary in the setting of significant comminution and/or bone loss. A trephine can be used to harvest cancellous graft from the anterior iliac crest through a small incision.
3. Complex fractures may require open reduction with both internal and external fixation to adequately stabilize the distal radius. The external fixator should be applied first to assist with intra-operative fragment reduction. In rare instances of extensive dorsal and volar comminution, both surfaces of the distal radius may require plating in addition to temporary external fixation.
4. It is not necessary to place a screw through every hole in a plate.
5. Provisional fixation with K-wires can be helpful (0.045 to 0.062 in).
6. For small, but critical bone fragments consider augmenting the fixation with screws and washers.
7. When placing screws in the distal radius, remember to accommodate for normal radial inclination and volar angulation to avoid inadvertent penetration into the joint.
8. Opening the extensor retinaculum in a step-cut fashion will facilitate subsequent closure by allowing the retinaculum to be reapproximated in a lengthened state.
9. Intravenous antibiotics should be given prior to tourniquet inflation.
10. Discuss with the patient the common potential complications associated with operative treatment of distal radius fractures.

What To Avoid

1. Avoid excessive retraction of the neurovascular structures.
2. Do not violate the volar capsule as injury to the volar radio-carpal ligaments may lead to carpal instability.

3. Avoid leaving the tendons in direct contact with the plate, which may cause tendon irritation and eventual rupture. In a volar approach, reattach the remaining pronator quadratus as a buffer over the plate. In a dorsal approach, elevate the fourth extensor compartment in a subperiosteal fashion, preserving both the periosteum and tendon sheath. A strip of the extensor retinaculum can be used as an interpositional material between the radial wrist extensors and dorsal plate.
4. Do not be overly aggressive in the elderly patient population. Internal fixation of osteoporotic bone can be difficult and the fixation tenuous. Low-demand elderly individuals often tolerate deformity better than younger patients.

Postoperative Care Issues

1. A well-padded gauze dressing is applied at the conclusion of the case. The wrist is supported in a volar plaster splint with the digits left free.
2. If fracture stability is a concern, a sugar tong splint can be applied with the forearm in neutral position.
3. A temporary arm sling is useful especially in the setting of regional anesthesia.
4. The drain is usually removed prior to discharge on the first postoperative day.
5. Digital motion should be encouraged immediately after surgery. Some patients may benefit from the assistance of an occupational therapist.
6. Do not neglect elbow and shoulder mobilization exercises.
7. If stable internal fixation is achieved, guarded wrist motion may begin within 2 weeks of surgery.
8. In the setting of concomitant external fixation, the fixator can often be removed 4 to 5 weeks postoperatively.

Operative Technique

Dorsal approach

1. Position the patient supine with the involved extremity resting over a hand table. Place a well-padded pneumatic tourniquet around the upper arm.

2. Rotate the operating room table to permit access for both an assistant and the fluoroscopy unit.

3. Prepare and drape the extremity in the usual sterile fashion. Include either iliac crest in the surgical field if autogenous bone grafting is anticipated.

4. A dorsal exposure can be achieved through several intercompartmental intervals. The most common interval used is between the second and fourth extensor compartments. A longitudinal skin incision is made in line with Lister's tubercle (**Fig. 15–1**).

5. During dissection, carefully identify and preserve small veins and branches of the dorsal radial sensory nerve.

6. The third extensor compartment should be fully released and the extensor pollicis longus tendon retracted radially.

7. The second and fourth extensor compartments are elevated as units by subperiosteal dissection. The second extensor compartment tendons and the extensor pollicis longus are retracted radially. The fourth extensor compartment tendons are retracted in an ulnar direction. Do not violate the sheath surrounding the fourth extensor compartment tendons (**Figs. 15–2A and 2B**).

8. Visualization of the distal radius can be maximized with self-retaining retractors, hand-held retractors, or penrose drains placed around the tendon units.

9. If exposure of the radio-carpal interval is necessary, the dorsal wrist capsule is incised either transversely or longitudinally.

10. A Freer elevator and dental probe are useful in elevating the fracture fragments. Finger-trap traction or external fixation can also facilitate fracture fragment reduction.

11. Consideration should be given toward autogenous bone grafting if a substantial defect exists. Smaller defects may be effectively filled with a bone substitute material.

12. If needed, provisional stabilization of the fracture fragments can be achieved with K-wires.

13. Depending on the fracture pattern, a T-shaped plate or other low-profile plate is contoured and secured to bone with cortical screws (**Fig. 15–3**). Special buttress pins are available with the pi-plating system to help stabilize the reconstructed articular surface.

14. Fluoroscopic images should be obtained throughout the procedure to evaluate fracture reduction, plate/screw position, and fracture stability.

Volar approach

1. Patient positioning and preparation are identical to that described for dorsal plating.

2. Blunt retractors are recommended to avoid injury to neurovascular structures.

3. The distal radius can be exposed from either the radial or ulnar side of the volar forearm.

Radial-sided exposure

The radial approach involves developing the interval between the flexor carpi radialis tendon and radial artery. The exposure permits preservation of the pronator quadratus muscle, but provides only limited visualization of the ulnar corner of the distal radius. A separate incision for median nerve decompression is recommended to avoid injury to the palmar cutaneous branch of the median nerve.

a. A longitudinal skin incision is made between the flexor carpi radialis tendon and radial artery. The tendon sheath is opened and the interval between the tendon and radial artery is developed.

b. The flexor tendons and median nerve are gently retracted ulnarly to expose the pronator quadratus. This muscle is divided along its radial and distal margins with preservation of a small cuff of tissue for later repair (**Fig. 15–4**). Care is taken not to detach the origin of the volar radio-carpal ligaments and to avoid vigorous retraction of the radial artery and median nerve.

c. Elevating the pronator quadratus from a radial to ulnar direction will provide exposure to the fracture site.

Ulna-sided exposure

The ulnar approach is extensile and involves developing the interval between the flexor carpi ulnaris tendon/ulnar neurovascular bundle and the contents of the carpal canal. The exposure permits carpal tunnel decompression, forearm fascial release, and good visualization of the ulnar corner of the distal radius. However, a large portion of the pronator quadratus muscle is often destroyed and the tip of the radial styloid is poorly visualized.

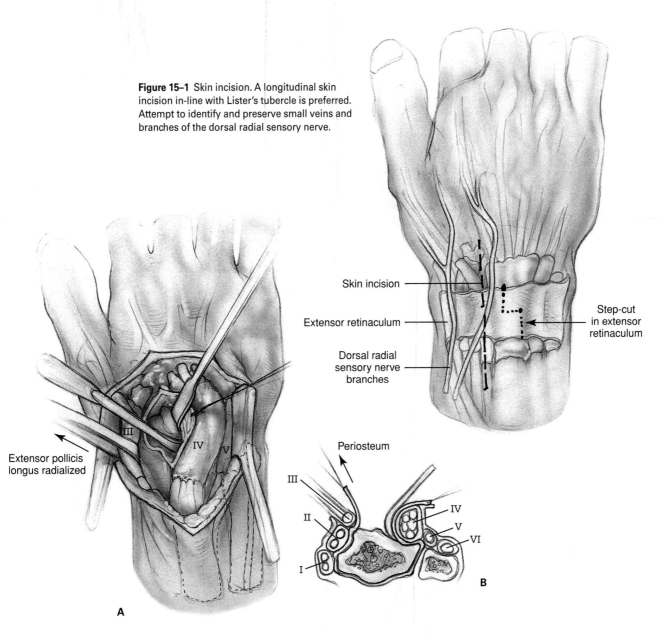

Figure 15–1 Skin incision. A longitudinal skin incision in-line with Lister's tubercle is preferred. Attempt to identify and preserve small veins and branches of the dorsal radial sensory nerve.

Skin incision

Extensor retinaculum

Dorsal radial sensory nerve branches

Step-cut in extensor retinaculum

Periosteum

III

II

I

IV

V

VI

B

Extensor pollicis longus radialized

III

IV

V

A

Figure 15–2 Dorsal exposure. **(A)** The third extensor compartment should be fully released and the extensor pollicis longus tendon retracted radially with the radial wrist extensors. **(B)** The fourth extensor compartment is elevated as a unit by subperiosteal dissection and retracted in an ulnar direction. Do not violate the sheath surrounding the tendons.

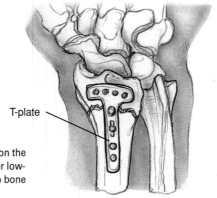

T-plate

Figure 15–3 T-shaped plate. Depending on the fracture pattern, a T-shaped plate or other low-profile plate is contoured and secured to bone with cortical screws.

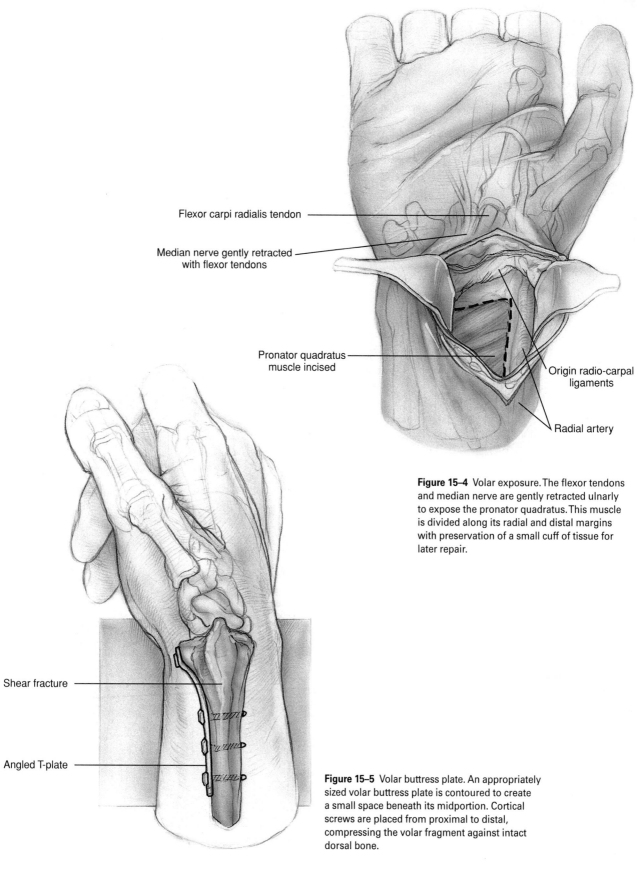

Flexor carpi radialis tendon

Median nerve gently retracted
with flexor tendons

Pronator quadratus
muscle incised

Origin radio-carpal
ligaments

Radial artery

Figure 15–4 Volar exposure. The flexor tendons and median nerve are gently retracted ulnarly to expose the pronator quadratus. This muscle is divided along its radial and distal margins with preservation of a small cuff of tissue for later repair.

Shear fracture

Angled T-plate

Figure 15–5 Volar buttress plate. An appropriately sized volar buttress plate is contoured to create a small space beneath its midportion. Cortical screws are placed from proximal to distal, compressing the volar fragment against intact dorsal bone.

a. A longitudinal incision is made through palmar skin overlying the carpal canal. The incision is extended proximally across the wrist in an ulnar direction. When the radial border of the flexor carpi ulnaris tendon is reached, the incision is angled obliquely toward the mid-line of the volar forearm.

b. The palmar fascia and transverse carpal ligament are opened in-line with the skin incision, exposing the carpal canal. The forearm fascia is released proximally along the radial border of the flexor carpi ulnaris tendon.

c. The interval between the flexor carpi ulnaris tendon/ulnar neurovascular bundle and the carpal tunnel tendons is developed and the structures within the carpal canal are gently retracted radially.

d. The pronator quadratus muscle is incised longitudinally and a segment is removed for exposure of the distal radius.

4. An appropriately sized volar buttress plate is contoured to create a small space beneath its midportion. Cortical screws are placed from proximal to distal, compressing the volar fragment against intact dorsal bone (**Fig. 15–5**). If there is dorsal comminution, the volar plate acts only as a passive restraint and should be contoured to the presumed shape of the pre-injured radius.

5. In assessing intra-articular fracture reduction, avoid opening the volar wrist capsule. Evaluate the reduction with fluoroscopy and plain radiographs. A small dorsal arthrotomy or diagnostic wrist arthroscopy may be helpful in equivocal cases.

Closure

1. Repair the deep soft tissues with 4-0 or 5-0 absorbable suture (volar approach: pronator quadratus; dorsal approach: extensor retinaculum). Ensure that there is a soft-tissue barrier between the plate and overlying tendons.

2. Do not repair the extensor pollicis longus tendon sheath when closing the extensor retinaculum. The extensor pollicis longus tendon should be positioned superficial to the repaired extensor retinaculum.

3. After closing the deep structures, release the tourniquet and apply pressure.

4. The wound is copiously irrigated and small bleeding vessels are electrocoagulated.

5. A drain is frequently placed to minimize the risk of hematoma formation.

6. The skin edges are reapproximated with either interrupted sutures or a subcuticular closure.

7. A compressive dressing and splint should be applied.

8. The patient is transferred to the recovery room, once deemed stable by the anesthesiologist.

9. In cases where excessive swelling precludes primary closure, the wound can either be covered with a split-thickness skin graft or the skin edges temporarily secured with sterile elastic bands. When the swelling subsides, the patient is returned to the operating room for delayed primary wound closure.

Suggested Readings

Cole RJ, Bindra RR, Evanoff BA, et al. Radiographic evaluation of osseous displacement following intra-articular fractures of the distal radius: reliability of plain radiography versus computed tomography. *J Hand Surg* 1997;22A:792–800.

Hanel DP. Volar plate fixation of distal radius fractures. *Atlas Hand Clin* 1997;2:1–24.

Ring D, Jupiter JB. Dorsal fixation of the distal radius using the pi plate. *Atlas Hand Clin* 1997;2:25–44.

Ring D, Jupiter JB. Open reduction internal fixation of the distal radius. In: Gellman H, ed. *Fractures of the Distal Radius*. Chicago, IL: AAOS Monograph Series, 1998, pp. 37–53.

CHAPTER 16

Distal Radius Fractures

External Fixation

Franklin Chen and David M. Kalainov

Indications

1. Unstable extra-articular fractures with metaphyseal comminution
2. Unstable intra-articular fractures
3. Fractures requiring re-reduction after initial closed treatment
4. In conjunction with open reduction and internal fixation for intra-operative distraction or as supplemental fixation
5. Open fractures with extensive soft tissue injury

Contraindications

1. Stable fractures amenable to cast immobilization
2. Associated ipsilateral fractures prohibiting secure placement of fixator pins
3. Patient noncompliance or severe coexisting medical illness

Preoperative Preparation

1. Standard AP/lateral/oblique plain radiographs
2. Identify fracture pattern and degree of comminution.
3. Evaluate entire extremity for associated injuries (e.g., scaphoid fracture, distal radioulnar joint instability, median nerve contusion/compression).
4. When initially treating a fracture by closed reduction and casting, obtain frequent radiographic follow-up to assess for fracture displacement.

Special Instruments, Position, and Anesthesia

1. Supine position
2. Hand table
3. Upper extremity pneumatic tourniquet
4. Standard or mini-fluoroscopy unit
5. Routine orthopedic instruments
6. External fixation systems are abundant. Familiarize yourself with one system and understand its capabilities and limitations.
7. Ensure availability of internal fixation plates, K-wires (0.045- and 0.062-in), and a powered wire driver if supplemental fixation is anticipated.
8. Small Bennett and Hohman retractors are helpful for soft-tissue retraction. A Freer elevator is useful not only for retraction but also for periosteal elevation.
9. The procedure can be performed under regional or general anesthesia.
10. Prepare the iliac crest if autogenous bone grafting is anticipated.

Tips and Pearls

1. K-wires can provide additional stability to the fracture. Recent studies have suggested that K-wire supplementation may allow for earlier fixator removal and wrist motion.
2. In the situation of a depressed intra-articular fracture, external fixation for ligamentotaxis combined

with local bone grafting is useful. The impacted graft will provide structural support and may permit earlier fixator removal.

3. Preoperative antibiotics should be administered prior to tourniquet inflation.

4. The fixator should be positioned to minimize interference with thumb motion. In addition, AP and lateral radiographic views of the distal radius should be unobstructed by the pins, connecting bars, and clamps.

5. Although no universal criteria have been established, in general, loss of reduction with radial shortening greater than 5 mm, radial inclination less than 15 degrees, sagittal angulation more than 15 degrees dorsal or more than 20 degrees volar, or articular incongruity greater than 2 mm should prompt one to consider abandoning cast treatment. Some authors have suggested 10 degrees as the acceptable upper limit for dorsal angulation.

6. Remember that the frame is only as strong as its weakest link; there is no need to use larger diameter pins in the radius if smaller ones are used in the metacarpal.

7. Inform the patient of the common potential complications associated with distal radius fractures and the use of external fixation.

8. If signs of worsening median nerve compression are present, perform a concurrent carpal tunnel release. Carpal tunnel pressures have been shown to increase with progressive wrist flexion in the treatment of Colles' fractures.

9. Have available an appropriate wrench or similar instrument for postoperative adjustment and tightening of the frame in the follow-up period.

What To Avoid

1. Do not place the pins percutaneously. This may increase the risk of cutaneous sensory nerve injury.

2. Do not leave the wrist in over-distraction as this will greatly increase the potential for finger stiffness and delayed union.

3. Avoid excessive ulnar deviation and/or flexion. If such positioning is necessary to maintain alignment, supplemental fixation should be considered.

4. Avoid tight closure of the skin around the pins as this will lead to skin irritation.

5. Avoid tethering tendons and muscles with the pins.

Postoperative Care Issues

1. A light compressive dressing is applied around the pin sites and is changed at the first follow-up visit.

2. Overnight hospitalization for observation may be indicated.

3. Immediate finger motion is emphasized and assistance from an occupational therapist may be helpful in the early postoperative period.

4. Do not neglect range of motion activities for the forearm, elbow, and shoulder.

5. Remove stitches after 10 days.

6. Obtain follow-up radiographs at 1, 3, and 6 weeks.

7. The timing of fixator removal is controversial. Generally, the fixator is kept in place for approximately 6 weeks. Earlier removal can occur in the setting of bone grafting and/or supplemental fixation.

Operative Technique

1. With the patient supine, ensure good access to the dorsal-radial aspect of the wrist.

2. The extremity is prepared and draped free in the usual sterile fashion. The planned incision sites are shaved.

3. The primary surgeon is seated at the patient's axilla. The fluoroscopy unit is positioned for easy access to the surgical field, either at the end of the hand table extension or opposite the primary surgeon.

4. First perform a closed reduction maneuver, then proceed with frame application; 10 to 12 pounds of finger-trap traction can be helpful.

5. The tourniquet should be inflated prior to pin placement.

6. Pins should be oriented 35 to 45 degrees from the frontal plane to avoid interference with thumb motion. Constructing the frame at this angle will also permit unobstructed lateral radiographs of the distal radius.

7. Distal pin placement is performed through either two stab incisions or a single longitudinal incision (**Figs. 16–1A and 1B**).

a. When dissecting down to the bone, care should be taken to avoid damage to dorsal veins and branches of the radial sensory nerve.

b. Visualize the central portion of the index metacarpal to facilitate sound bicortical purchase during pin placement.

c. Pin guides included with the external fixator system are generally used to assist in pre-drilling and pin placement.

d. The AO/ASIF system allows for metacarpal pins to be placed at a converging angle to maximize bone purchase (a converging angle of 40 to 60 degrees is recommended). Many newer fixator systems necessitate pin placement perpendicular to the metacarpal shaft.

e. The more proximal of the 2 pins can also be engaged into the radial cortex of the third metacarpal for additional purchase strength. This will often require placement of all fixator pins in line with the frontal plane.

f. Avoid tethering the first dorsal interosseous muscle when placing pins.

8. Proximal pin placement is generally in the middle to distal portion of the radius.

a. The proximal pins should be oriented in the same plane as the distal pins (35 to 45 degrees from the frontal plane).

b. An open approach is recommended as blind pin placement risks injury to the radial sensory nerve and branches of the lateral antebrachial cutaneous nerve. The incision is generally 4 to 5 cm in length, centered at the junction of the middle and distal one-thirds of the radius.

c. The interval between the extensor carpi radialis longus and extensor carpi radialis brevis tendons is identified and developed. The abductor pollicis longus and the extensor pollicis brevis tendons are frequently visualized at the distal end of the incision (**Fig. 16–2**).

d. The dorsal and volar margins of the radial shaft should be exposed to ensure central placement of the pins.

e. Templates or guides can be used to facilitate pre-drilling and pin placement.

9. Verify bicortical fixation of all 4 fixator pins with fluoroscopy.

10. Irrigate the wounds and close the skin edges loosely with interrupted sutures.

11. Deflate the tourniquet.

12. Assemble the fixator frame onto the pins, taking into account radiographic accessibility to the fracture site.

13. Before tightening the fixator, make final adjustments to the fracture reduction.

a. At this stage, K-wires can be used as joysticks for fracture manipulation and also as supplemental fixation.

b. Fine tuning of fracture alignment is possible with most fixator systems.

c. The ideal position of the wrist is neutral flexion/extension and radial/ulnar deviation. If excessive flexion or ulnar deviation is required to maintain fracture alignment, supplemental fixation is recommended (**Fig. 16–3**).

d. Check the carpus under fluoroscopy for over-distraction. The radiocarpal interval should be no more than 1 to 2 mm wider than the midcarpal interval on the AP projection. The carpal height index (CHI) can also be helpful in determining over-distraction. Caution is advised in over-reliance upon radiographic parameters, however, as recent investigators have questioned their reliability.

e. Make sure that the fingers can be easily flexed to a complete fist as an additional check against over-distraction.

14. If K-wires have been placed, the exposed tips are either bent or capped.

15. Check the skin around the pins for excessive tension and make relaxing skin incisions as necessary.

16. A light compressive dressing is applied and the patient is transferred to the recovery room once stable.

17. A postoperative sling can be used for comfort. Instructions are given to begin early finger motion and to elevate and ice the wrist to reduce postoperative swelling.

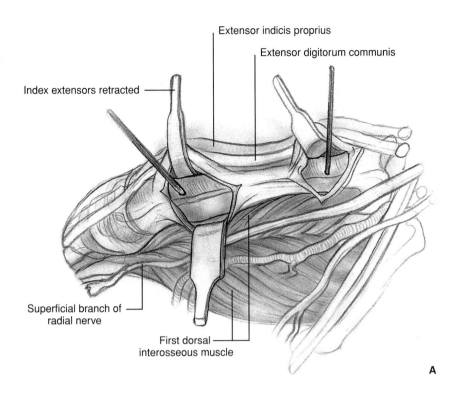

Extensor indicis proprius

Extensor digitorum communis

Index extensors retracted

Superficial branch of
radial nerve

First dorsal
interosseous muscle

A

Figure 16–1 (A) Distal pin placement. Distal pin placement is
performed through either two stab incisions or a single longitudinal
incision. When dissecting down to the bone, care should be taken
to avoid damage to dorsal veins and branches of the radial sensory
nerve. **(B)** Distal pin placement. Seat the pins at a converging angle
of 40 to 60 degrees to maximize metacarpal bone purchase. Orient
both pins 35 to 45 degrees from the frontal plane to avoid interference
with thumb motion.

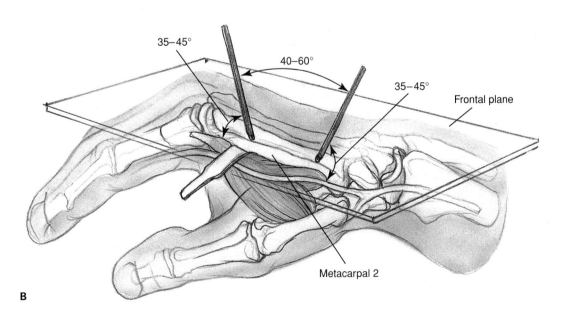

35–45°

40–60°

35–45°

Frontal plane

Metacarpal 2

B

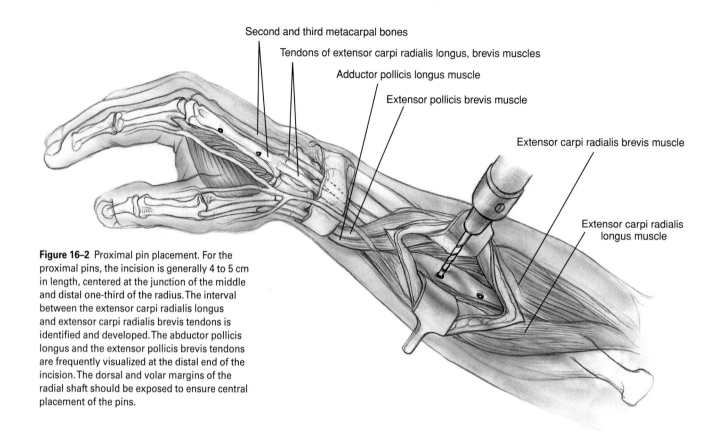

Second and third metacarpal bones

Tendons of extensor carpi radialis longus, brevis muscles

Adductor pollicis longus muscle

Extensor pollicis brevis muscle

Extensor carpi radialis brevis muscle

Extensor carpi radialis longus muscle

Figure 16–2 Proximal pin placement. For the proximal pins, the incision is generally 4 to 5 cm in length, centered at the junction of the middle and distal one-third of the radius. The interval between the extensor carpi radialis longus and extensor carpi radialis brevis tendons is identified and developed. The abductor pollicis longus and the extensor pollicis brevis tendons are frequently visualized at the distal end of the incision. The dorsal and volar margins of the radial shaft should be exposed to ensure central placement of the pins.

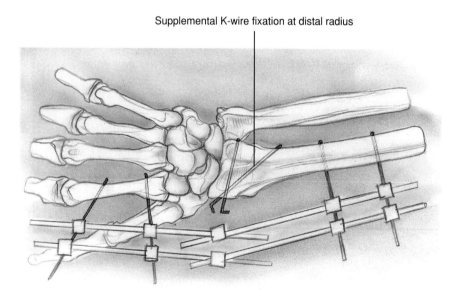

Supplemental K-wire fixation at distal radius

Figure 16–3 External fixator placement. The ideal position of the wrist is neutral flexion/extension and radial/ulnar deviation. If excessive flexion or ulnar deviation is required to maintain fracture alignment, supplemental K-wire fixation is recommended.

Suggested Readings

Gelberman RH, Szabo RM, Mortensen WW. Carpal tunnel pressures and wrist position in patients with Colles' fractures. *J Trauma* 1984;24:747–749.

Graham TJ. Surgical correction of malunited fractures of the distal radius. *J Am Acad Orthop Surg* 1997;5:270–281.

Gupta R, Bozentka DJ, Bora FW. The evaluation of tension in an experimental model of external fixation of distal radius fractures. *J Hand Surg* 1999;24A:108–112.

Kaempffe FA, Wheeler DJ, Peimer CA, et al. Severe fractures of the distal radius: effect of amount and duration of external fixator distraction on outcome. *J Hand Surg* 1993;18A:33–41.

Leung KS, Shen WY, Tsang HK, et al. An effective treatment of comminuted fractures of the distal radius. *J Hand Surg* 1990;15A:11–17.

McQueen M, Caspers J. Colles fracture: does the anatomical result affect the final function? *J Bone Joint Surg* 1988;70B:649–651.

Putnam MD, Fischer MD. Treatment of unstable distal radius fractures: methods and comparison of external distraction and ORIF versus external distraction-ORIF neutralization. *J Hand Surg* 1997;22A:238–251.

Seitz WH Jr. External fixation of distal radius fractures: indications and technical principles. *Orthop Clin North Am* 1993;24:255–264.

Wolfe SW, Lorenze MD, Austin G, et al. Load-displacement behavior in a distal radial fracture model: the effect of simulated healing on motion. *J Bone Joint Surg* 1999;81A:53–59.

CHAPTER 17

Extensor Tendon Repair

Michael S. Bednar

Indications

1. Extensor tendon laceration in zones 1 through 8 (**Figs. 17–1 and 17–2**)
2. Following incision of extensor tendon for exposure of proximal phalanx (Chamay approach)

Contraindications

1. Lacerations in zone 6 proximal to the raffe and lacerations in zones 7 and 8 greater than 10 to 14 days old (myostatic contracture of the muscle will keep the tendon from being pulled out to its normal length; if a repair is attempted with excessive tension, the repair will be too tight)
2. Closed rupture of extensor tendon in zone 1 (mallet finger) or zone 3 (acute boutonniere deformity)
3. Crush injury with loss of tendon (requires primary or delayed grafting, depending on status of skin)
4. Infected wound (need to debride prior to placing sutures in tendon)

Preoperative Preparation

1. Document status of preoperative neurovascular examination.
2. If a delayed primary repair is to be performed (within 10 to 14 days), the wound is initially irrigated and closed. The extremity is splinted with the wrist in 20 degrees of extension and the fingers fully extended.

Special Instruments, Position, and Anesthesia

1. The patient is positioned supine on the operating table. The arm is positioned on an arm board.
2. An upper arm tourniquet is applied with cast padding.
3. The procedure may be done with general or regional anesthesia (regional is preferred to help protect he repair while the patient awakens from anesthesia).
4. Routine small joint orthopaedic surgical instruments are required. A Bunnell tendon retriever or #8 pediatric feeding tube may be required if the tendon has retracted proximally.

Tips and Pearls

1. Extensor tendons are thin. The average thickness is 0.5 to 0.8 mm over the phalanges and 1.5 to 1.8 mm over the metacarpals. Care must be taken in handling the tissue to avoid shredding it.
2. Distal to the raffe, the extensor tendon will not gap more than a few millimeters. Rather than pulling the ends of the tendon toward each other, hyperextend the joints slightly to create a tension-free repair. Because the tendon ends are easily visualized in zones 1 through 5, most of these repairs can be done in the emergency room.
3. Proximal to the raffe (zones 6 through 8), the proximal tendon may retract. Because of this retraction and the requirement to make a proximal incision,

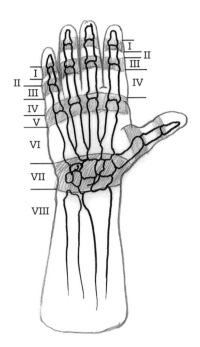

Figure 17–1 Extensor tendon zones. Note that odd numbered zones overly the joints.

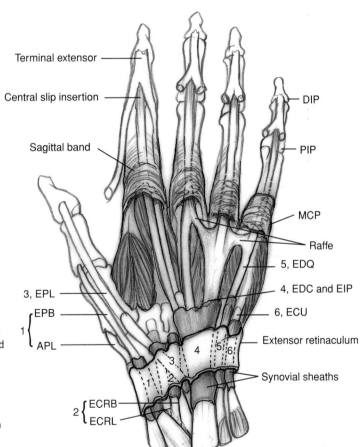

Terminal extensor

Central slip insertion

Sagittal band

DIP

PIP

MCP

Raffe

5, EDQ

3, EPL

4, EDC and EIP

EPB

6, ECU

1

APL

Extensor retinaculum

4

5 6

3

Synovial sheaths

1 2

ECRB

2

ECRL

Figure 17–2 Extensor mechanism of the hand and wrist. There are six extensor compartments at the wrist (zone 7). The extensor tendons of the middle, ring, and small fingers are interconnected in zone 6 by the raffe. Proximal migration of the extensor tendon is prevented when the tendon is cut distal to the raffe. APL = abductor pollicis longus; ECRB = extensor carpi radialis brevis; ECRL = extensor carpi radialis longus; ECU = extensor carpi ulnaris; EDC = extensor digitorum communis; EDQ = extensor digiti quinti; EIP = extensor indicis proprius; EPB = extensor pollicis brevis; EPL = extensor pollicis longus.

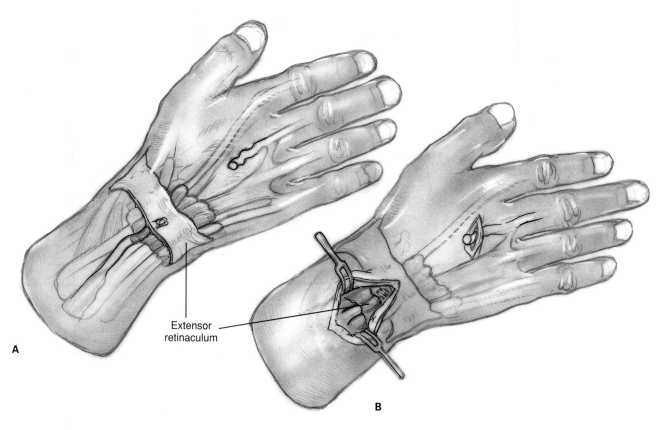

Extensor
retinaculum

Figure 17–3 **(A)** Proximal extensor tendon laceration. When the
extensor tendon is cut proximal to the raffe, the proximal tendon
end is usually found under the extensor retinaculum. **(B)** Proximal
exploratory incision. If the tendon end cannot be grasped proximally
and pulled distally, a second incision is made proximal to the
retinaculum and the tendon end retrieved.

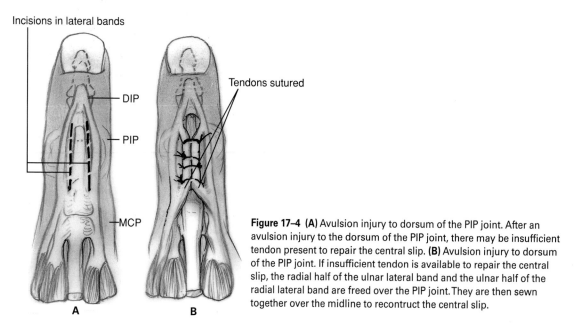

Incisions in lateral bands

DIP

Tendons sutured

PIP

MCP

Figure 17–4 **(A)** Avulsion injury to dorsum of the PIP joint. After an
avulsion injury to the dorsum of the PIP joint, there may be insufficient
tendon present to repair the central slip. **(B)** Avulsion injury to dorsum
of the PIP joint. If insufficient tendon is available to repair the central
slip, the radial half of the ulnar lateral band and the ulnar half of the
radial lateral band are freed over the PIP joint. They are then sewn
together over the midline to recontruct the central slip.

most repairs in this location are done in the operating room.

What To Avoid

1. Do not shred the extensor tendon.
2. Do not overtighten the repair. At zone 3, shortening the tendon by as little as 3 mm will cause significant loss of flexion at the PIP joint.

Postoperative Care Issues

1. Immobilization of the repair site is required for 4 weeks.
2. For zone 1 and 2 repairs, only the distal interphalangeal (DIP) joint is splinted in extension.
3. For zone 3 and 4 repairs, the DIP and proximal interphalangeal (PIP) joints are splinted in extension.
4. For zones 5 through 8, the wrist is splinted in 30 degrees of extension, the MP joint in full extension, but active motion is permitted of the PIP and DIP joints.

Operative Technique

1. Place the patient supine. Extend the arm on an arm board. Place an upper arm tourniquet over cast padding on the proximal limb.
2. Prepare and drape the limb in the usual sterile fashion.
3. Exsanguinate the limb with an elastic or Esmarch bandage. Inflate the tourniquet to 250 mm Hg.
4. At any zone, adequate visualization of the tendon ends is required. If necessary, extend the wound. Take care to avoid longitudinal incisions over the joint creases.
5. In zones 1 through 5, the tendon ends are usually in close proximity. Approximate the tendon ends by hyperextending the joints.
6. In zones 6 through 8, the proximal tendon may have retracted (**Fig. 17–3A**). For lacerations in zone 6, the tendon end is usually under the extensor retinaculum.

a. Retrieve the proximal tendon end by grasping it with a Bunnell tendon retriever.
b. If unsuccessful, make an incision proximal to the extensor retinaculum (proximal to Lister's tubercle) over the extensor digitorum comminus (**Fig. 17–3B**).
c. Identify the lacerated tendon. Attempt to pass the lacerated tendon into the distal wound.
d. If unsuccessful, pass a #8 pediatric feeding tube from the proximal wound into the distal wound.
e. Sew the lacerated tendon to the tube with a single suture.
f. Pull the tube with the tendon distally.
g. Hold the tendon in place by piercing it with a 25 gauge, 1½-in needle.

Repair

7. Repair the tendon.

a. In zones 1 through 4, since the tendons are thin, perform the repair with a 4-0 braided, nonabsorbable suture in a figure eight or vertical mattress fashion.
b. In zones 5 through 8, since the tendons are thicker, perform the repair with a 4-0 braided, nonabsorbable suture in a Kessler or modified Kessler-Tajima fashion. A two-strand (one-loop) repair is adequate for extensor tendon repairs.
c. In zone 3, if inadequate tendon is present to repair the central slip, one-half of each lateral band is split and sewn together over the midline to reconstruct the tendon (**Figs. 17–4A and 4B**).

Closure

8. Close the skin with 4-0 nylon.
9. Cover the wound with a nonadherent dressing.
10. Release the tourniquet.
11. Apply the postoperative dressing.

a. For zones 1 through 4, apply a bulky finger dressing with the DIP and PIP joints in full extension.
b. For zones 5 through 8, apply a bulky dressing and splint with the wrist in 30 degrees of extension and the metacarpophalangeal (MP), PIP, and DIP joints in full extension.

c. If the extensor pollicis longus is repaired proximal to the interphalangeal (IP) joint, apply a bulky dressing and splint with the wrist in 30 degrees of extension, the CMC joint in extension and adduction, and the MCP and IP joints in extension.

12. Transfer the patient to the recovery room with the arm elevated above the level of the heart.

Suggested Readings

Aulicino PL. Extensor tendon injuries. In: Light TR, ed. *Hand Surgery Update 2*. Rosemont, IL: American Academy of Orthopaedic Surgery, 1999, pp. 149–158.

Dolye JR. Extensor tendons—acute injuries. In: Green DP, Hotchkiss RN, Pederson WC, eds. *Green's Operative Hand Surgery*. 4th ed. New York, NY: Churchill Livingstone, 1999, pp. 1950–1987.

CHAPTER 18

Flexor Tendon Repair

Michael S. Bednar

Indications

1. Flexor tendon laceration in zones I through V **(Fig. 18–1)**
2. Flexor digitorum profundus avulsion
3. Flexor tendon rupture

Contraindications

1. Flexor tendon lacerations or avulsions greater than 7 to 10 days old in which a myostatic contracture of the muscle has developed
2. Crush injury with tendon loss (requires primary or two-stage grafting depending on the status of skin, pulleys, and bones)
3. Infected wound (need to debride prior to placing sutures in tendon)

Preoperative Preparation

1. Document status of preoperative neurovascular examination.
2. If a delayed primary repair is performed (within 10 to 14 days), the wound is initially irrigated and closed. The extremity is splinted with the wrist in 30 degrees of flexion and the metacarpophalangeal (MCP) joints in 50 degrees of flexion.

Special Instruments, Position, and Anesthesia

1. The patient is positioned supine on the operating table. The arm is positioned on an arm board.
2. An upper arm tourniquet is applied with cast padding.
3. The procedure may be done with general or regional anesthesia (regional anesthesia is preferred to help protect the repair while the patient awakens from anesthesia).
4. Routine small-joint orthopaedic surgical instruments are required. A Bunnell tendon retriever or #8 pediatric feeding tube may be required if the tendon has retracted proximally.

Tips and Pearls

1. The diagnosis of a flexor tendon laceration can often be made by observation. Loss of the normal cascade of the digits, with extension of the involved finger, indicates a flexor laceration. In addition, loss of the tenodesis effect or loss of passive flexion with active extension of the wrist also indicates a laceration. Finally, if the flexor tendon is intact, compression of the flexor muscles in the forearm should cause the finger to flex.

2. When testing the flexor digitorum superficialis (FDS) tendon of an involved finger, all other fingers must be in full extension. This prevents the flexor digitorum profundus (FDP) tendon from flexing the PIP joint. Remember that in some patients, the FDS of the ring and small fingers have a common muscle belly. Therefore, if the FDS of the small finger does not appear to be working, allow the ring and small fingers to flex at the same time while holding the index and middle in extension.

3. Adequate exposure is essential to achieve optimal visualization of the tendons, pulleys, and neurovascular structures.

4. If possible, repair both the FDS and FDP tendons.

5. Zone II flexor tendon repairs must be done while preserving the A2 and A4 pulleys. The most difficult repairs are those occurring at, or near, the pulleys. If possible, suture the tendon proximal to the pulley by flexing the DIP joint. If this cannot be done, the tendon is pulled distal to the pulley, the core sutures placed, and repair passed back proximally (Figs. 18–1 and 18–2).

6. The proximal end of the tendon may be hard to find when it retracts. Wrist flexion and distal massage of the flexor muscles may improve tendon visualization. In addition, one or two passes with the Bunnell tendon passer can assist in retrieving the tendon from the proximal sheath. However, repeated attempts are discouraged as they can lead to scarring in the sheath.

7. If necessary, depending on the laceration level, the proximal tendon end can be identified proximal to the carpal tunnel or in the mid palm. A number 8 pediatric feeding tube can be passed from the finger wound to the proximal incision. The proximal tendon end is then sewn to the feeding tube and the tube pulled distally. Once the core suture is placed, the tendon is again pulled proximally, the suture to the feeding tube is cut, and the tube withdrawn from the finger.

What To Avoid

1. Avoid touching the epitenon with forceps. Wherever the epitenon is grabbed, this becomes a potential site for development of adhesions.

2. Avoid cutting the A2 or A4 pulleys. This can produce a flexion contracture and limit flexion excursion, which limits active flexion (Fig. 18–2).

3. Avoid advancing the tendon more than 1 cm. If a larger gap is present, a tendon graft is required. Advancement of the FDP tendon more than 1 cm will weaken the adjacent profundi tendons because of their common origin (quadriga effect).

Postoperative Care Issues

1. Motion at the tendon repair site is required to minimize adhesion formation. However, excessive motion can result in repair gapping or rupture.

2. Early mobilization techniques use passive flexion and active extension of the digit in a protective dorsal blocking splint. The splint holds the wrist in 20 degrees of flexion and the MCP joint in 50 degrees of flexion. With the modified Duran technique the distal interphalangeal (DIP), proximal interphalangeal (PIP), and MCP joints are passively flexed by the contralateral hand and actively extended. In the Kleinert technique, passive flexion is accomplished by a rubber band attached to a hook glued to the fingernail. Passive flexion is continued for 4 to 5 weeks after surgery. Composite flexion then begins; the splint is removed and the patient extends the wrist and flexes the fingers.

   a. Passive finger extension is begun in postoperative week 6.

   b. Strengthening is begun in postoperative week 8.

   c. Strengthening and unrestricted use is begun in postoperative weeks 10 through 12.

3. With the development of the four strand flexor tendon repair (see Operative Technique, below), active finger flexion begins in the first postoperative week. Patients are allowed to actively extend the wrist and passively flex the fingers. Digital flexion is maintained for about 5 s. Other parts of the protocol are essentially unchanged.

Operative Technique

1. Place the patient supine. Extend the arm on an arm board. Place an upper arm tourniquet over cast padding on the proximal limb.

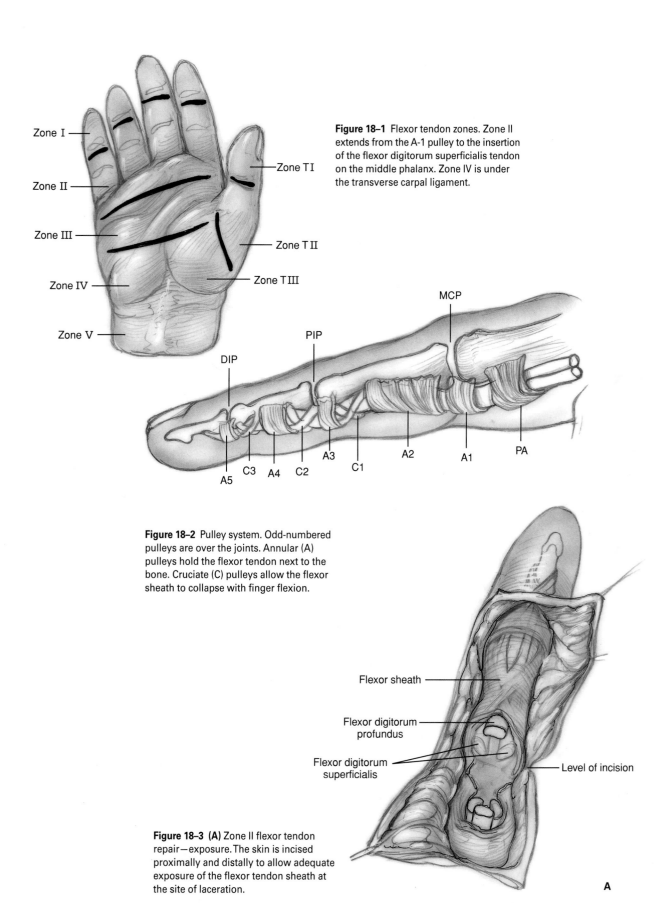

Figure 18–1 Flexor tendon zones. Zone II extends from the A-1 pulley to the insertion of the flexor digitorum superficialis tendon on the middle phalanx. Zone IV is under the transverse carpal ligament.

Zone I
Zone II
Zone III
Zone IV
Zone V
Zone T I
Zone T II
Zone T III

MCP
PIP
DIP
A5 C3 A4 C2 C1 A3 A2 A1 PA

Figure 18–2 Pulley system. Odd-numbered pulleys are over the joints. Annular (A) pulleys hold the flexor tendon next to the bone. Cruciate (C) pulleys allow the flexor sheath to collapse with finger flexion.

Flexor sheath
Flexor digitorum profundus
Flexor digitorum superficialis
Level of incision

Figure 18–3 (A) Zone II flexor tendon repair—exposure. The skin is incised proximally and distally to allow adequate exposure of the flexor tendon sheath at the site of laceration.

A

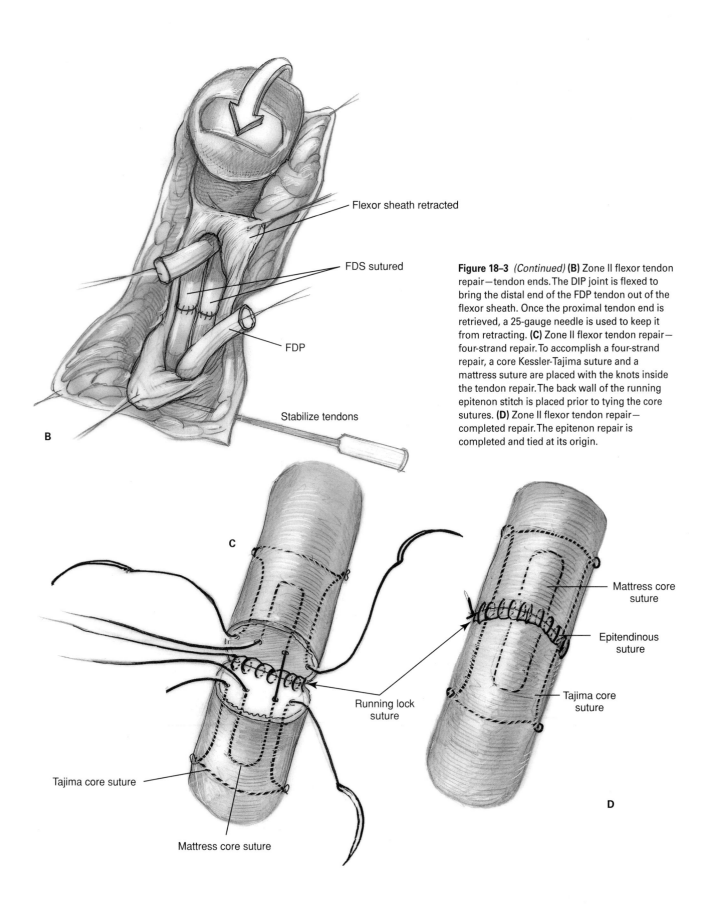

Flexor sheath retracted

FDS sutured

FDP

Stabilize tendons

B

Figure 18–3 *(Continued)* **(B)** Zone II flexor tendon repair—tendon ends. The DIP joint is flexed to bring the distal end of the FDP tendon out of the flexor sheath. Once the proximal tendon end is retrieved, a 25-gauge needle is used to keep it from retracting. **(C)** Zone II flexor tendon repair—four-strand repair. To accomplish a four-strand repair, a core Kessler-Tajima suture and a mattress suture are placed with the knots inside the tendon repair. The back wall of the running epitenon stitch is placed prior to tying the core sutures. **(D)** Zone II flexor tendon repair—completed repair. The epitenon repair is completed and tied at its origin.

C

Tajima core suture

Mattress core suture

Running lock suture

Mattress core suture

Epitendinous suture

Tajima core suture

D

2. Prepare and drape the limb in the usual sterile fashion.

3. Exsanguinate the limb with an elastic or Esmarch bandage. Inflate the tourniquet to 250 mm Hg.

4. At any zone, adequate visualization of the tendon ends is required. If necessary, extend the wound. In zones 1 and 2, wound extension is either by Brunner zigzag incisions or with a midlateral incision (**Fig. 18–3A**). In zones 3 and 4, Brunner incisions are preferred.

5. Protect the neurovascular structures, the A2 and A4 pulleys and the transverse carpal ligament when involved in the incision. If possible, also preserve the A1, A3, and A5 pulleys (**see Fig. 18–2**).

6. Make a window in the flexor sheath at the site of the laceration. Bring the tendon ends to this site (**Fig. 18–3B**). Identification of the proximal tendon end is discussed in Tips and Pearls, above. At least 1 cm of tendon must be exposed through the window for placement of the core sutures. If an inadequate amount of tendon is exposed, bring the tendon end through the adjacent window for sutures placement. Take care to re-establish the anatomic relationship between the FDS and FDP tendons in zone 2.

7. Consider holding the tendon ends in position by passing a 25-gauge needle through the tendon and pulley. First place core sutures into each end of the tendon. Many different types of core sutures have been described. One well-described method (Strickland) uses a 3-0 or 4-0 braided, non-absorbable sutures in a modified Kessler-Tajima fashion (**Fig. 18–3C**).

   a. Place the first core suture through the cut end of the tendon on either the radial or ulnar side. The suture should exit the tendon approximately 1 cm from the end.

   b. Pass the suture through a small portion of the tendon to lock it at this site.

   c. Pass the suture transversely across the tendon. Lock it on the other side before passing it back out the cut end.

   d. Repeat the process on the opposite end of the lacerated tendon.

   e. Place the dorsal half of a running epitenon stitch. Use a 6-0 nylon to capture the distal 3 to 4 mm of the epitenon (**Fig. 18–3C**).

   f. Place a second core suture in a mattress fashion. Place one 3-0 or 4-0 braided, nonabsorbable suture similarly to the Kessler-Tajima stitch. The difference is the suture is not locked in the corners and the same suture is placed into the proximal and distal ends of the tendon. This leaves one knot instead of two inside the tendon repair site.

   g. Tie the core sutures. Complete the palmar half of the epitenon suture. Take care to maintain the wrist and fingers in flexion after the sutures are tied (**Fig. 18–3D**).

8. Repair the flexor sheath with 6-0 nylon.

9. Close the skin wound with nonabsorbable sutures.

10. Apply a bulky dressing and splint with wrist in 30 degrees of flexion and the MCP joints in 60 degrees of flexion.

11. Transfer the patient to the recovery room with the arm elevated above the level of the heart.

Suggested Readings

Cannon NM, Strickland JW. Therapy following flexor tendon surgery. *Hand Clin* 1985;1:147–165.

Kleinert HE, Cash SL. Current guidelines for flexor tendon repair within the fibroosseous tunnel: indications, timing, and techniques. In: Hunter JM, Schneider LH, Mackin EJ, eds. *Tendon Surgery in the Hand*. St. Louis, MO: C.V. Mosby, 1987, pp. 118–125.

Strickland JW. Flexor tendons—acute injuries. In: Green DP, Hotchkiss RN, Pederson WC, eds. *Green's Operative Hand Surgery*. 4th ed. New York, NY: Churchill Livingston, 1999, pp. 1851–1897.

CHAPTER 19

Fifth Metacarpal Fracture

Operative Repair

David M. Kalainov and Franklin Chen

Indications

1. Inadequate closed reduction

   a. Head: greater than 1 mm to 2 mm articular step-off, collateral ligament avulsion fracture with more than 2 mm displacement, malrotation
   b. Neck (Boxer's Fracture): greater than 50 degrees apex dorsal angulation (relative), palmar prominence of the metacarpal head, malrotation
   c. Shaft: greater than 20 to 30 degrees apex dorsal angulation, more than 3 to 4 mm shortening, less than 50% bone apposition, malrotation
   d. Base: greater than 1 to 2 mm articular step-off, carpometacarpal joint subluxation/dislocation, malrotation

2. Adequate closed reduction obtained but not maintained by cast, splint, or functional brace
3. Open fracture
4. Comminuted fracture (relative)
5. Segmental bone loss
6. Multiple metacarpal fractures (relative)
7. Concomitant soft-tissue injury requiring frequent access to the wound (e.g., burn)
8. Tendon repair necessitating early metacarpophalangeal joint motion (relative)

Contraindications

1. Stable, reduced fracture
2. Patient noncompliance or severe coexisting medical illness
3. Nonfunctional hand (relative)

Preoperative Preparation

1. Standard AP/lateral/oblique plain radiographs of the injured hand
2. Special imaging studies

   a. Brewerton view—head fractures
   b. CT or tomograms—articular injuries

3. Characterize the fracture

   a. Location: head, neck, shaft, base
   b. Pattern of injury: transverse, oblique, spiral, comminuted, segmental bone loss
   c. Degree and direction of displacement
   d. Stability
   e. Soft-tissue integrity

4. Document the neurovascular status and evaluate the extremity for associated trauma.

5. Plan the method of fixation: K-wires, interfragmentary screws, plate and screws, external fixation, tension-band wiring, cerclage wiring.

6. Discuss with the patient the common potential complications associated with operative treatment of metacarpal fractures.

Special Instruments, Position, and Anesthesia

1. Supine position with a hand table extension
2. Upper arm pneumatic tourniquet set at 250 mm Hg
3. Regional or general anesthesia
4. Low-power loop magnification (2.5×)
5. Basic hand tray and routine orthopedic instruments (e.g., tissue scissors, retractors, dental probe, sharp pointed reduction clamp, periosteal elevator, Freer elevator, curettes, osteotomes, mallet)
6. Standard or mini-fluoroscopy unit
7. Powered wire driver and K-wires (0.028 to 0.062 in)
8. Internal fixation set with 2-mm and 2.7-mm screws and plates (one quarter tubular, DCP, T-shaped, L-shaped, mini condylar); smaller screws for articular injuries (1.0 to 1.5 mm)
9. 26-gauge malleable wire, external fixation set, and mini suture anchors if indicated

Tips and Pearls

1. Intravenous antibiotics are best administered prior to tourniquet inflation.
2. Open fractures should be thoroughly cleaned prior to stabilizing.
3. Several techniques of fracture fixation are possible; the simplest method requiring the least amount of soft-tissue disruption is preferred.
4. When placing K-wires percutaneously, insert the tip by hand against bone and confirm the position under image intensification. Attach the powered wire driver as a second step. This lends more control than positioning the pin and wire driver together as a unit.

5. K-wires should cross either proximal or distal to the fracture site. Wires crossing at the level of the fracture may lead to distraction and interfere with bone healing.

6. Basic principles of lag screw fixation are important when stabilizing spiral and long oblique shaft fractures with interfragmentary screws.

   a. The fracture length should be at least twice the diameter of the metacarpal shaft to accommodate two or more screws.

   b. Each screw should be positioned at least two thread diameters away from the nearest cortical margin and directed along a plane that bisects both the fracture line and longitudinal axis of the metacarpal.

   c. Prominent screw heads should be countersunk.

7. A plate can be applied in a neutralizing, bridging, buttress, or compression mode. If a T-shaped or L-shaped plate is selected, fix the proximal portion of the plate to bone before the straight portion to avoid creating a rotational deformity.

8. Consider early bone grafting and soft-tissue coverage for fractures with significant bone loss and soft-tissue destruction.

9. Small amounts of cancellous bone graft can be harvested from the distal radius. Larger quantities of cancellous graft and corticocancellous structural graft can be obtained from the anterior iliac crest.

10. Clinically assess the fracture reduction after adequate stabilization and before all wires/screws are placed.

    a. Passively flex and extend the wrist. The tenodesis effect will lead to partial finger extension when the wrist is flexed and to partial finger flexion when the wrist is extended. The small finger should remain well-aligned with the ring finger without overlap and all finger tips should point toward the scaphoid tubercle in flexion.

    b. Compare the plane of the finger nails with the uninjured hand with the digits in extension. The alignment of the finger nails should be nearly equivalent.

11. In rare instances of metacarpal head destruction, skeletal traction or immediate silicone implant arthroplasty may be indicated.

What To Avoid

1. Avoid capturing the collateral ligaments and extensor mechanism in the fixation.
2. Review the course of the ulnar nerve motor and sensory branches. Avoid inadvertent injury with percutaneous pinning and open techniques.
3. Preserve dorsal veins if possible during dissection.
4. Prevent unnecessary stripping of the periosteum and interosseous muscles.
5. Refrain from releasing the origin of the collateral ligaments from the metacarpal head.
6. Avoid prominent hardware beneath the skin which may impede tendon excursion and result in finger stiffness, pain, and cosmetic deformity.

Postoperative Care Issues

1. Apply a light dressing and immobilize the wrist and hand in an ulnar-gutter plaster splint.
2. Change the dressing after 3 to 5 days. If swelling permits, arrange for fabrication of a forearm-based thermoplastic splint. Include the wrist in 20 degrees of extension and the proximal phalanges of the ring and small fingers in 60 degrees of flexion at the metacarpophalangeal joints ("safe position").
3. Consider buddy taping or a protective wrist splint without inclusion of the fingers if the fixation is solid (e.g., interfragmentary screws, external fixation).
4. Remove skin sutures at 7 to 10 days.
5. Begin motion of the small finger as soon as possible to lessen the risk of tendon adhesions and joint contracture.

   a. If the fixation is secure, begin full active finger range of motion at the first postoperative visit.
   b. If the fixation is secure but the fracture is at risk of displacement, begin gentle, limited passive metacarpophalangeal joint motion.
   c. If the fixation is tenuous, avoid motion at the metacarpophalangeal joint for a period of 2 to 3 weeks.

   d. If pins exiting the metacarpophalangeal joint interfere with motion, delay motion at this joint until the pins are removed.
   e. Emphasize early active interphalangeal joint motion in all cases.

6. Address superficial pin-tract infections, which may develop during the course of treatment, with a 7-day course of an oral antibiotic.
7. Remove pins and external fixation devices 4 to 6 weeks postoperatively if there is clinical and radiographic evidence of healing.
8. Initiate grip strengthening and work towards restoring full finger motion after pin removal.
9. Discontinue protective splinting 6 to 8 weeks postoperatively.
10. Consider removing buried implants after fracture union if the hardware is irritating and/or prominent.

Operative Technique

Closed reduction and percutaneous pinning

1. Head fractures: an open approach is recommended.
2. Neck and shaft fractures

   a. Reduce by applying longitudinal distraction and upward pressure against the metacarpal head through the flexed proximal phalanx. Shaft fractures will require counter pressure against the fracture apex.
   b. Manipulate the fracture percutaneously with a towel clip or fracture clamp to assist with reduction.
   c. Stabilize with one of the following techniques:

      i. Crossed K-wires: pass two pins in a retrograde fashion, starting at the retrocondylar fossae of the metacarpal head. Cross the pins proximal or distal to the fracture line, penetrating the far cortices (**Fig. 19–1A**).
      ii. Intramedullary K-wires: introduce several pins in an anterograde fashion through a small hole at the base of the metacarpal. Cut the ends of the pins short and bury in the canal (**Fig. 19–1B**). Alternatively, drill one or two intramedullary pins retrograde through the nonarticular margin(s) of the metacarpal head (**Fig. 19–1C**).

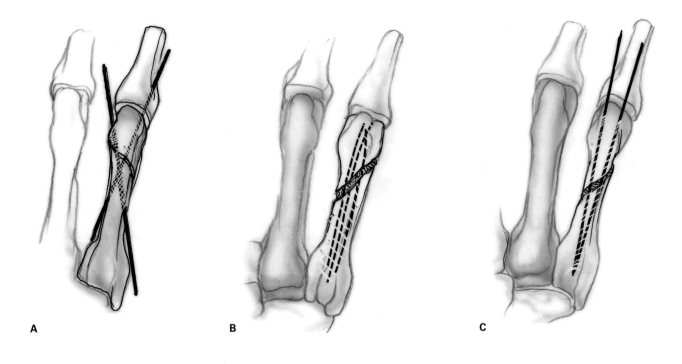

A   B   C

Figure 19–1 Techniques of percutaneous pinning. **(A)** Crossed K-wires; **(B,C)** Intramedullary K-wires; **(D)** Transverse K-wires; **(E)** Diverging K-wires.

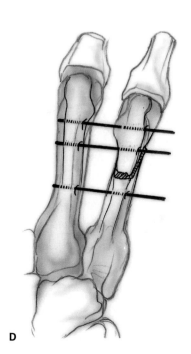

D

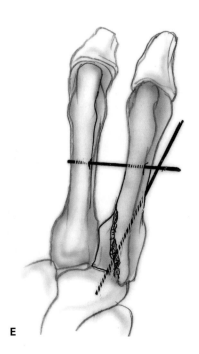

E

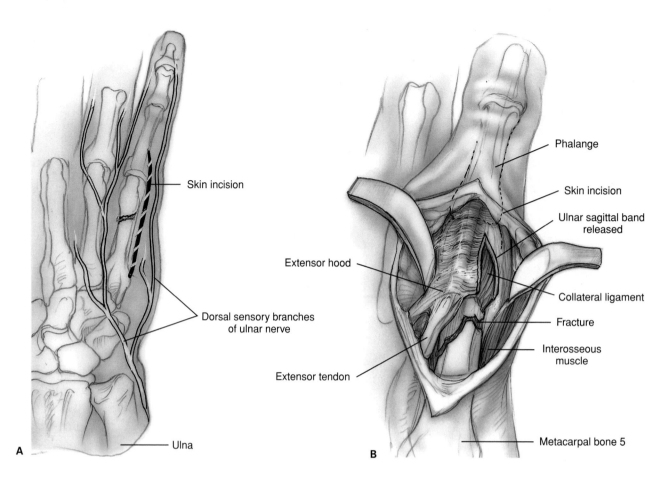

Figure 19–2 Exposure of head and neck fractures. **(A)** A longitudinal incision is made over the fracture, offset to one side. **(B)** The ulnar sagittal band is released and the extensor tendons are retracted. Minimal stripping of the periosteum and interosseus muscles is performed when exposing the fracture. The collateral ligaments are preserved.

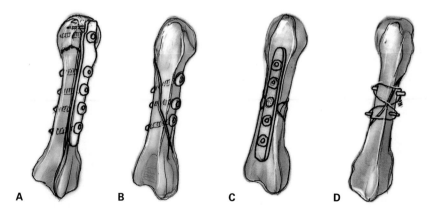

Figure 19–3 Methods of open stabilization. **(A)** Mini condylar plate; **(B)** Interfragmentary screws; **(C)** Straight plate; **(D)** K-wires and tension band.

iii. Transverse K-wires: place one pin proximal and one or two pins distal to the fracture, securing the ends in the adjacent metacarpal (**Fig. 19–1D**). If the fracture pattern is oblique or spiral, consider limiting fixation to the injured metacarpal, placing two or more pins perpendicular to the fracture line.

3. Base fractures

a. Reduce by applying longitudinal distraction and digital pressure against the metacarpal base.

b. Stabilize with one of the following techniques:

   i. Diverging K-wires: place two pins through the base of the fifth metacarpal, one passing into the base of the fourth metacarpal and the other into the hamate. Acceptable fixation is usually achieved without spearing the fragment(s) (**Fig. 19–1E**).

   ii. Intramedullary K-wire: place one pin retrograde through the metacarpal head with the metacarpophalangeal joint flexed. Drive the pin down the metacarpal shaft and across the carpometacarpal joint into the carpus. Advancing the pin proximally into the metacarpal canal will leave the metacarpophalangeal joint free for early motion.

Open reduction and internal fixation

1. Head and neck fractures

a. Make a dorsal longitudinal incision over the fifth metacarpophalangeal joint. Offset to one side in an effort to decrease adhesion formation between the skin and extensor tendons (**Fig. 19–2A**).

b. Release the radial or ulnar sagittal band, leaving a cuff of tissue for later repair (**Fig. 19–2B**). If the radial sagittal band is incised, the junctura tendinum interconnecting the ring and small finger extensor tendons may also require division.

c. Retract the extensor tendons and identify and preserve the metacarpophalangeal joint collateral ligaments.

d. Clean debris from the fracture site and reduce the fragments. Stabilize intra-articular head fractures with screws if possible to permit early joint motion.

e. Address neck fractures by pinning, tension band wiring, or plating. The mini condylar plate is useful for neck fractures with intra-articular extension and is ideally positioned on the lateral surface of the bone (**Fig. 19–3A**).

f. A mini suture anchor is recommended for fixation of displaced collateral ligament avulsion injuries. Alternatively, an intraosseous wiring technique may be employed.

2. Shaft and base fractures

a. Make a longitudinal incision over the fracture site, offset to one side, and retract the extensor tendons.

b. Split the periosteum longitudinally and expose the fracture subperiosteally. Preserve the attachment of the extensor carpi ulnaris tendon proximally.

c. Clean debris from the fracture site and reduce the fragments.

d. Stabilize spiral and long oblique shaft fractures with at least two interfragmentary screws (**Fig. 19–3B**).

e. Treat comminuted shaft fractures and shaft fractures necessitating bone graft with straight plates. Secure the plates dorsally with at least two screws (four cortices) at both ends of the fracture (**Fig. 19–3C**). T-shaped, L-shaped, and mini condylar plates are indicated for metacarpal fractures at the proximal diaphyseal metaphyseal junction or base. Short oblique shaft fractures are ideally treated with a single lag screw and neutralization plate.

f. Consider cerclage or tension-band wiring for fractures found difficult to stabilize by other methods. One or two K-wires supplemented by a 26-gauge wire loop affords a fairly stable construct (**Fig. 19–3D**).

External fixation

1. Consider for any fifth metacarpal fracture with significant bone loss, comminution, soft-tissue injury, or infection.

2. Place one or two pins proximal and one or two pins distal to the zone of injury. Position the pins through small mid-lateral incisions to avoid impaling the extensor tendons.

3. Assemble clamps and connecting bars onto the pins, bring the fracture out to length, reduce the fragments, and tighten the construct.

4. If significant displacement persists, consider concomitant open reduction with supplemental K-wire/screw fixation. Subchondral defects should be bone grafted; larger defects may necessitate structural grafting.

Closure

1. Reapproximate the periosteum over the implants if possible using 4-0 resorbable sutures.

2. If the junctura tendinum and one or both sagittal bands have been divided, repair with 4-0 non-resorbable sutures.

3. After repairing the deep structures, release the tourniquet and apply pressure to the wound.

4. Copiously irrigate the wound and coagulate small bleeding vessels with bipolar cautery.

5. Reapproximate the skin edges with either interrupted sutures or a subcuticular closure.

6. Cut pins external to the skin surface and bend or cap the ends.

7. Apply a light dressing and ulnar gutter splint.

8. Support the arm in a temporary sling in the setting of regional anesthesia.

Suggested Readings

Faraj AA, Davis TRC. Percutaneous intramedullary fixation of metacarpal shaft fractures. *J Hand Surg* 1999;24B:76–79.

Foster RJ. Stabilization of ulnar carpometacarpal dislocations or fracture dislocations. *Clin Orthop* 1996;327:94–97.

Freeland AE, Jabaley ME. Stabilization of fractures in the hand and wrist with traumatic soft tissue and bone loss. *Hand Clin* 1988;4:425–436.

Greene TL, Noellert RC, Belsole RJ. Treatment of unstable metacarpal and phalangeal fractures with tension band wiring techniques. *Clin Orthop* 1987;214:78–84.

Gropper PT, Bowen V. Cerclage wiring of metacarpal fractures. *Clin Orthop* 1984;188:203–207.

Jupiter JB, Axelrod TS, Belsky MR. Fractures and dislocations of the hand. In: Browner BD, Jupiter JB, Levine AM, Trafton PG, eds. *Skeletal Trauma*. 2nd ed. Vol. 2. Philadelphia, PA: W.B. Saunders, 1998, pp. 1249–1269.

Lane CS. Detecting occult fractures of the metacarpal head: the Brewerton view. *J Hand Surg* 1977;2:131–133.

Njus N. Percutaneous pin fixation of the diaphysis of the metacarpals. In: Blair WF, ed. *Techniques in Hand Surgery*. Baltimore, MD: Williams & Wilkins, 1996, pp. 229–238.

Parsons SW, Fitzgerald JAW, Shearer JR. External fixation of unstable metacarpal and phalangeal fractures. *J Hand Surg* 1992;17B:151–155.

Stern PJ. Fractures of the metacarpals and phalanges. In: Green DP, Hotchkiss RN, Pederson WC, eds. *Green's Operative Hand Surgery*. 4th ed. Vol. 1. Philadelphia, PA: Churchill Livingstone, 1999, pp. 711–732.

Section Four

Hip and Femur

CHAPTER 20

Total Hip Arthroplasty

Hybrid and Uncemented

Douglas E. Padgett

Indications

The prime indications for total hip arthroplasty are relief of hip pain and improvement of hip function as a result of any disabling hip condition. These conditions include:

1. Osteoarthritis
2. Inflammatory arthritis (rheumatoid arthritis, psoriatic arthritis, etc.)
3. Posttraumatic arthritis
4. Osteonecrosis

Contraindications

1. Active sepsis (absolute)
2. Active causalgia/reflex dystrophy (absolute)
3. Neuropathic joint (relative)
4. Insufficient musculature about the hip girdle (relative)
5. Inability or unwillingness to adhere to postoperative precautions (relative)

Preoperative Preparation

1. Complete history and physical examination. Record location, quality and activities associated with hip pain. Also document gait pattern, leg length, and range of motion.
2. Appropriate medical and anesthetic evaluation.
3. Document preoperative neurovascular status.
4. Radiographs including anteroposterior (AP) of the pelvis, true or "frog leg" lateral of affected hip, and AP and lateral of lumbar spine.
5. The preoperative radiographs should be assessed in conjunction with the appropriate hip prosthetic templates to determine approximate sizes for both the acetabular and femoral components. Existing acetabular bone stock, as well as any deficiencies in the dome or rim of the acetabulum influence acetabular component size. Femoral templating helps determine:

   a. Level of femoral neck resection
   b. Femoral component size
   c. Distances from fixed points on the femur to the center of hip rotation in order to help optimize postoperative limb length
   d. If femoral implant adequately reconstructs femoral offset and proper hip mechanics

Special Instruments, Position, and Anesthesia

1. The preferred patient position for a posterolateral approach to the hip joint is the lateral decubitus position. Adequate padding of the axilla is necessary to avoid injury to the brachial plexus. While the patient must be secure on the operation room table, avoid excessive tightening of pelvic posts,

which can compromise the neurovascular status of the "down-leg" (**Fig. 20–1**).

2. All pressure points should be padded.

3. The procedure can be done with general, epidural, or long-acting spinal anesthesia. There is some evidence that epidural anesthesia decreases the risk of deep-vein thrombosis as well as decreases blood loss during total hip arthroplasty.

4. Instruments required for total hip arthroplasty include self-retaining retractors, straight and bent Hohman-type retractors, a femoral neck elevator to facilitate exposure of the proximal femur, and battery powered reamers and power saws. In addition, the specific instruments, broaches and trial components unique to the prosthesis to be implanted should be available.

5. Consider using enclosed helmets and body exhausts, which may help minimize the risk of perioperative sepsis.

6. Intravenous antibiotics appropriate for the hospital's bacterial flora should be administered prior to tourniquet inflation and continued for at least 24 hours after surgery.

Tips and Pearls

1. Extensile exposure is essential for success. The use of short or "mini" incisions is to be avoided as it may compromise component insertion.

2. The inability to anteriorly translate the femur enough to achieve adequate visualization of the acetabulum is usually due to insufficient release of the gluteus maximus tendon at its femoral insertion and/or of the reflected head of the rectus femoris tendon at its insertion site into the supra-acetabulum.

3. Preoperative measurements (level of neck resection, distance from lesser trochanter to center of hip rotation) should be reassessed during surgery since radiographic magnification may vary as much as 10 to 15%.

4. Ensure that all significant osteophytes are identified and removed at the time of surgery. Medial acetabular osteophytes can result in lateralization of the cup that may affect abductor mechanics. Osteophytes located on the acetabular rim or on the

femoral neck can cause impingement leading either to decreased hip motion and/or to hip instability.

5. Assess the stability of the hip prior to closure. Pay particular attention to impingement from either osteophytes or the prosthetic femoral neck on the rim of the acetabular component. Stability often reflects the adequacy of reconstruction of both length and offset. Failure to restore offset, especially in large individuals, may result in impingement and hip instability. Hip motions evaluated should include:

   a. Hip flexion of 90 degrees without rotation (simulating sitting in a chair)
   b. Hip flexion of 45 degrees, hip adduction of 15 degrees, and internal rotation of 15 degrees (simulating sleeping position)
   c. Hip extension, abduction and external rotation to assess anterior instability

What To Avoid

1. Because of the problems associated with infection, great care is taken to minimize this complication. Operating room traffic should be minimized, and preoperative antibiotics administered.

2. Avoid a vertical or retroverted alignment of the acetabular component.

3. Avoid over-reaming the acetabulum and removing excessive bone. Conversely avoid under-reaming the acetabulum and using excessive force during component impaction, thereby increasing the risk of acetabular fracture. Controlled acetabular reaming is preferred. If the press-fit stability of the acetabular component is not satisfactory, the use of a supplemental acetabular fixation screw is recommended.

4. Avoid a varus or retroverted alignment of the femoral component.

5. Avoid excessive broaching or reaming of the femur especially when cement fixation of the femoral component is planned. Over zealous removal of cancellous bone will weaken the bone-cement interface and may predispose to early component loosening. Femoral preparation should be performed in a controlled methodical fashion.

6. Avoid excessive force during femoral preparation for an uncemented femoral component. Preparation of the femur for an uncemented femoral component requires patience in order to minimize the risk of fracture.

   If a fracture occurs, it is vital to assess component stability. If a fracture is recognized during either broaching or implant insertion, remove the broach or implant and expose the fracture. Consider obtaining intraoperative radiographs. If the stem will adequately bypass the fracture (at least 1.5 cortical diameters), then the femur should be cerclaged with either 16-gauge chrome cobalt wires or 2.0-mm cables. At this point, the broach or final implant can be reinserted. If the implant is axially or torsionally unstable, a larger implant may be required. If stability is questionable, consider insertion of a cemented stem.

7. Avoid inserting an undersized *uncemented* femoral component. Use of an implant that is too small may compromise initial implant stability, thereby resulting in implant motion and possibly predisposing to early failure. Preoperative templating is useful to help indicate the approximate size of the implant to be inserted. If there is a significant discrepancy between the preoperative projected implant size and the apparent intraoperative implant size, consider obtaining intraoperative radiographs. The leading cause for undersizing the femoral stem is not positioning it sufficiently lateral in the trochanteric bed and thus placing the stem in varus.

Postoperative Care Issues

1. While not mandatory, a suction-type drain can be used and normally, safely discontinued the morning after surgery.
2. Thromboembolic precautions are recommended. Options include intraoperative heparin, aspirin, warfarin, low-molecular weight heparin, and intermittent pneumatic compression.
3. Weight-bearing status may depend on the method of femoral component fixation: full weight bearing with cement fixation; partial weight bearing with uncemented fixation.
4. "Hip precautions" such as avoiding excessive hip flexion and/or hip rotation should be reviewed with the patient.

Operative Technique (Posterolateral Approach)

Approach

1. Position the patient in the lateral decubitus position. Pad all pressure points including the axilla. While the patient must be secure on the operation room table, avoid excessive tightening of pelvic posts, which can compromise the neurovascular status of the "down-leg" **(Fig. 20–1)**.
2. Prepare and drape the limb in the hospital's standard sterile fashion.
3. Make a straight lateral incision approximately 15 cm in length. Center the incision over the lateral shaft of the femur. The incision should start approximately 5 cm proximal to the tip of the greater trochanter and extend distally about 10 cm.
4. Carry the dissection directly through the subcutaneous tissue. Maintain adequate hemostasis. Identify the fascia lata.
5. Incise the fascia lata longitudinally. Bluntly split the fibers of the gluteus maximus at the proximal pole of the fascia lata.
6. Insert a self-retaining retractor. Partially release the femoral insertion of the gluteus maximus tendon with the electrocautery. This greatly facilitates anterior translation of the femur that will be necessary for acetabular preparation. Attempt to avoid the small perforating branches of the profunda femoris artery.
7. While gently rotating the hip internally, identify the piriformis and conjoined tendons. Incise them at their insertion on the posterolateral femur with an electrocautery. Tag the tendon ends with nonabsorbable suture **(Fig. 20–2)**.
8. Place a cobra ("Aufranc") retractor around the inferior femoral neck between the posterior hip joint capsule and the quadratus femoris. Retracting the muscle fibers of the quadratus femoris inferiorly helps expose the entire posterior capsule. Retract the gluteus medius superiorly with a thin, bent Hohman or other retractor.
9. Perform a trapezoidal-shaped posterior capsulotomy. Tag the proximal and distal corners of the capsule with nonabsorbable sutures.
10. Dislocate the hip by gently internal rotating and adducting the femur.

11. With the leg held in internal rotation (foot pointing toward the ceiling), use an electrocautery to strip the capsule and soft tissue off the posterior femur (which now points up) until the lesser trocahnter is visible.

12. Determine the optimal site for the femoral neck osteotomy based on both the preoperative radiographic measurements and the intraoperative anatomic landmarks. Use an oscillating saw to make the femoral neck osteotomy (**Fig. 20–3**). Remove the femoral head and save it on the back table. Occasionally, there is a need for an autogenous bone graft in primary hip arthroplasty, and the femoral head is a convenient bone source.

13. Place retractors around the acetabulum. Anteriorly, place a curved pointed acetabular retractor to translate the femur anteriorly. Superiorly, impact a large smooth Steinman pin to retract the abductor mass. Posteriorly, insert a wide Hohman-type retractor into the tuberosity of the ischium. Take care not to place this retractor through the posterior acetabular wall and into the acetabular fossa. Inferiorly, insert a cobra retractor after releasing the transverse acetabular ligament. Should exposure be difficulty, check to ensure that both the distal insertion of the gluteus maximus tendon on the femur and the retained superior capsule and tendon of the reflected head of the proximal rectus femoris have been adequately released. If these structures are tight, insufficient anterior translation of the femur makes acetabular exposure difficult.

Acetabular preparation

14. Remove remnants of acetabular labrum from the acetabular brim. Next remove the pulvinar (fibrofatty material medially). Take care to avoid the ascending branch of the obturator artery when removing the inferior pulvinar near the transverse acetabular ligament. If a large medial osteophyte is present, the pulvinar may not visible. This means that acetabular reaming needs to proceed medially down to the true medial aspect of the acetabulum.

15. Use power acetabular reamers to prepare the acetabulum (**Fig. 20–4**). Start with a small reamer (commonly, about 40 mm in diameter) and ream medially to the floor of the acetabulum. Do not penetrate the medial wall; merely go down to this level. If identification of the medial wall is difficult, use a power drill to make a small hole through the medial wall. After drilling to a depth of about 3 to 5 mm, use a depth gauge to assess the bone thickness. If the remaining medial wall is thicker than 3 to 5 mm, a portion of the medial osteophyte probably persists and further reaming should be performed. A review of the preoperative radiographs can be useful at this time.

16. Once the proper depth of the acetabulum has been reached, concentrically enlarge the acetabulum in 1 to 2 mm increments using sequentially larger reamers. Direct the reamers so they ream approximately at an angle of 40 degrees of lateral opening (abduction) and 20 degrees of forward flexion (anteversion). Check the integrity of the acetabular columns and medial wall after each successive reamer is used.

17. Continue sequential reaming until bleeding cancellous bone is encountered around the dome and walls of the acetabulum.

18. When inserting an acetabular component without the use of acrylic bone cement, the decision to under-ream (insertion of a prosthesis larger than the last reamer) or ream line-to-line is up to the individual surgeon. Under-reaming often results in an excellent initial "snug fit" of the acetabular component and minimizes the need for supplemental screw fixation. However, the under-reaming increases the possibility of acetabular fracture during component insertion. Line-to-line reaming allows easier implant insertion but often requires the use of supplemental cancellous screw fixation. It is mandatory to remember the "safe zones" for acetabular screw insertion when placing these screws. In general, screws in the posterosuperior quadrant have been shown to have the lowest risk of neurovascular injury.

19. Place the hemispherical acetabular component's shell onto the insertion device and then impact it into the acetabulum. Take care to insert the shell in approximately 40 degrees of abduction (slightly horizontal) and 20 degrees of anteversion. Commercial alignment devices are helpful in determining proper alignment of the component, but they are not "fool proof." Ensure that the shell seats completely and fully medial in the acetabulum after impaction. Insufficiently seated components are at

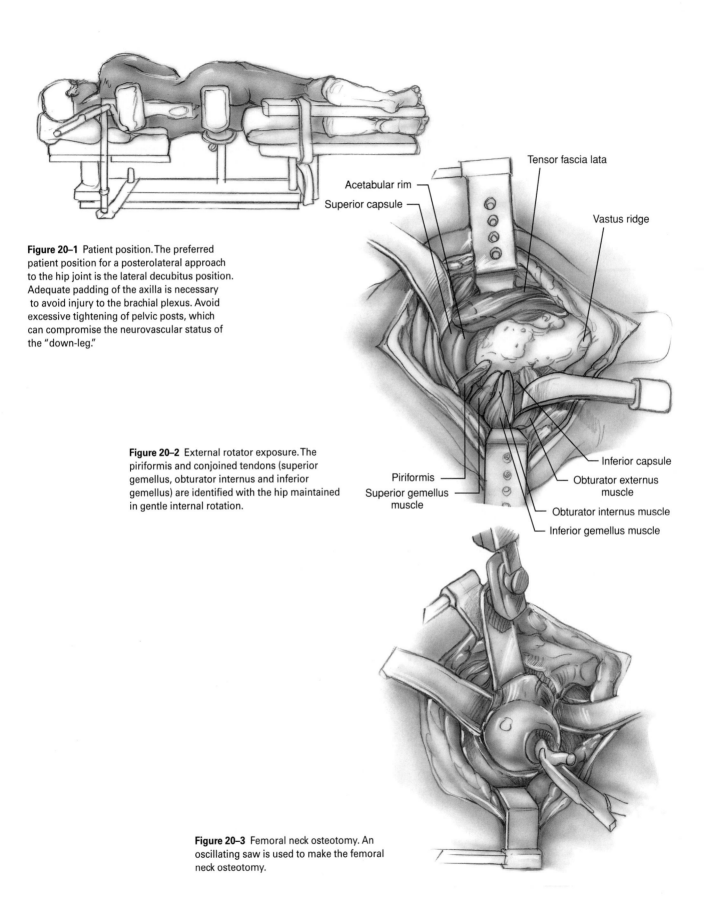

Figure 20–1 Patient position. The preferred patient position for a posterolateral approach to the hip joint is the lateral decubitus position. Adequate padding of the axilla is necessary to avoid injury to the brachial plexus. Avoid excessive tightening of pelvic posts, which can compromise the neurovascular status of the "down-leg."

Figure 20–2 External rotator exposure. The piriformis and conjoined tendons (superior gemellus, obturator internus and inferior gemellus) are identified with the hip maintained in gentle internal rotation.

Tensor fascia lata

Acetabular rim

Superior capsule

Vastus ridge

Inferior capsule

Piriformis

Superior gemellus muscle

Obturator externus muscle

Obturator internus muscle

Inferior gemellus muscle

Figure 20–3 Femoral neck osteotomy. An oscillating saw is used to make the femoral neck osteotomy.

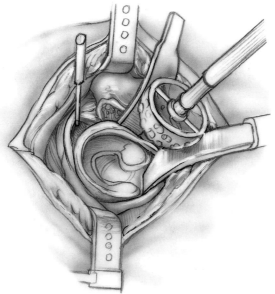

Figure 20–4 Acetabular reaming. Power acetabular reamers are used to prepare the acetabulum. Note the position of the retractors. A curved pointed acetabular retractor is used to translate the femur anteriorly. A large smooth Steinman pin is used to retract the abductor mass superiorly. A cobra retractor is positioned inferiorly. A wide Hohman-type retractor can be inserted into the tuberosity of the ischium posteriorly (not shown).

Figure 20–5 Acetabular component insertion. The acetabular component's shell is impacted into the acetabulum. In general, the goal is to insert the shell in approximately 40 degrees of abduction (slightly horizontal) and 20 degrees of anteversion.

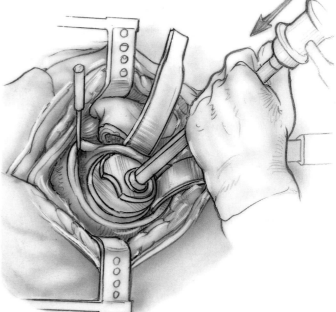

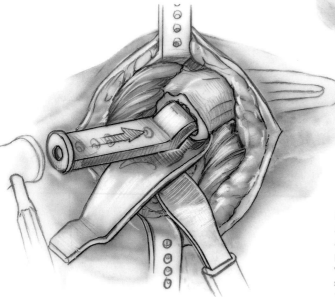

Figure 20–6 Femoral canal broaching. Sequentially larger broaches are impacted into the femoral canal until a reasonably snug fit is achieved. As with reaming, do not "over-broach." During broaching, pay attention to the alignment of the broach in all planes (varus-valgus, flexion-extension, and rotation). In general, insert the broaches so they rotational align with the natural femoral neck. This is usually 12 to 15 degrees of anteversion.

risk for change in orientation in the early postoperative period (**Fig. 20–5**).

20. Insert the polyethylene liner. The use of standard flat-faced liners or elevated liners depends on the surgeon's preference. Remember that elevated liners generally help enhance hip stability in only one direction. Conversely, they may be a source of impingement in the opposite direction. Therefore, careful assessment is required when positioning and inserting elevated liners.

21. Remove the acetabular retractors.

Femoral preparation

22. Hold the leg in 90 degrees of hip flexion, 90 degrees of internal rotation, and 15 to 20 degrees of adduction. Place a femoral neck retractor under the proximal femur, which helps exposure by lifting the femur out of the wound. Place a bent Hohman retractor underneath the abductor mass and retract the muscle cephalad. Place a cobra ("Aufranc") retractor underneath the inferior femoral neck and retract the soft tissues and psoas tendon.

23. Remove the soft tissue from the lateral femoral neck. This soft tissue represents the remains of the short external rotators. Use a box osteotome or gouge to remove remnants of bone from the superior femoral neck. However, take care not to remove bone from the greater trochanter. Adequate lateral access to the trochanteric bed is essential to minimize the tendency of inserting the broach and implant in varus.

24. Gently insert a straight canal finder by hand into the femoral canal. Gentle insertion is essential, especially in patients with severe osteoporosis, since perforation of the femoral cortex can occur with surprising ease. Pay particular attention to the direction that the canal finder takes as it seats within the femoral canal. Assess the degree of flexion/extension as well as varus/valgus. This indicates the natural morphology of the femur.

Cemented stem

a. Consider using axial reamers to enlarge the distal diaphysis until the cortex is encountered. The use of axial reamers depends on individual surgeon's preference. However, if reamers are used, care should be taken to avoid excessive reaming.

b. Broach the proximal femur with sequentially larger broaches until a reasonably snug fit occurs (**Fig. 20–6**). As with reaming, do not "over-broach." A good cancellous bone bed is essential to optimize fixation at the bone-cement interface. During broaching, pay attention to the alignment of the broach in all planes (varus-valgus, flexion-extension, and rotation). If axial reamers were used, insert the broaches in the same varus-valgus and flexion-extension planes as the axial reamers. In general, insert the broaches so they rotational align with the natural femoral neck. This is usually 12 to 15 degrees of anteversion. If the host bone has abnormal version, consider inserting a smaller prosthesis at the appropriate rotation to optimize hip alignment and stability. Insufficient anteversion may result in hip instability.

c. Insert the final trial broach or the trial implant. Place a modular trial femoral head on the taper. Commonly, start with the standard ("plus zero") femoral head length. Measure the distance from the lesser trochanter to the center of hip rotation. Depending on the patient's anatomy, this measurement is usually within a few millimeters of the distance measured on the preoperative radiographs. If the intraoperative measurement is longer than anticipated, *do not resect additional bone from the femoral neck at this time.* Rather, perform a trial reduction and assess hip stability, component orientation, and soft tissue tension. If necessary one can go back and resect more neck; the converse is not true. If the intraoperative measurement is shorter than anticipated, consider using a longer femoral head.

d. Perform a trial hip reduction. If necessary, change the length of the femoral head. Remember that extremely long modular neck components with "wide modular skirts" effectively bulk up the neck-trunion region and can be a source of impingement. However, they are required in certain clinical situations.

   i. Assess the combined orientation of the femoral and acetabular components.

   ii. Pay special attention to possible sites of impingement including impingement of prosthetic neck on the socket or impingement of the femoral component on osteophytes.

iii. Assess component stability. Examine the hip at: 90 degrees of hip flexion-simulating sitting; flexion, adduction and internal rotation simulating the fetal sleeping position; and in extension, abduction and external rotation, assessing for any evidence of anterior instability. The performance of the "push-pull" (shuck test) test to determine myofascial tension appears to be less reliable.

iv. Assess leg lengths. While restoring "normal" extremity length is desirable, it is not always possible. It may be necessary to accept some degree of leg length inequality in order to optimize component fit, soft tissue tension, and hip stability.

e. After the optimal femoral head length is determined, dislocate the hip and remove the trial components. Return the hip to its starting position of flexion and internal rotation.

f. Replace the femoral retractors. Measure the femoral canal for a distal cement plug. Insert the plug so it resides in the femoral canal approximately 2 cm distal to where the end of the stem will sit. This helps ensure adequate distal cement. Upon reaching the correct insertion depth, check the fit of the plug by pushing it further distally. It should feel tight. Do not pull back on the plug. Our concern is distal advancement of the plug, not that it will fail by backing retrograde out of the femur. If the plug is loose, remove and place the next larger size.

g. Irrigate the femoral canal with a pulsatile jet lavage system. Remove all loose cancellous bone. Pack the femoral canal with either vaginal packing or sponge. If needed, consider using an epinephrine soaked sponge, which can decrease the amount of blood in the femoral canal. The goal is to obtain a clean, dry bone bed for interdigitation with the cement.

h. Mix the acrylic cement. Consider a vacuum-mixing technique to enhance cement consistency and reduce overall cement porosity. In general, 80 grams of methylmethacrylate is sufficient for an adult femur. However, 120 grams may be needed in larger canals. It is preferable to have extra cement than not enough.

i. Use a cement gun to insert the cement when it reaches a "doughy" state and no longer adheres to the surgical gloves. Push the cement nozzle down to, but not past, the cement plug. Introduce the cement by applying slow, steady pressure to the cement gun. Allow the cement pressure to gently push the gun out of the canal. Remove the gun when the femur is full of cement. Break off the nozzle. Attach the proximal pressurizer to the gun and place it against the upper femur. Pressurize the cement with slow, steady pressure (**Fig. 20–7**). Commonly, this causes marrow extrusion out of nutrient foramina of the proximal femur.

j. Insert the stem along the same axis and at the same alignment as the broaches were inserted. In addition, take care to replicate component version. Use predominately manual force when inserting the cement, rather than using a mallet. Additional cement pressurization is usually apparent at the time. Use a mallet to fully seat the implant the last few millimeters down to the level of the neck osteotomy. Perform a final check of axial and torsional orientation (**Fig. 20–8**).

k. Excise excess cement. Until cement polymerization is complete, keep motion of the stem-femur composite to a minimum.

l. Clean and dry the modular taper. Insert the appropriate modular head based on the trial reduction.

m. Reduce the hip and reassess hip stability (**Fig. 20–9**).

Uncemented stem

The exact technique for preparing the femur prior to inserting an uncemented stem depends greatly on the specific instruments unique to each individual hip system. Therefore, the following steps should be used as a general operative guide for implanting an uncemented femoral stem; however, the exact procedure for specific femoral components should be checked with the manufacturer's suggested technique manual.

a. If required, use sequential larger axial reamers until cortical engagement is detected. Preoperative templating is a good indicator to the extent of canal reaming required. Avoid over-reaming.

b. Use sequential broaches to prepare the femoral canal. Broaching should be methodical since attempts at rapid canal preparation can result in disastrous consequences. Use firm mallet blows to gradually enlarge the canal with sequentially larger

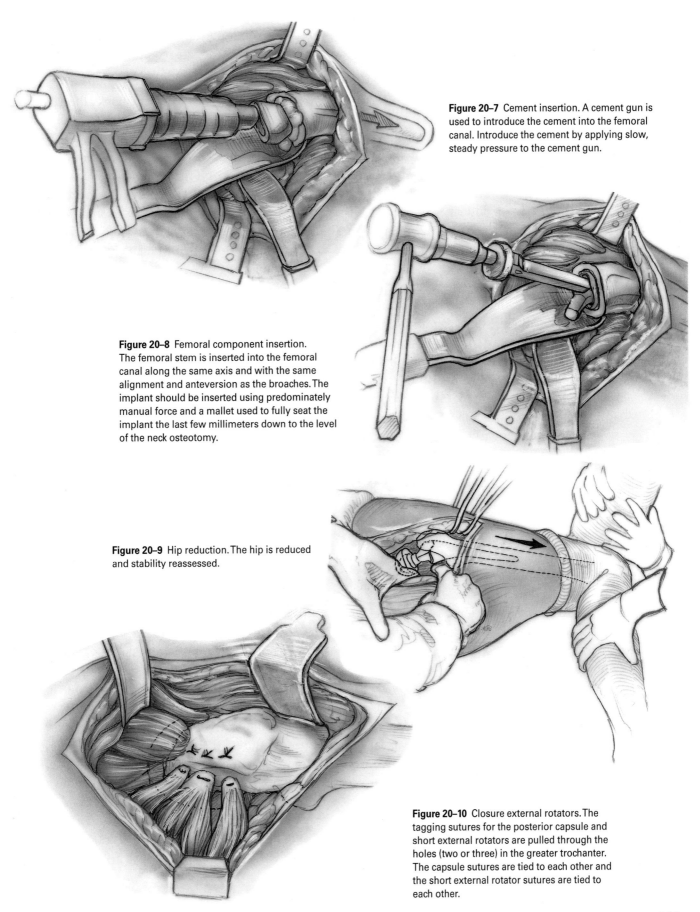

Figure 20–7 Cement insertion. A cement gun is used to introduce the cement into the femoral canal. Introduce the cement by applying slow, steady pressure to the cement gun.

Figure 20–8 Femoral component insertion. The femoral stem is inserted into the femoral canal along the same axis and with the same alignment and anteversion as the broaches. The implant should be inserted using predominately manual force and a mallet used to fully seat the implant the last few millimeters down to the level of the neck osteotomy.

Figure 20–9 Hip reduction. The hip is reduced and stability reassessed.

Figure 20–10 Closure external rotators. The tagging sutures for the posterior capsule and short external rotators are pulled through the holes (two or three) in the greater trochanter. The capsule sutures are tied to each other and the short external rotator sutures are tied to each other.

131

broaches. Use the broach to assess both axial and torsional stability. If there is obvious motion of the broach within the canal (exceeding 1 to 2 mm), then insert the next larger broach (**Fig. 20–6**).

    i. For straight stems, insert the broaches so they rotational align with the natural femoral neck. This is usually 12 to 15 degrees of anteversion. Insufficient anteversion may result in hip instability. If the host bone has abnormal version, consider inserting a smaller cemented prosthesis at the appropriate rotation to optimize hip alignment and stability (a rare occurrence).

    ii. For anatomic (curved) stems, the broaches will "conform" to the natural morphology and version of the proximal femur. Do not attempt to rotate the broaches into either anteversion or retroversion. If the host bone has abnormal version, consider inserting a smaller cemented prosthesis at the appropriate rotation to optimize hip alignment and stability (a rare occurrence).

c. When using the apparent final broach, carefully assess hip stability and femoral cortical integrity. If a fracture is identified, use the steps previously outlined for management.

d. Place a modular trial femoral head on the taper. Commonly, start with the standard ("plus zero") femoral head length. Measure the distance from the lesser trochanter to the center of hip rotation. Depending on the patient's anatomy, this measurement is usually within a few millimeters of the distance measured on the preoperative radiographs. If the intraoperative measurement is longer than anticipated, *do not resect additional bone from the femoral neck at this time.* Rather perform a trial reduction and assess hip stability, component orientation, and soft tissue tension. If necessary one can go back and resect more neck; the converse is not true. If the intraoperative measurement is shorter than anticipated, consider using a longer femoral head.

e. Perform a trial hip reduction. If necessary, change the length of the femoral head. Remember that extremely long modular neck components with "wide modular skirts" effectively bulk up the neck-trunion region and can be a source of impingement. However, they are required in certain clinical situations.

    i. Assess the combined orientation of the femoral and acetabular components.

    ii. Pay special attention to possible sites of impingement, including impingement of prosthetic neck on the socket or impingement of the femoral component on osteophytes.

    iii. Assess component stability. Examine the hip at: 90 degrees of hip flexion-simulating sitting; flexion, adduction and internal rotation simulating the fetal sleeping position; and in extension, abduction and external rotation assessing for any evidence of anterior instability. The performance of the "push-pull" (shuck test) test to determine myofascial tension appears to be less reliable.

    iv. Assess leg lengths. While restoring "normal" extremity length is desirable, it is not always possible. Restoration of leg length is even more difficult than with cemented femoral stems since implant height is dictated almost exclusively by the extent of component fit and fill within the canal. Some degree of leg length modification can be achieved by use of the modular heads. However, it may be necessary to accept some degree of leg length inequality in order to optimize component fit, soft tissue tension, and hip stability.

f. After the optimal femoral head length is determined, dislocate the hip and remove the trial components. Return the hip to its starting position of flexion and internal rotation.

g. Replace the femoral retractors. Irrigate the femoral canal with a pulsatile jet lavage system.

h. Confirm implant size on the packaging prior to opening. Insert the real implant with a series of steady mallet blows. Avoid rapid or excessive force when inserting the component since this can predispose to fracture. During implant insertion, allow ample time for the femur to adapt to the implant being impacted because the visco-elastic properties of bone will allow some bone expansion and facilitate insertion.

Commonly, the real implant is 1 to 2 mm larger than the final broach due to the thickness of the porous coating. The discrepancy between trial and real implant varies greatly between manufacturers and is based upon manufacturing tolerances, implant design, and type of porous coating. Familiarity with the system being utilized is essential.

The prosthesis is fully seated when the implant appears stable and no longer moves axially into the femur with mallet blows. The final position often results in the implant being either proud or countersunk a few millimeters. The key is to achieve optimal stability of the component in the femoral canal. Do not compromise component stability by incompletely inserting the implant. Leg length can be adjusted by use of the appropriate modular heads. Conversely, do not attempt to use excessive force to "countersink" an implant that is fully seated but proud a few millimeters (**Fig. 20–8**).

i. Following stem insertion, reassess proximal cortical integrity. If a fracture is identified, use the steps previously outlined for management.

j. Evaluate the final position of the stem and reassess which length of modular femoral head is most appropriate. If necessary, perform a trial reduction with trial modular femoral heads placed on the real implant.

k. Clean and dry the modular taper. Gently impact the appropriate modular head on the modular taper of the real implant.

l. Reduce the hip. Recheck hip stability in both flexion and extension. If stability is adequate, begin closure (**Fig. 20–9**).

Closure and transfer

25. Irrigate the wound with copious antibiotic irrigation.
26. Maintain appropriate hemostasis.
27. If a suction drain is utilized, place it subfacial through a separate incision that exits the anterolateral thigh at the distal extent of the incision. Take care throughout the closure to minimize the risk of inadvertently sewing in the drain.
28. Make two drill holes in the posterolateral aspect of the greater trochanter approximately 1 cm apart (it may be easier to make these drill holes prior to reducing the hip).
29. Pull the tagging sutures of the posterior capsule and short external rotators through the holes. Tie the capsule sutures to each other; then tie the short external rotator sutures to each other (**Fig. 20–10**).
30. If possible, repair the quadratus femoris muscle-tendon.
31. Repair the tendinous insertion of the gluteus maximus with absorbable sutures.
32. Close the deep fascial layer in a meticulous fashion with multiple absorbable sutures (normally zero or number one).
33. Close the subcutaneous tissue in a layered fashion with interrupted absorbable sutures (normally number one, zero and 2-0 sutures).
34. Close the skin with staples, nylon, or prolene.
35. Apply a sterile dressing and a compressive bandage to the hip.
36. Transfer the patient off the operating table taking care to avoid excessive hip rotation or flexion. Transfer the patient to recovery room.
37. Obtain a radiograph in the recovery room to ensure the hip is reduced.

Suggested Readings

Huo MH, Waldman BJ. Cemented total hip replacement. In: Craig EV, ed. *Clinical Orthopaedics.* Baltimore, MD: Lippincott Williams & Wilkins, 1999, pp. 522–534.

Nestor BJ, Buly RL. Cementless total hip arthroplasty. In: Craig EV, ed. *Clinical Orthopaedics.* Baltimore, MD: Lippincott Williams & Wilkins, 1999, pp. 535–548.

Pellicci PM, Padgett DE. *Atlas of Total Hip Replacement.* New York, NY: Churchill Livingstone, 1995.

Sharrock NE, Minco R, Urquhart B, Salvati EA. The effect of two levels of hypotension on intraoperative blood loss during total hip arthroplasty performed under lumbar epidural anesthesia. *Anesth Analg* 1993;76(3):580–584.

CHAPTER 21

Internal Fixation of Hip Fracture

Steven H. Stern

Indications

Compression screw and side plate
1. Intertrochanteric hip fracture (**Fig. 21–1A**)
2. Low femoral neck fracture ("base of neck" fracture)

Multiple cannulated screws
1. Impacted femoral neck fracture (**Fig. 21–1B**)
2. Displaced femoral neck fracture (in younger patient after "satisfactory" reduction)

Contraindications
1. Medical contraindications
2. Nonambulatory patient (relative—must individualize)

Preoperative Preparation
1. Hip radiographs
2. Appropriate medical and anesthetic evaluation
3. Document status of preoperative neurovascular examination

Special Instruments, Position, and Anesthesia
1. The patient is placed supine on the fracture table (**Fig. 21–2**).
2. All pressure points should be padded.
3. The procedure can be done with general, spinal or epidural anesthesia.

Tips and Pearls
1. Assess the adequacy of the fracture reduction after positioning the patient on the fracture table, but prior to prepping and draping. Use fluoroscopy in two planes to evaluate the reduction.
2. Most intertrochanteric fractures can be reduced with longitudinal traction and internal rotation.
3. Femoral neck fractures may require live fluoroscopy to aid reduction.
4. Administer intravenous antibiotics appropriate for the hospital's bacterial flora prior to skin incision.
5. Take care to ensure adequate padding of the feet and lower extremities.
6. Position the noninjured extremities so they do not interfere with the fluoroscopy. Commonly, the contralateral lower extremity is positioned in a flexed and abducted position. The ispilateral upper extremity is taped across the anterior chest wall.

What To Avoid
1. If possible, avoid a varus hip reduction.
2. For intertrochanteric fractures, attempt to avoid medial displacement of the proximal fragment and concurrent lateral displacement of the femoral shaft.
3. For impacted femoral neck fractures, avoid excessive traction, which could serve to disimpact the fracture fragments.

4. Avoid placing the cannulated screws below the level of the lesser trochanter. This can result in a "stress riser" in the lateral femoral cortex and increase the risk of a subtrochanteric fracture.

5. Avoid allowing the guidepin to penetrate through the femoral head into the soft tissues of the pelvis.

Postoperative Care Issues

1. When medically possible, attempt to mobilize the patient in the postoperative period. If the medical condition permits, the patient should be placed in a sitting position as expeditiously as possible.

2. Consider utilizing some form of deep-vein thrombosis prophylaxis. Options include warfarin, low-molecular weight heparin, and intermittent pneumatic compression.

3. Depending on the fracture stability, adequacy of the reduction and the patient's bone quality, ambulation can commence either with non-weight bearing (NWB), toe-touch weight bearing (TTWB) or weight bearing as tolerated (WBAT).

4. Reassessment of the distal neurovascular examination should be done after surgery.

Operative Technique

Compression screw and side plate

1. Position the patient supine on the fracture table. The patient should be positioned directly against the groin post. Pad the extremities. Most fractures can be reduced with a combination of traction and internal rotation. The degree of internal rotation can be assessed by evaluating knee rotation (**Fig. 21–2**).

2. Prior to prepping and draping the patient, evaluate the fracture using biplanar fluoroscopy. It is important prior to draping to assess the patient's position to ensure that the fluoroscopic C-arm adequately obtains satisfactory AP and lateral hip images. Optimize the fracture reduction at this time.

3. Prepare and drape the patient and extremity per the hospital's standard sterile protocol. Commonly, a large plastic drape ("shower curtain") is utilized.

4. Obtain an AP hip fluoroscopic image to assist in positioning the skin incision. Place a metal clamp or Steinman pin on the anterior thigh so it serves as a visible landmark on the fluoroscopic image.

5. Make a skin incision along the lateral aspect of the thigh. Palpate the femur to ensure that the incision is positioned in the femur's AP mid-point. The skin incision should be approximately 15 cm in length. The incision's proximal pole should extend 1 to 2 cm proximal to the lesser trochanter (**Fig. 21–3**).

6. Carry the dissection directly through the subcutaneous tissue. Maintain adequate hemostasis. Identify the tensor fascia lata (**Fig. 21–4**).

7. Sharply incise the tensor fascia lata longitudinally. Place retractors deep to the tensor fascia lata. Identify the vastus lateralis.

8. Retract the vastus lateralis anteriorly. Sharply incise the fascia of the vastus lateralis longitudinally. This incision is positioned to allow dissection through the posterior one-third of the vastus lateralis. Take care to incise only the fascia and not the muscle (**Fig. 21–5**).

9. Use a periosteal elevator to bluntly dissect through the muscle fibers of the vastus lateralis. Carry the dissection down to the femur. Place a Bennett retractor over the anterior femur so it lies against the medial femoral cortex. Use it to retract the soft tissues medially to enhance visualization (**Fig. 21–6**).

10. Use a medium- (~3.5 mm—commonly, the drill bit that will be used later in the procedure for the cortical screws is used) size drill bit to locate the optimal starting point on the lateral femoral cortex for the compression screw. Optimize the superior-inferior starting hole position by evaluating AP fluoroscopic hip images. Generally, the starting hole should be at or below the level of the lesser trochanter. Palpate the femur to ensure that the starting hole is midway between the anterior and posterior femoral cortex (**Fig. 21–6**).

11. Drill the hole through the lateral femoral cortex. First start drilling perpendicular to the bone's long axis to gain purchase in the lateral femoral cortex. Then drill a "sloppy" hole by aiming the drill at the approximate angle desired for the compression screw. The "sloppy" hole enhances accurate placement of the guidepin in the next step.

12. Introduce the guidepin into the hole in the lateral femoral cortex. Drill the guidepin through the femoral neck and into the femoral head. The

guidepin can be positioned utilizing either a hand or power drill. In addition, the guidepin can either be positioned through a preset angle guide (commonly 130, 135, or 140 degrees) or positioned by hand in the femoral head. The author's preference is to hand position the guidepin.

13. Use biplanar fluoroscopic images to optimize the guidepin's position in the femoral head. Ideally, position the guidepin so it is centered in the femoral head on both the AP and lateral fluoroscopic images. In general, guidepin placement that is slightly inferior on the AP view and slightly posterior on the lateral view is acceptable. Attempt to avoid superior or anterior guidepin position (**Figs. 21–7A and 7B**).

14. After optimal guidepin position is obtained, drill the guidepin deeper into the femoral head so its tip is within a few millimeters of the subchondral bone.

15. Measure the length of the guidepin within the femur with the depth gauge. Measure the guidepin's angle with the angle-measuring guide. Ideally, an anatomic or slight valgus pinning is desired (135 degrees or greater). However, some patients' bony anatomy or fracture patterns do not make this possible.

16. Set the reamer so it will not ream deeper than the measured depth of the guidepin.

17. Under fluoroscopic control, ream over the guidepin. Allow the reamer to follow along the guidepin's path. Check fluoroscopic images to ensure that the guidepin has not inadvertently advanced deeper into the femoral head.

18. Remove the reamer. If the guidepin is inadvertently removed with the reamer, reinsert it into the center of the already drilled channel. Use biplanar fluoroscopy to ensure that the reinserted guidepin is correctly repositioned.

19. Place the appropriate size compression screw and side plate on the operative field. The compression screw should be the length measured by the depth gauge. The side plate is commonly a four-hole plate with the angle measured with the angle guide.

20. Inset the compression screw over the guidepin. Depending on the surgeon's preference, the side plate can be prepositioned on the screwdriver or can be inserted as a separate step later in the procedure. Use the biplanar fluoroscopy to ensure that the compression screw is properly inserted along the guidepin's track. Since most intertrochanteric fractures occur in osteoporotic bone, it is rarely necessary to tap the bone prior to inserting the compression screw.

21. Insert the side plate over the compression screw until it rests against the lateral femoral cortex. Many compression screws only allow the side plate to be inserted at a specific rotation angle. In these cases, ensure that the compression screw is rotated correctly during insertion. Ensure that the side plate is fully seated against the lateral femoral cortex and the compression screw is visible within the barrel of the side plate.

22. Clamp the side plate to the femur.

23. Drill a bicortical hole with the 3.5-mm drill bit through one of the side plate's holes. Avoid plunging the drill through the bone's medial cortex because of risk of injury to the medially neurovascular structures. Use a depth gauge to measure the length of the screw hole.

24. Insert a 4.5-mm cortical screw. The goal is to achieve bicortical fixation with one or two screw threads across the femur's medial cortex. The tip of the screw should be palpable along the femur's medial cortex (**Fig. 21–8**).

25. Repeat the same process for each of the other screw holes.

26. Assess the final position of the side plate and screws with the biplanar fluoroscopy (**Figs. 21–9A and 9B**). *Some surgeons insert a locking screw within the compression screw to aid in compression. Many surgeons forego this step.*

27. Copiously irrigate the wound. Maintain excellent hemostasis. If needed, place a drain through a separate stab incision. However, in many procedures a drain is not required.

28. Close the fascia of the vastus lateralis with a running #1 or 0 absorbable suture.

29. Close the fascia lata with interrupted #1 or 0 absorbable sutures.

30. Close the subcutaneous tissue with absorbable sutures. Close the skin with staples. Apply a compression dressing.

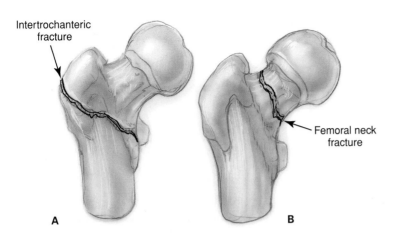

Figure 21–1 **(A)** Intertrochanteric fracture. **(B)** Femoral neck fracture.

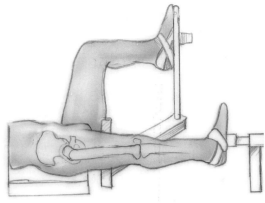

Figure 21–2 Patient position. The patient should be positioned directly against the groin post. Take care to ensure that the patient's position allows adequate clearance for the fluoroscopy. The ipsilateral arm is placed across the chest. The foot of the involved extremity is placed in a well-padded fracture boot. Ensure that all pressure points are well padded. Position the extremity to optimize the fracture reduction.

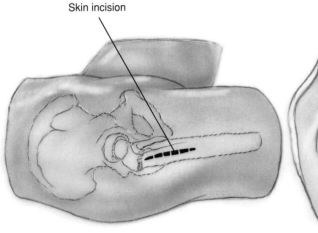

Figure 21–3 Skin incision. The incision's proximal pole should extend 1 to 2 cm proximal to the lesser trochanter. It extends distally along the lateral aspect of the thigh. The length of the incision depends on which procedure is being performed. Insertion of a compression screw and side plate requires a longer incision than does insertion of multiple cannulated screws.

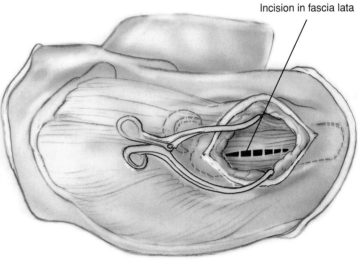

Figure 21–4 Superficial dissection. The fascia lata should be identified directly below the subcutaneous tissue. The fascia lata should be incised longitudinally in line with the skin incision.

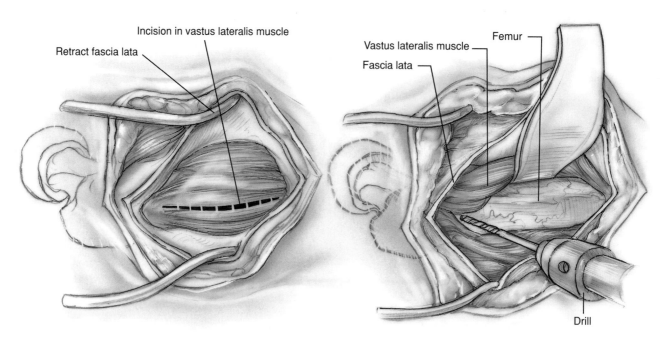

Figure 21–5 Deep dissection. The fascia of the vastus lateralis should be identified directly below the fascia lata. The fascia of the vastus lateralis should be incised longitudinally in line with the skin incision.

Figure 21–6 Starting hole for guidepin. A Bennett retractor is placed over the anterior femur so it lies against the medial femoral cortex. It retracts the soft tissues medially to enhance visualization. Note the position of the starting hole for the compression screw is at or below the level of the lesser trochanter.

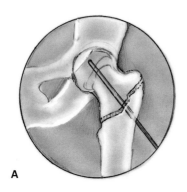

A

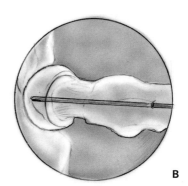

B

Figure 21–7 (A) Guidepin position (AP). Assess the position of the guidepin with biplanar fluoroscopy. Ideally, the guidepin should be positioned in the center of the femoral head on the AP fluoroscopic images. In general, guidepin placement that is slightly inferior on the AP view is acceptable. Attempt to avoid a superior guidepin position. **(B)** Guidepin position (lateral). Ideally, the guidepin should be positioned in the center of the femoral head on the lateral fluoroscopic images. In general, guidepin placement that is slightly posterior on the lateral view is acceptable. Attempt to avoid an anterior guidepin position.

Multiple cannulated screws

1. Position the patient supine on the fracture table. The patient should be positioned directly against the groin post. Pad the extremities. For impacted femoral neck fractures, avoid excessive traction, which could disimpact the fracture fragments. The degree of hip rotation can be assessed by evaluating knee rotation (**Fig. 21–2**).

2. Prior to prepping and draping the patient, evaluate the fracture using biplanar fluoroscopy. It is important prior to draping to assess the patient's position to ensure that the fluoroscopic C-arm adequately obtains satisfactory AP and lateral hip images. Optimize the fracture reduction at this time.

3. Prepare and drape the patient and extremity per the hospital's standard sterile protocol. Commonly, a large plastic drape ("shower curtain") is utilized.

4. Obtain an AP hip fluoroscopic image to assist in positioning the skin incision. Place a metal clamp or guidepin on the anterior thigh so it serves as a visible landmark on the fluoroscopic image.

5. Make a skin incision along the lateral aspect of the thigh. Palpate the femur to ensure that the incision is positioned in the femur's anteroposterior midpoint. The skin incision should be long enough for placement of three screws. The incision's proximal pole should extend 1 to 2 cm proximal to the lesser trochanter (**Fig. 21–3**).

6. Carry the dissection directly through the subcutaneous tissue. Maintain adequate hemostasis. Identify the fascia lata (**Fig. 21–4**).

7. Sharply incise the tensor fascia lata longitudinally. Place retractors deep to the tensor fascia lata. Identify the vastus lateralis.

8. Retract the vastus lateralis anteriorly. For most fractures, it is not necessary to incise the fascia of the vastus lateralis.

9. Place the guidepin for the cannulated screw through the vastus lateralis directly onto the lateral femoral cortex. Optimize the superior-inferior position by evaluating AP fluoroscopic hip images. The guidepin should be at or above the level of the lesser trochanter. Avoid positioning the guidepin below the level of the lesser trochanter. In general, most fractures can be fixed with three screws placed in a triangular configuration with the apex of the triangle inferior. Commonly, the guidepin for the inferior screw is the first one inserted.

10. Use a power drill to insert the guidepin through the femoral neck and into the femoral head. Use biplanar fluoroscopic images to optimize the guidepin's position in the femoral head. Ideally, position the first guidepin so it is in the inferior portion of the femoral head on the AP fluoroscopic images and in the center of the femoral head on the lateral fluoroscopic images.

11. After optimal guidepin position is obtained, drill the guidepin deeper into the femoral head so its tip is within a few millimeters of the subchondral bone.

12. Insert two more guidepins utilizing either a "freehand" technique or by inserting the guidepins through a triangular template guide. Commonly, a triangular configuration with the apex of the triangle inferior is employed. Therefore, one pin should be slightly superior-anterior and one pin superior-posterior to the initial inferior guidepin. Use biplanar fluoroscopy to optimize the position of these guidepins within the femoral head.

13. Check to ensure that all of the guidepins are drilled within the femoral head so the tip is within a few millimeters of the subchondral bone. Starting with the inferior guidepin, measure the length of the guidepin within the femur with a depth gauge.

14. Insert the appropriate length cannulated screw over the guidepin. If self-tapping screws are utilized or if the bone is significantly osteoporotic, it is not necessary to overdrill the lateral femoral cortex. However, if needed, make a starting hole in the lateral femoral cortex with a cannulated drill inserted over the guidepin.

15. Insert the screws so they are fully seated. Check to ensure that all of the screw threads lie in the proximal femoral head fragment. Ideally, when the screw is fully seated, none of the threads should lie across the fracture.

16. Using a similar technique, insert the other two screws over the remaining two guidepins.

17. Assess the final position of the screws with the biplanar fluoroscopy (**Figs. 21–10A and 10B**).

18. Copiously irrigate the wound. Maintain excellent hemostasis. In most procedures a drain is not required.

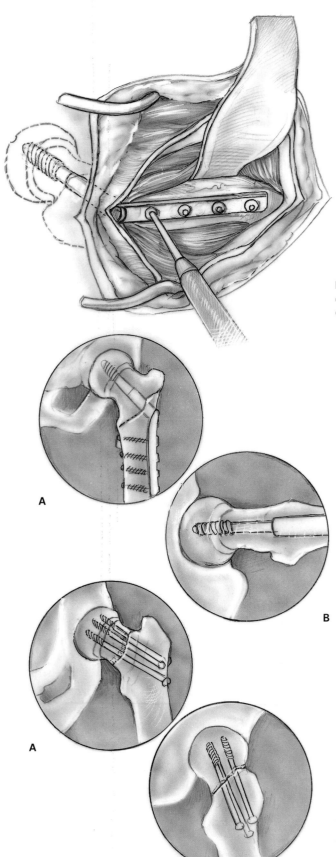

Figure 21–8 Screw insertion. The side plate is placed over the compression screw and against the lateral femoral cortex. Multiple cortical screws (commonly 4) are used to fix the side plate to the bone.

Figure 21–9 (A) Final hardware alignment—compression screw and side plate (AP). Anteriorposterior view showing the position of the compression screw and side plate in place. This is assessed with the biplanar fluoroscopy. **(B)** Final hardware alignment—compression screw and side plate (Lateral). Lateral view showing the position of the compression screw in place. This is assessed with the biplanar fluoroscopy.

Figure 21–10 (A) Final hardware alignment—multiple cannulated screws (AP). AP view showing the position of the multiple cannulated screws in place. This is assessed with the biplanar fluoroscopy. Avoid positioning the screws below the level of the lesser trochanter. In general, most fractures can be fixed with 3 screws placed in a triangular configuration with the apex of the triangle inferior. **(B)** Final hardware alignment—multiple cannulated screws (lateral). Lateral view showing the position of the multiple cannulated screws in place.

19. Close the fascia lata with interrupted #1 or 0 absorbable sutures.

20. Close the subcutaneous tissue with absorbable sutures. Close the skin with staples. Apply a compression dressing.

Suggested Readings

Bartlett CS III, Buly, RL, Helfet, DL. Intertrochanteric and subtrochanteric fractures of the proximal femur. In: Craig EV, ed. *Clinical Orthopaedics*. Baltimore, MD: Lippincott Williams & Willkins, 1999, pp. 439–478.

Brennan, MJ. Intertrochanteric femur fractures. In: Levine AM, ed. *Orthopaedic Knowledge Update: Trauma*. Rosemont, IL: American Academy of Orthopaedic Surgeons, 1996, pp. 121–126.

Cornell, CN. Intracapsular fractures of the femoral neck. In: Craig EV, ed. *Clinical Orthopaedics*. Baltimore, MD: Lippincott Williams & Willkins, 1999, pp. 479–490.

Proceedings of the American College of Chest Physicians 5th Consensus on Antithrombotic Therapy. *Chest* 1998; 114(Suppl 5):439S–769S.

Turen, CH. Intracapsular hip fractures. In: Levine AM, ed. *Orthopaedic Knowledge Update: Trauma*. Rosemont, IL: American Academy of Orthopaedic Surgeons, 1996, pp. 113–120.

CHAPTER 22

Hip Fracture

Hemiarthroplasty

Douglas E. Padgett

Indications

1. Displaced femoral neck fractures not appropriate for reduction and internal fixation
2. Displaced low femoral neck fractures ("base of neck") not appropriate for reduction and internal fixation

Contraindications

1. Proximal femoral fracture in the setting of active sepsis: either acute osteomyelitis or acute suppurative arthritis (absolute)
2. Proximal femoral fracture in the setting of neuropathic joint (relative)
3. Proximal femoral fracture in patients unable or unwilling to comply with postoperative protocols that minimize the risk of hip dislocation (relative)
4. Decubitus wounds contiguous with the planned surgical incision (relative)

Preoperative Preparation

Fractures of the proximal femur are a sentinel event in the life of any patient. Femoral neck fractures in patients under the age of 50 usually result either from high-energy trauma or in association with significant metabolic bone disease that has weakened the femur. Femoral neck fractures in the elderly are usually not high-energy injuries, but frequently occur in patients with significant medical cormorbidities. Elderly patients with these fractures are at a significant risk for morbidity and/or mortality in the perioperative period. These facts should always be remembered when treating a patient with a proximal femoral fracture.

1. Complete history and physical examination
2. Appropriate medical and anesthetic evaluation
3. Document preoperative neurovascular status.
4. Examine and document the status of the skin's integrity since many of the patients are at risk for postoperative decubitus ulcers.
5. Radiographs including anteroposterior (AP) of the pelvis and lateral of the proximal femur. Occult fractures may not be apparent on plain radiographs and require either magnetic resonance imaging (MRI) or bone scintingraphy to diagnose a fracture.
6. The preoperative radiographs should be assessed in conjunction with the appropriate hip prosthetic templates to determine approximate component sizes. Preoperative templating should be performed to determine:
   a. Level of femoral neck resection
   b. Femoral component size
   c. Distances from fixed points on the femur to the center of hip rotation in order to help optimize postoperative limb length
   d. If the femoral implant adequately reconstructs femoral offset and proper hip mechanics

e. Approximate size of bipolar head to be utilized. With current modular systems, the size of the bipolar cup determines the femoral head size (22, 26, or 28 mm) that allows adequate polyethylene thickness.

Special Instruments, Position, and Anesthesia

1. The patient is placed in the lateral decubitus position with the affected hip upward. Adequate padding of the axilla is necessary to avoid injury to the brachial plexus. While the patient must be secure on the operating room table, excessive tightening of pelvic posts should be avoided, since this can compromise the neurovascular status of the "down-leg" (Fig. 22–1).

2. All pressure points should be padded.

3. The procedure can be done with general, epidural, or long-acting spinal anesthesia. There is some evidence that epidural anesthesia decreases the risk of deep-vein thrombosis as well as decreasing blood loss during total hip arthroplasty (presumably by a reduction in pelvic venous pressure). In addition, postoperative analgesia may be administered via the epidural catheter.

4. Instruments required for hemiarthroplasty include self-retaining retractors, straight and bent Hohman-type retractors, a femoral neck elevator to facilitate exposure of the proximal femur, and power saws. In addition, the specific instruments, broaches, and trial components unique to the prosthesis to be implanted should be available.

5. Consider using enclosed helmets and body exhausts, which may help minimize the risk of perioperative sepsis.

6. Intravenous antibiotics appropriate for the hospital's bacterial flora should be administered prior to tourniquet inflation and continued for at least 24 h after surgery.

Tips and Pearls

1. Accurate re-establishment of the preoperative leg length is difficult to accomplish in the setting of a displaced femoral neck fracture. On occasion, the approximate leg length can be estimated based upon the opposite extremity.

2. Due to the edema associated with an acute hip fracture, some of the tissue planes adjacent to the posterior capsule can be difficult to identify. If necessary, consider taking down the posterior capsule and short external rotator tendons as one large flap.

3. The use of a ligamentum teres knife (a curved blade) is useful in aiding extraction of the femoral head from the acetabulum.

4. If the bone is extremely osteoporotic, consider using only broaches for femoral preparation (to compact the cancellous bone) rather than a combination of broaching and reaming (which tends to remove the cancellous bone bed).

5. The size of the bipolar head is determined by feel. Consider measuring the diameter of the excised femoral head. This serves as a rough guide for the appropriate size of the bipolar head. The trial bipolar head should fit easily into the acetabular socket. However, there should be a slight suction fit of the trial component.

6. Optimizing stability with bipolar hemiarthroplasty is essential. In situations where there is a large fixed flexion contracture with adduction, altering surgical approach to an anterior or anterolateral (Hardinge) approach can be considered.

7. The use of cement for femoral component fixation is recommended for treatment of the majority of these fractures.

What To Avoid

1. Because of the problems associated with infection, great care is taken to minimize this complication. Operating room traffic should be minimized, and preoperative antibiotics administered.

2. Avoid "overstuffing" the acetabulum socket with an oversized bipolar component. This may be a source of postoperative groin pain or increase the risk of component dislocation in some patients.

3. Avoid compromising cement technique in order to "rush through" the case. An adequate cement mantel is critical for success in both total hip arthroplasty

as well as bipolar hemiarthroplasty. Adhere to appropriate methods of canal preparation and cement pressurization during surgery.

4. Avoid excessive broaching or reaming of the femur especially when cement fixation of the femoral component is planned. Over-zealous removal of cancellous bone will weaken the bone-cement interface and may predispose to early component loosening. Femoral preparation should be performed in a controlled methodical fashion.

5. Do not excessively antevert or retrovert the femoral component. Careful assessment of the femur's inherent torsion is an excellent indicator of amount of anteversion with which to insert the stem.

6. Avoid a varus or retroverted alignment of the femoral component.

Postoperative Care Issues

1. While not mandatory, a suction type drain can be used and normally safely discontinued the morning after surgery.

2. Thromboembolic precautions are recommended. Options include intraoperative heparin, aspirin, warfarin, low-molecular weight heparin, and intermittent pneumatic compression.

3. The use of a hip abduction splint or hip abduction slings attached to overhead suspension is useful to avoid untoward motions of the limb, which may compromise hip stability. Many patients undergoing hip hemiarthroplasty are elderly and have a tendency for confusion and disorientation, which increases the risk of dislocation. Consider using a knee immobilizer to help minimize the risk of dislocation, as it maintains the knee in an extended position, thereby making hip flexion difficult. Thus, the chance that the hip will be placed in a hyperflexed position, which predisposes it to dislocation, is reduced.

4. Weight-bearing status is dependent upon fixation, integrity of the trochanter, as well as the presence of any other associated fractures. This information must be conveyed to the physical therapy staff and nursing staff. Full weight bearing is most common with cement fixation.

5. Precautions such as avoiding excessive hip flexion and/or hip rotation should be reviewed with the patient.

Operative Technique

Approach

1. Position the patient in the lateral decubitus position. Pad all pressure points including the axilla. While the patient must be secure on the operation room table, avoid excessive tightening of pelvic posts, which can compromise the neurovascular status of the "down-leg" (**Fig. 22–1**).

2. Prepare and drape the limb in the hospital's standard sterile fashion.

3. Make a straight lateral incision approximately 15 cm in length. Center the incision over the lateral shaft of the femur. The incision should start approximately 5 cm proximal to the tip of the greater trochanter and extend distally about 10 cm.

4. Carry the dissection directly through the subcutaneous tissue. Maintain adequate hemostasis. Identify the fascia lata.

5. Incise the fascia lata longitudinally. Bluntly split the fibers of the gluteus maximus at the proximal pole of the fascia lata.

6. Insert a self-retaining retractor. Partially release the femoral insertion of the gluteus maximus tendon with the electrocautery. This greatly facilitates anterior translation of the femur that will be necessary for acetabular preparation. Attempt to avoid the small perforating branches of the profunda femoris artery.

7. Place a cobra ("Aufranc") retractor around the inferior femoral neck between the posterior hip joint capsule and the quadratus femoris. Place a bent Hohman retractor around the superior femoral neck between the hip capsule and the gluteal muscles. Retracting the muscle fibers of the quadratus femoris inferiorly and the gluteus minimus superiorly helps expose the entire posterior capsule.

8. Due to the intrascapular edema and hematoma as well as shortening of the femoral neck from the fracture, the short external rotators may be difficult to identify as a distinct layer. Use either the

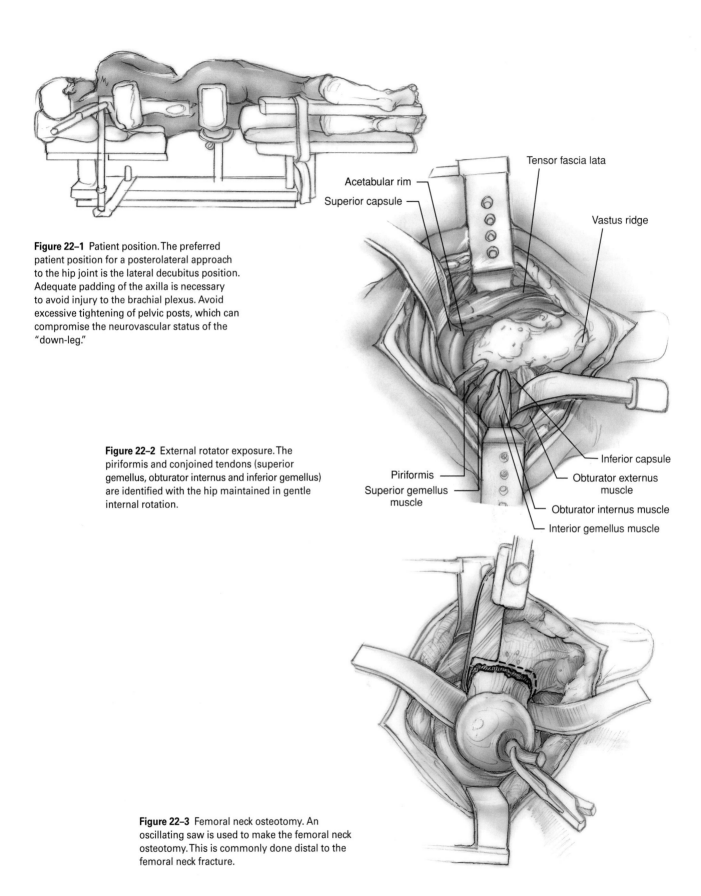

Figure 22–1 Patient position. The preferred patient position for a posterolateral approach to the hip joint is the lateral decubitus position. Adequate padding of the axilla is necessary to avoid injury to the brachial plexus. Avoid excessive tightening of pelvic posts, which can compromise the neurovascular status of the "down-leg."

Figure 22–2 External rotator exposure. The piriformis and conjoined tendons (superior gemellus, obturator internus and inferior gemellus) are identified with the hip maintained in gentle internal rotation.

Acetabular rim
Superior capsule
Tensor fascia lata
Vastus ridge
Inferior capsule
Obturator externus muscle
Obturator internus muscle
Interior gemellus muscle
Piriformis
Superior gemellus muscle

Figure 22–3 Femoral neck osteotomy. An oscillating saw is used to make the femoral neck osteotomy. This is commonly done distal to the femoral neck fracture.

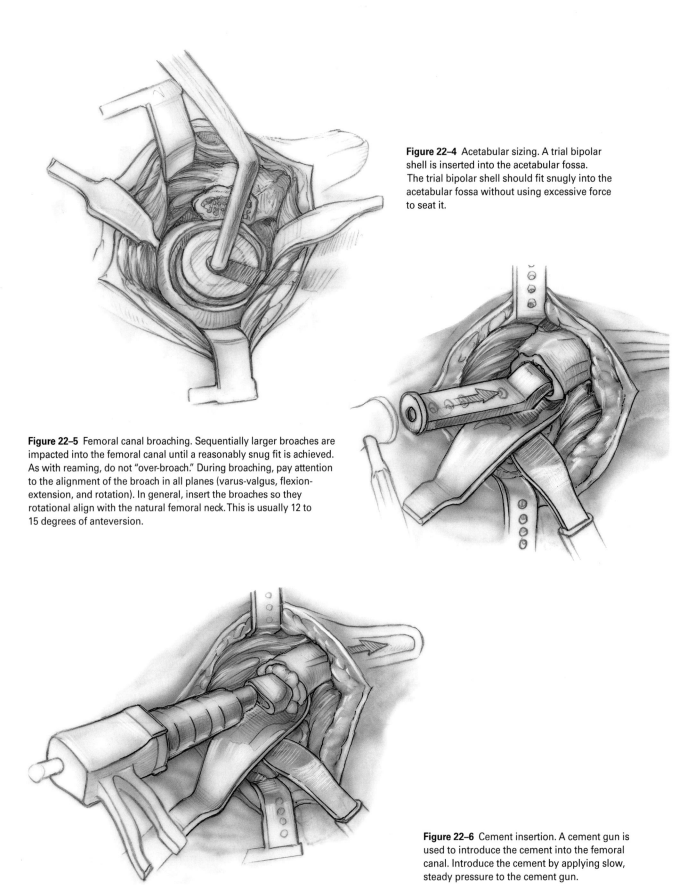

Figure 22–4 Acetabular sizing. A trial bipolar shell is inserted into the acetabular fossa. The trial bipolar shell should fit snugly into the acetabular fossa without using excessive force to seat it.

Figure 22–5 Femoral canal broaching. Sequentially larger broaches are impacted into the femoral canal until a reasonably snug fit is achieved. As with reaming, do not "over-broach." During broaching, pay attention to the alignment of the broach in all planes (varus-valgus, flexion-extension, and rotation). In general, insert the broaches so they rotational align with the natural femoral neck. This is usually 12 to 15 degrees of anteversion.

Figure 22–6 Cement insertion. A cement gun is used to introduce the cement into the femoral canal. Introduce the cement by applying slow, steady pressure to the cement gun.

electrocautery or a knife to make a large posterior flap, trapezoidal in shape, which includes both the short external rotators and the posterior joint capsule. Tag the ends of the flap with nonabsorbable suture for later reattachment (**Fig. 22–2**).

9. Expose the fractured femoral neck by gently flexing, adducting, and internally rotating the femur. The femoral head will remain in the acetabular fossa.

10. With the leg held in internal rotation, use an electrocautery to strip the capsule and soft tissue off the posterior femur (which now points up) until the lesser trochanter is visible.

11. Determine the optimal site for the femoral neck osteotomy based on both the preoperative radiographic measurements and the intraoperative anatomic landmarks. Use an oscillating saw to make the femoral neck osteotomy. Even if the fracture has occurred at the precise level where the neck is to be resected, recut the femoral neck so the osteotomy has a smooth surface (**Fig. 22–3**).

12. Insert acetabular retractors or use a femoral bone hook to expose the retained femoral head within the acetabular fossa.

Acetabular preparation

13. Remove the femoral head from the acetabular fossa. If the femoral head is difficult to extract due to the ligamentum teres, cut the ligament with either a curved scalpel (teres knife) or with the Bovie electrocautery.

14. Assess the degree, if any, of arthritic changes on the femoral head and acetabular socket. If frank arthritic changes are seen, consider proceeding directly with a total hip arthroplasty. However, for most displaced femoral neck fractures, hemiarthroplasty is the preferred procedure.

15. Inspect, but do not resect the acetabular labrum. It is beneficial in adding stability to the hemiarthroplasty. Similarly, do not remove the pulvinar unless it is hypertrophic and interferes with seating of the bipolar component.

16. Insert trial bipolar shells into the acetabular fossa. Measure the diameter of the resected femoral head. The size of the resected femoral head serves as a reasonable approximation for the size of the appropriate bipolar head. The trial bipolar shell should fit snugly into the acetabular fossa without excessive

force needed to seat it. An excessively tight shell can be a source of postoperative groin pain and increase the risk of dislocation. Conversely, a shell that is "too loose" may result in excessive motion at the bipolar-acetabular interface and be a source of acetabular cartilage degeneration and postoperative pain. Record the size of the bipolar shell to be utilized (**Fig. 22–4**).

Femoral preparation

17. Hold the leg in 90 degrees of hip flexion, 90 degrees of internal rotation, and 15 to 20 degrees of adduction. Place a femoral neck retractor under the proximal femur, which helps exposure by lifting the femur out of the wound. Place a bent Hohman retractor underneath the abductor mass and retract the muscle cephalad. Place a cobra ("Aufranc") retractor underneath the inferior femoral neck and retract the soft tissues and psoas tendon.

18. Remove the soft tissue from the lateral femoral neck. This soft tissue represents the remains of the short external rotators. Use a box osteotome or gouge to remove remnants of bone from the superior femoral neck. However, take care not to remove bone from the greater trochanter. Adequate lateral access to the trochanteric bed is essential to minimize the tendency of inserting the broach and implant in a varus position.

19. Gently insert a straight canal finder by hand into the femoral canal. Gentle insertion is essential, especially in patients with severe osteoporosis, since perforation of the femoral cortex can occur with surprising ease. Pay particular attention to the direction that the canal finder takes as it seats within the femoral canal. Assess the degree of flexion/extension as well as varus/valgus. This indicates the natural morphology of the femur.

20. Consider using axial reamers to enlarge the distal diaphysis until the cortex is encountered. The use of axial reamers depends on individual surgeon's preference. However, if reamers are used, care should be taken to avoid excessive reaming.

21. Broach the proximal femur with sequentially larger broaches until a reasonably snug fit occurs (**Fig. 22–5**). By definition, the femurs in patients with hip fractures have some degree of metabolic bone disease and thus are at increased risk for further

fractures. As with reaming, do not "over-broach." A good cancellous bone bed is essential to optimize fixation at the bone-cement interface. During broaching, pay attention to the alignment of the broach in all planes (varus-valgus, flexion-extension, and rotation). If axial reamers were used, insert the broaches in the same varus-valgus and flexion-extension planes as the axial reamers. In general, insert the broaches so they align rotationally with the natural femoral neck. This usually involves inserting them so there is 12 to 15 degrees of anteversion. If the host bone has abnormal version, consider inserting a smaller prosthesis at the appropriate rotation to optimize hip alignment and stability. Insufficient anteversion may result in hip instability.

22. Insert the final trial broach or the trial implant. The final broach should fit snugly into the femoral canal but not compromise cortical integrity.

23. Place a modular trial femoral head on the taper. Commonly, start with the standard ("plus zero") femoral head length. Measure the distance from the lesser trochanter to the center of hip rotation. Depending on the patient's anatomy, this measurement is usually within a few millimeters of the distance measured on the preoperative radiographs. If the intraoperative measurement is longer than anticipated, *do not resect additional bone from the femoral neck at this time.* Rather, perform a trial reduction and assess hip stability, component orientation, and soft tissue tension. If necessary one can go back and resect more neck; the converse is not true. If the intraoperative measurement is shorter than anticipated, consider using a longer femoral head.

24. With the appropriate head-neck combination in place, insert a trial bipolar shell onto the femoral component and perform a trial hip reduction. If necessary, change the length of the femoral head.

25. During the trial reduction, assess the ease of reduction, concentricity of the bipolar shell, and construct stability.

   a. Pay special attention to possible sites of impingement including impingement of prosthetic neck on the socket or impingement of the femoral component on osteophytes.

   b. Assess component stability. Examine the hip at: 90 degrees of hip flexion simulating sitting; flexion, adduction and internal rotation simulating the fetal sleeping position; and in extension, abduction and external rotation assessing for any evidence of anterior instability. Performing the "push-pull" (shuck test) test to determine myofascial tension appears to be less reliable.

   c. Assess leg lengths. While restoring "normal" extremity length is desirable, it is not always possible. It may be necessary to accept some degree of leg length inequality in order to optimize component fit, soft tissue tension and hip stability.

26. After the optimal femoral head length is determined, dislocate the hip and remove the trial components. Return the hip to its starting position of flexion and internal rotation.

27. Replace the femoral retractors. Measure the femoral canal for a distal cement plug. Insert the plug so it resides in the femoral canal approximately 2 cm distal to where the end of the stem will sit. This helps ensure adequate distal cement. Upon reaching the correct insertion depth check the fit of the plug by pushing it further distally. It should feel tight. Do not pull back on the plug. The main concern is distal advancement of the plug, rather than concerns about whether it will fail by backing retrograde out of the femur. If the plug is loose, remove and place the next larger size.

28. Irrigate the femoral canal with a pulsatile jet lavage system. Remove all loose cancellous bone. Pack the femoral canal with either vaginal packing or sponge. If needed, consider using an epinephrine-soaked sponge, which can decrease the amount of blood in the femoral canal. The goal is to obtain a clean, dry bone bed for the interdigitation with the cement.

29. Mix the acrylic cement. Consider a vacuum mixing technique to enhance cement consistency and reduce overall cement porosity. In general, 80 g of methylmethacrylate is sufficient for an adult femur. However, 120 g may be needed in larger canals. It is preferable to have extra cement than not enough.

30. Use a cement gun to insert the cement when it reaches a "doughy" state and no longer adheres to

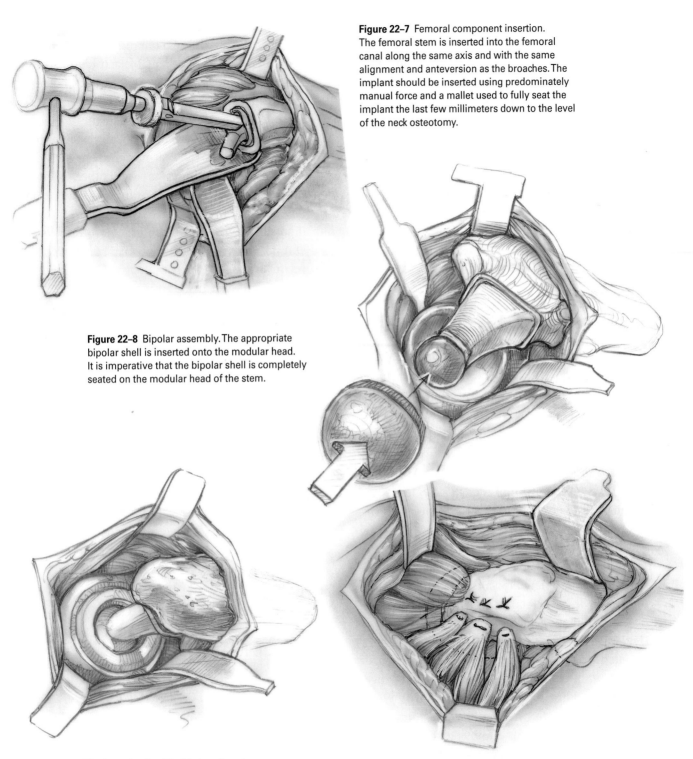

Figure 22–7 Femoral component insertion. The femoral stem is inserted into the femoral canal along the same axis and with the same alignment and anteversion as the broaches. The implant should be inserted using predominately manual force and a mallet used to fully seat the implant the last few millimeters down to the level of the neck osteotomy.

Figure 22–8 Bipolar assembly. The appropriate bipolar shell is inserted onto the modular head. It is imperative that the bipolar shell is completely seated on the modular head of the stem.

Figure 22–9 Bipolar reduction. The hip is reduced and stability reassessed.

Figure 22–10 Closure external rotators. The tagging sutures for the posterior capsule and short external rotators are pulled through the holes (two or three) in the greater trochanter. The capsule sutures are tied to each other and the short external rotator sutures are tied to each other.

the surgical gloves (**Fig. 22–6**). Push the cement nozzle down to, but not past, the cement plug. Introduce the cement by applying slow, steady pressure to the cement gun. Allow the cement pressure to gently push the gun out of the canal. Remove the gun when the femur is full of cement. Break off the nozzle. Attach the proximal pressurizer to the gun and place it against the upper femur. Insert the cement with slow, steady pressure. Commonly, this causes marrow extrusion out of nutrient foramina of the proximal femur. The anesthesia team should be alerted when femoral cementing commences. Some patients may respond to cement insertion with hypotension and/or hypoxemia and require appropriate resuscitation.

31. Insert the stem along the same axis and at the same alignment that the broaches were inserted (**Fig. 22–7**). In addition, take care to replicate component version. Use predominately manual force when inserting the component, rather than using a mallet. Additional cement pressurization is usually apparent at the time. Use a mallet to fully seat the last few millimeters of the implant down to the level of the neck osteotomy. Perform a final check of axial and torsional orientation.

32. Excise excess cement. Until cement polymerization is complete, keep motion of the stem-femur composite to a minimum.

33. Clean and dry the modular taper. Insert the appropriate modular head based on the trial reduction. Insert the appropriate bipolar shell onto the modular head. It is imperative that the bipolar shell completely seat on the modular head of the stem (**Fig. 22–8**).

34. Irrigate the acetabular fossa. Inspect the acetabular fossa to ensure that there is no evidence of retained bone debris, loose acrylic cement, or soft tissue.

35. Reduce the bipolar hemiarthroplasty into the acetabulum. Perform a final assessment of the component position and hip stability (**Fig. 22–9**).

Closure

36. Irrigate the wound with copious antibiotic irrigation.
37. Maintain appropriate hemostasis.
38. If a suction drain is utilized, place it subfacial through a separate incision that exits the anterolateral thigh at the distal extent of the incision. Take care throughout the closure to minimize the risk of inadvertently sewing in the drain. Make two drill holes in the posterolateral aspect of the greater trochanter approximately 1 cm apart (it may be easier to make these drill holes prior to reducing the hip).

39. Pull the tagging sutures on the short external rotators and posterior capsular flap through the holes. Tie the capsule sutures to each other; then tie the short external rotator sutures to each other (**Fig. 22–10**).

40. If possible, repair the quadratus femoris muscle-tendon. In some instances, there may be sufficient tissue for reattachment. It can enhance the extent of the posterior soft tissue envelope.

41. Repair the tendinous insertion of the gluteus maximus with absorbable sutures.

42. Close the deep fascial layer in a meticulous fashion with multiple absorbable sutures (normally 0 or #1).

43. Close the subcutaneous tissue in a layered fashion with interrupted absorbable sutures (normally number 1, 0, and 2-0 sutures).

44. Close the skin with staples, nylon, or prolene.

45. Apply a sterile dressing and a compressive bandage to the hip.

46. Transfer the patient off the operating table taking care to avoid excessive hip rotation or flexion. Transport the patient to recovery room.

47. Obtain a radiograph in the recovery room to ensure the hip is reduced.

Suggested Readings

Cornell CN. Intracapsular fractures of the femoral neck. In: Craig EV, ed. *Clinical Orthopaedics*. Baltimore, MD: Lippincott Williams & Wilkins, 1999, pp. 479–490.

Pellicci PM, Padgett DE. *Atlas of Total Hip Replacement*. New York, NY: Churchill Livingstone, 1995.

Sharrock NE, Minco R, Urquhart B, Salvati EA. The effect of two levels of hypotension on intraoperative blood loss during total hip arthroplasty performed under lumbar epidural anesthesia. *Anesth Analg* 1993;76(3):580–584.

CHAPTER 23

Intramedullary Rodding of Femoral Shaft Fractures

Scott D. Cordes

Indications

1. Closed displaced femoral shaft fractures
2. Open grade 1 or 2 femoral shaft fractures (can be done acutely after a thorough irrigation and debridement of the open wound)

Contraindications

1. Gross wound contamination
2. Nonviable soft tissue envelope
3. Proximal or distal shaft fractures with significant metaphyseal extension

Preoperative Preparation

1. Appropriate extremity radiographs including hip and knee joints
2. Template radiographs to ensure that femoral nails of the appropriate length and diameter are available
3. Neurovascular exam with emphasis on assessing arterial blood flow and distal nerve function
4. Assessment of the skin and soft tissues; evaluate for compartment syndrome.

Special Instruments, Position, and Anesthesia

1. General or regional anesthesia; avoid long-acting regional anesthesia because they make assessment of compartment syndrome difficult.
2. Position patient supine on a fracture table.
3. Check the fluoroscopy prior to draping the patient to ensure that it is in working order and that the C-arm can be positioned to obtain adequate AP and lateral images from the hip to the knee.

Tips and Pearls

1. Position the patient on the fracture table with adequate leg and torso adduction. The exact amount of adduction depends on patient size and body habitus. Extremity adduction allows optimal access to the piriformis fossa and minimizes rod impingement during insertion.
2. Make sure the skin over the entry point for the distal screws is not "draped out" of the operative field.
3. Make sure adequate radiographs of the femoral neck have been obtained and reviewed. Concurrent femoral neck fractures are not uncommon and can be difficult to detect.

4. A controlled, steady force on the awl is required because of the dense bone in the piriformis fossa. Avoid allowing the awl to slip off the bone or cut out posteriorly.

5. Initial passage of the blunt tip guide rod can be difficult through the proximal third of the femur. Consider "choking up" on the blunt-tipped guide rod with the T-handle or vise grip. This will make rod passage easier with less chance of bowing or bending of the guide rod.

What To Avoid

1. Attempt to avoid internal or external rotational malalignment of the fracture when impacting the femoral nail. The patella should be directed toward the ceiling to grossly adjust the rotational alignment of the limb. Reconfirm alignment prior to distal locking.

2. Avoid reckless passes with the guide rod. Slow meticulous passage across the fracture site using proprioceptive feel is imperative.

3. Avoid allowing the guide rod to "back out" past the fracture site during reaming.

Postoperative Care Issues

1. Initially, most patients are allowed to ambulate either non-weight bearing (NWB) or toe-touch weight bearing (TTWB).

2. Depending on the stability of the fracture, protected weight bearing can be advanced approximately 6 weeks after surgery. This is dependent on radiographic evaluation and clinical symptoms.

Operative Technique

1. Transport the patient to the operating room. Appropriate anesthesia is administered.

2. After adequate anesthesia is achieved, position the patient on a fracture table with adequate leg and torso adduction. The exact degree of extremity adduction depends on patient size and body habitus. Adduction allows optimal access to the piriformis fossa and minimizes rod impingement during insertion. Care should be taken to ensure that the patient's position allows adequate clearance for the fluoroscopy. Pad all bony prominences. Place the ipsilateral arm across the chest. Place the foot of the involved extremity in a well-padded fracture boot (**Fig. 23–1**).

3. Apply longitudinal traction through the fracture boot. If a tibial traction has been inserted, remove the pin. Prep the pin with betadine. Cut the pin with a bolt cutter flush with the skin and remove the traction pin from the opposite side with a hand drill. Apply sterile dressing. Alternatively, if a tibial traction pin has been inserted, it can be used to apply longitudinal traction. If the pin is used for traction, remove it at the end of the procedure as outlined above.

4. Evaluate the reduction using fluoroscopy in both the anteroposterior (AP) and lateral projection. Typically, some residual posterior "sag" at the fracture site is visualized on the lateral projection. If necessary, improve fracture alignment by supporting the fracture fragments with a supporting buttress (i.e., a standard crutch placed beneath the thigh at the level of the fracture). On occasion, manual manipulation of the thigh can unlock or improve the alignment of fracture fragments that are difficult to reduce.

5. Prepare and drape the extremity in the usual sterile fashion. Prep the leg from the iliac crest to a level just distal to the knee. If the standard translucent curtain is not long enough to cover this region, apply a translucent adhesive drape. This can be applied circumferentially around the distal half of the femur with the main translucent curtain being placed over the center of the hip to ensure satisfactory sterile draping of the entire length of the femur and hip.

Approach

6. Make a longitudinal skin incision starting at the tip of the greater trochanter and extending proximally 8 to 10 cm (**Fig. 23–2**).

7. Dissect through the soft tissues down to the fascia. Split the fascia longitudinally in a line parallel to the skin incision.

8. Digitally split the fibers of the gluteus maximus to the level of the piriformis fossa. Palpate the piriformis fossa to conform its location (**Fig. 23–3**).

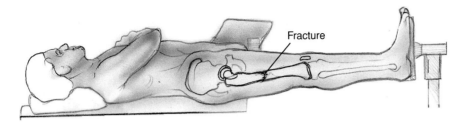

Fracture

Figure 23–1 Patient position. The patient is positioned on a fracture table with adequate leg and torso adduction. Adduction allows optimal access to the piriformis fossa and minimizes rod impingement during insertion. Take care to ensure that the patient's position allows adequate clearance for the fluoroscopy. The ipsilateral arm is placed across the chest. The foot of the involved extremity is placed in a well-padded fracture boot.

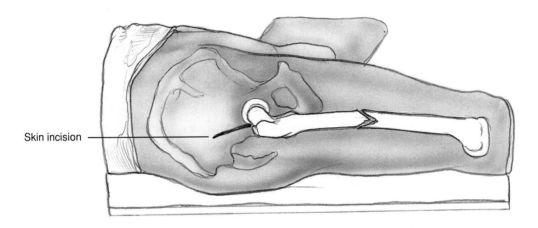

Skin incision

Figure 23–2 Skin incision. The longitudinal skin incision starts at the tip of the greater trochanter and extends proximally 8 to 10 cm.

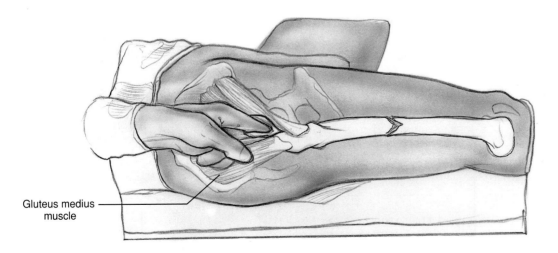

Gluteus medius muscle

Figure 23–3 Muscle dissection. The fibers of the gluteus maximus are digitally split down to the level of the piriformis fossa. The fossa should be palpated to confirm its location.

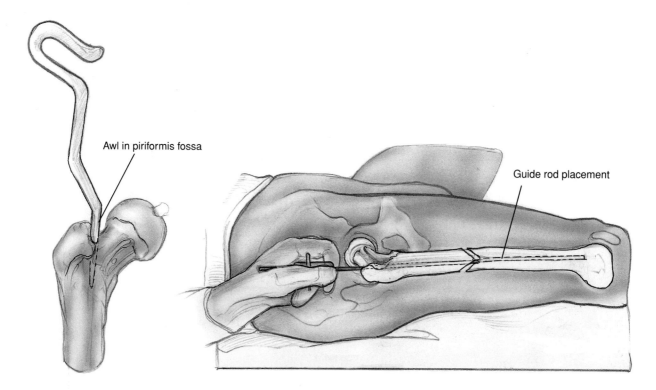

Figure 23–4 Awl introduction. The awl is passed through the previously identified entry point in the piriformis fossa. The awl is kept parallel to the long axis of the femur.

Figure 23–5 Guide rod passage. The blunt tip guide rod is gently passed down the long axis of the femur across the fracture site. Use proprioceptive sensation while passing the guide rod across the fracture fragments.

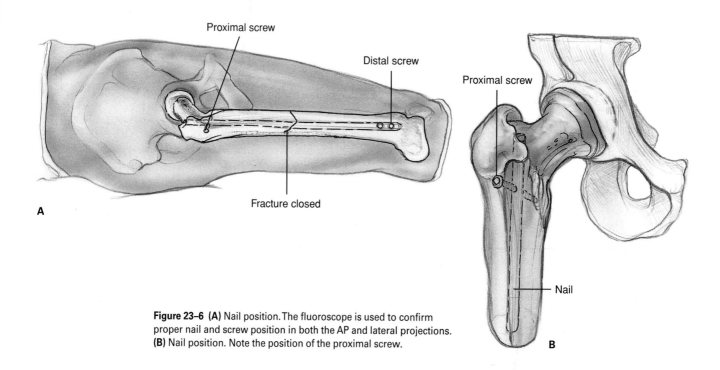

Figure 23–6 (A) Nail position. The fluoroscope is used to confirm proper nail and screw position in both the AP and lateral projections. **(B)** Nail position. Note the position of the proximal screw.

Guide rod insertion

9. Insert an awl into the piriformis fossa (**Fig. 23–4**). Keep the awl parallel to the long axis of the femur. Depending on the patient's size, extremity adduction may be required to ensure a satisfactory entry point for the awl. Use biplanar fluoroscopy to confirm the awl is aligned properly. Alternatively, in younger individuals, the bone in this region can be extremely dense and a cannulated drill passed over a guide pin may be needed to initiate the starting hole in the piriformis fossa.

10. Insert a blunt tip guide rod into the femoral canal through the hole in the piriformis fossa. A T-handle holder or vice grip and mallet can be used to assist in introduction of the guide rod. Depending on the fracture configuration, slightly bend the distal aspect of the guide rod to assist in passage across the fracture site.

11. Advance the blunt tip of the guide rod down the long axis of the femoral shaft to the level of the fracture. Use fluoroscopy to aid in passage of the guide rod across the fracture site. The guide rod should be advanced slowly, gently, and meticulously across the fracture site. Use proprioceptive feel to assist in passing the guide rod across the fracture site. The fracture table typically reduces the fracture well enough for easy passage of the guide rod. In difficult cases a supporting buttress, such as a crutch, can be placed posteriorly to correct for any residual angulation (posterior sag) at the fracture site (**Fig. 23–5**).

12. Use fluoroscopy to confirm the guide rod has been successfully passed across the fracture and is within the distal femoral canal. Insert the guide rod to the level of the patella.

13. Determine the length for the desired femoral nail. Place a radiopaque ruler over the anterior aspect of the thigh. Measure from the superior pole of the patella to the level of the piriformis fossa. Use spot imaged fluoroscopy proximally and distally to confirm the measured length.

Reaming

14. Commence reaming. Use a slow reaming speed to help minimize marrow embolization. Commonly, an 8-mm reamer is used initially. Increase reamer diameters in 0.5-mm increments. Ream the femoral canal 1.5 to 2 mm larger than the desired diameter of the femoral nail. The desired diameter of the femoral nail is determined based on preoperative X-ray measurements and "chatter" of the reamers.

15. Confirm the length and diameter of the desired femoral nail prior to it being unpackaged and placed on the operative field.

Guide rod exchange

16. Place the translucent exchange tube into the femoral canal by inserting it over the blunt tip guide rod. Use the fluoroscopy to confirm that the radiopaque marker at the end of the translucent exchange tube is correctly positioned well beyond the fracture site and well seated in the distal fragment.

17. Remove the blunt tip guide rod and replace it by inserting a smooth tip guide rod down the translucent exchange tube. Use fluoroscopy to confirm that the smooth tip rod is across the fracture site.

Nail insertion

18. Mount the femoral nail securely to the proximal targeting device. Inspect the femoral nail and targeting device to ensure it is mounted correctly. The proximal targeting device should be placed laterally and the anterior bow of the nail should correspond to the anterior bow of the femur.

19. Impact the femoral nail. Use occasional spot fluoroscopy images to confirm correct advancement of the nail across the fracture site and proper seating of the nail. When fully impacted, the proximal portion of the nail should be flush with the piriformis fossa to minimize mechanical irritation. The nail's distal end should roughly be at the level of the femur's epiphyseal scar, near the superior pole of the patella.

20. Remove the smooth tip guide rod. Alternatively, the smooth guide rod can be removed after passage of the nail across the fracture site, but prior to final nail impaction.

Proximal locking screws

21. Insert the drill guide sleeves for the proximal targeting device. Ensure that the sleeves are flush with the bone.

22. Make a bicortical drill hole under fluoroscopic guidance. Determine the desired length for the screw using the depth gauge or reading off of the drill bit.

23. Insert the appropriate proximal locking screw. Remove the proximal targeting device.

Distal locking screws

24. Adjust the fluoroscopy so it is exactly perpendicular to the long axis of the femur. Use the fluoroscopy to visualize the distal holes in the nail as perfect circles on the lateral image. If the nail holes appear as ellipses on the image, adjust the C-arm until perfect circles are obtained. Normally, only small C-arm adjustments are necessary to achieve flawless image circles.

25. Make a small longitudinal stab incision in the skin directly over the visualized nail holes seen on the fluoroscopic image. A ring forcep can be used to locate the appropriate spot.

26. Use a sharp tip Steinman pin or disposable trocar pin to make a starting entry point in the bone. A disposable sharp tip pin minimizes sliding away from the hole's epicenter. Center the pin's tip directly in the middle of the perfect circle seen on the fluoroscopy.

27. After this unicortical hole is established, make a bicortical drill hole through the nail. Alternately, use a radiolucent drill. Align the targeting device of the drill concentrically with the visualized circular hole in the nail. Use the drill to make a bicortical hole.

28. Similarly to the proximal screws, use a standard depth gauge to measure the desired screw length. Insert the appropriate length distal-locking screws.

29. If necessary, utilize a similar technique for additional distal-locking screws.

30. Use the fluoroscope to confirm proper nail and screw position in both the AP and lateral projections. Appropriately placed locking screws will obliterate the visualized holes in the femoral nail (**Fig. 23–6**).

Closure

31. Copiously irrigate the wounds (especially the proximal one) to remove any residual reaming at the level of the piriformis fossa. This may minimize later heterotopic bone formation.

32. Close the fascia with interrupted or figure eight O Vicryl.

33. Use a standard closure for the skin and subcutaneous tissue.

Suggested Readings

Jones, AL. Fractures of the femur. In: Levine AM, ed. *Orthopaedic Knowledge Update: Trauma*. Rosemont, IL: American Academy of Orthopaedic Surgeons, 1996, pp. 127–136.

Whittle, AP. In: Canale ST. *Campbell's Operative Orthopaedics*, 9th ed. St. Louis, MO: Mosby-Year Book, Inc., 1998, pp. 2136–2166.

Section Five

Knee and Leg

CHAPTER 24

Arthroscopy

Steven H. Stern

Indications

1. Symptomatic meniscal tear (medial or lateral)
2. Loose body
3. Osteochondritis dissecans
4. Septic knee
5. Evaluation of the articular cartilage and osteochondral structures of the knee
6. Arthritis (relative). Arthroscopy is an unpredictable procedure in treating mild to moderate arthritis or patellofemoral syndrome ("chondromalacia"). It is rarely beneficial in severe osteoarthritis unless there is a significant mechanical component causing the patient symptoms.

Contraindications

1. Unsatisfactory skin condition
2. History of knee reflex sympathetic dystrophy (relative)

Preoperative Preparation

1. Knee radiographs
2. Magnetic resonance imaging (MRI) depending on the patient's symptoms and the specific surgical procedure planned

Special Instruments, Position, and Anesthesia

1. The patient is placed supine on the operating room table.
2. All pressure points should be padded.
3. The procedure can be done with general, spinal, or local anesthesia with sedation.
4. A leg holder or lateral support post can be used.
5. A pneumatic thigh tourniquet should be placed as proximal as possible on the thigh. However, most standard arthroscopic procedures can successfully be completed without tourniquet inflation.
6. Standard arthroscopic instruments are needed. These should include an arthroscopic "shaver."
7. If a meniscal repair is contemplated, the instruments and implants for introduction of an absorbable fixation device should be available.

Tips and Pearls

1. Arthroscopy is most reliable for *symptomatic* mechanical problems within the knee such as meniscal tears and loose bodies. The results achieved with articular cartilage debridement for patellofemoral syndrome ("chondromalacia") or osteoarthritis or with menisectomy for asymptomatic or incidental meniscal tears are significantly less predictable. The best results occur when the

patient's preoperative symptoms and physical examination correlate with mechanical finding on a diagnostic study (i.e., MRI).

2. If a leg holder is utilized it should be positioned as proximal as possible on the thigh. If a lateral support post is utilized, it should be positioned just distal to the tourniquet on the proximal thigh.

3. In general, all procedures should commence with a systematic diagnostic inspection of the entire joint performed in a standard manner prior to any operative surgery. However, if a loose body is found, it is appropriate (and desirable) to immediately proceed with its removal while it is easily visualized. The author's preferred order for the systematic diagnostic inspection of the entire knee joint is: suprapatellar pouch, patellofemoral joint, lateral gutter, medial gutter, medial compartment, intercondylar notch, and lateral compartment.

4. Add epinephrine to the inflow bags to minimize bleeding.

5. Remember the arthroscope and camera move independently. The arthroscope should be positioned and rotated to optimize the field of view. The camera should then be rotated to insure correct picture orientation on the video monitor. The light cord inserts on the arthroscope 180 degrees from the scope's field of view (**Fig. 24–2**).

What To Avoid

1. Try to avoid multiple operations on the same knee for the same problem over a short time period.
2. Avoid violating the patella tendon with placement of the portals.
3. Attempt to minimize damage to the articular cartilage with the arthroscopic instruments and shavers.
4. Avoid leaving free meniscal debris floating within the joint after morselization of the meniscus.

Postoperative Care Issues

1. Consider injecting a local anesthetic (i.e., 0.25% bupivacaine) into the knee at the end of the procedure to minimize postoperative pain.

2. A compressive dressing should be placed at the end of surgery and is normally removed approximately 48 hours after the procedure.

3. In most cases, patients can weight-bear as tolerated (WBAT) after surgery. Most patients are able to discontinue crutches in the first week after surgery.

4. Range-of-motion and strengthening exercises can be initiated immediately after the procedure. Routine formal physical therapy is not required for all patients. Most patients can successfully rehabilitate with a home exercise program.

Operative Technique

Arthroscope insertion

1. Position the patient supine on the operating room table. Place a thigh tourniquet as proximal as possible on the thigh. While most cases can be performed without tourniquet inflation, the tourniquet can be inflated if bleeding impedes visualization.

2. Depending on surgeon preference, either a post or thigh holder can be used. Position the lateral post just distal to the thigh tourniquet. If a thigh holder is utilized, position it as proximal as possible.

3. Prepare and drape the limb in the hospital's standard sterile fashion.

4. Extend the knee and make a small stab wound superior and medial to the patellar. Ideally this should be medial to the quadriceps tendon (**Fig. 24–1**).

5. Introduce the inflow cannula into the joint utilizing the blunt obturator. Commonly, a "pop" can be felt as the obturator enters the knee capsule. Do not inflate the joint at this time, since the fluid will obscure the landmarks used in placement of the remaining portals.

6. Flex the knee. Identify the "soft spot" for the inferior lateral portal. This can be palpated as a soft indentation in the lateral retinaculum which lies just lateral to the patellar tendon at the level of the joint line. Many surgeons use the inferior pole of the patellar as a landmark. Make a small stab incision in this spot (the author prefers a horizontal incision). Inflate the joint (**Fig. 24–1**).

7. Introduce the cannula for the arthroscope through this portal. This is best done with the knee still

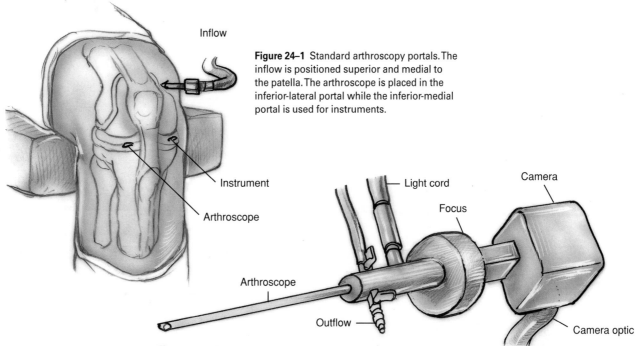

Inflow

Figure 24–1 Standard arthroscopy portals. The inflow is positioned superior and medial to the patella. The arthroscope is placed in the inferior-lateral portal while the inferior-medial portal is used for instruments.

Instrument

Arthroscope

Light cord

Camera

Focus

Arthroscope

Outflow

Camera optic

Figure 24–2 Arthroscope. Note the components of a common arthroscopic setup. The arthroscope is introduced into the joint through a cannula that allows either fluid outflow (pictured) or inflow. The arthroscope and camera rotate independently. The light cord inserts on the arthroscope 180 degrees from the scope's field of view.

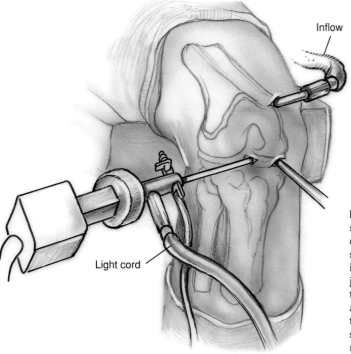

Inflow

Light cord

Figure 24–3 Medial compartment. Note the standard position for viewing the medial compartment. The knee is either extended or slightly flexed. The arthroscope is positioned in the medial compartment so it parallels the joint line and looks lateral (light cord is parallel to the joint line and going medial). The camera is adjusted so the picture is correctly oriented with the femur superior and the tibia inferior. A valgus stress can be applied to the tibia to "open" the medial compartment and improve visualization.

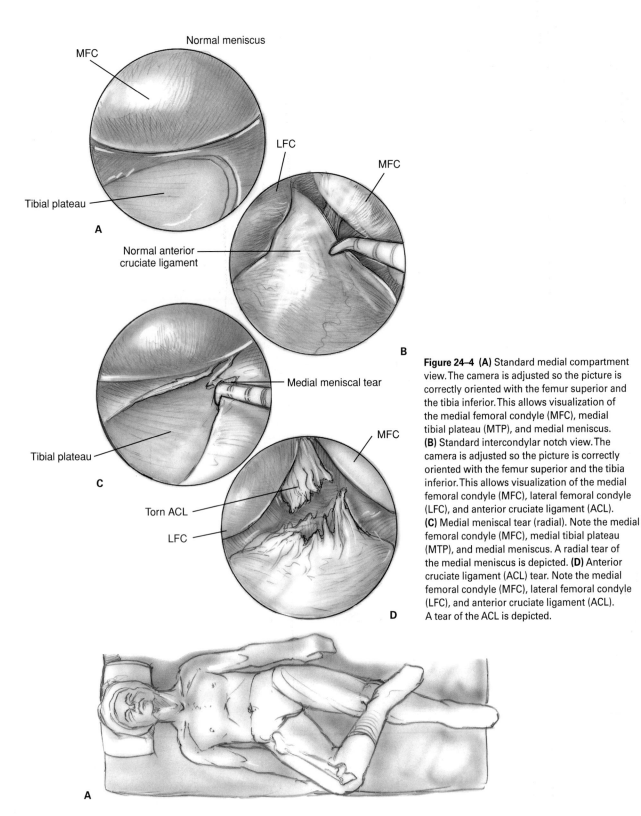

Figure 24–4 **(A)** Standard medial compartment view. The camera is adjusted so the picture is correctly oriented with the femur superior and the tibia inferior. This allows visualization of the medial femoral condyle (MFC), medial tibial plateau (MTP), and medial meniscus. **(B)** Standard intercondylar notch view. The camera is adjusted so the picture is correctly oriented with the femur superior and the tibia inferior. This allows visualization of the medial femoral condyle (MFC), lateral femoral condyle (LFC), and anterior cruciate ligament (ACL). **(C)** Medial meniscal tear (radial). Note the medial femoral condyle (MFC), medial tibial plateau (MTP), and medial meniscus. A radial tear of the medial meniscus is depicted. **(D)** Anterior cruciate ligament (ACL) tear. Note the medial femoral condyle (MFC), lateral femoral condyle (LFC), and anterior cruciate ligament (ACL). A tear of the ACL is depicted.

Figure 24–5 **(A)** "Figure four" position. The "figure four" position is used to view the lateral compartment. The knee is flexed and the hip externally rotated so the operative ankle lies on the anterior portion of the contralateral leg. This position improves visualization by "opening" the lateral compartment.

flexed. Aim for the intercondylar notch. Commonly, a "pop" can be felt as the cannula enters the knee capsule.

8. Insert the arthroscope into the knee joint through the cannula (**Fig. 24–2**). Extend the knee and position the arthroscope in the suprapatellar pouch.

9. Connect the outflow tubing to the arthroscopic cannula. The tubing can be attached to gravity drainage.

10. Identify the prior placed inflow cannula in the suprapatellar pouch to ensure that it is correctly positioned. Focus and color balance the arthroscope if this has not already been done.

Arthroscopic knee evaluation

➤ Commence a systematic evaluation of the knee joint. The author's preferred order for the systematic diagnostic inspection of the entire knee joint is: suprapatellar pouch, patellofemoral joint, lateral gutter, medial gutter, medial compartment, intercondylar notch, and lateral compartment.

➤ Remember the arthroscope and camera move independently. The arthroscope should be positioned and rotated to optimize the field of view. The camera should then be rotated to ensure correct picture orientation on the video monitor. Remember the light cord inserts on the arthroscope 180 degrees from the scope's field of view (**Fig. 24–2**).

11. Inspect the suprapatellar pouch.

12. Inspect the patellofemoral joint. Rotate the arthroscope downward to inspect the femur's trochlear groove, and rotate it upward to evaluate the patella.

13. Inspect the lateral gutter. Rotate the arthroscope so it is looking down and move it laterally over the top of the lateral femoral condyle. Enter the lateral gutter by raising the camera so the tip of the arthroscope moves posterior. Ensure that there are no loose bodies in the gutter.

14. Inspect the medial gutter. First return the arthroscope to the patellofemoral joint and then move it medially over the medial femoral condyle into the medial gutter.

15. Enter the medial compartment. Flex the knee and insert the arthroscope into the medial compartment. Optimize visualization by rotating the arthroscope so it parallels the joint line and looks lateral. Adjust the camera so the picture is oriented correctly. The femur should be superior and the tibia inferior on the video monitor (**Fig. 24–3**).

16. Make the instrumentation portal. Use a spinal needle to assist in placing this portal. Place the needle into the medial compartment by inserting it through the medial "soft spot." This is at the joint line just medial to the patellar tendon. Check the intra-articular position of the needle to ensure it is correctly positioned. Ideally the needle should enter the joint just superior to the medial meniscus and easily be moveable to the other knee compartments.

17. Inspect the medial compartment (**Fig. 24–4A**). Place a valgus stress on the knee against the lateral post or thigh holder. This improves visualization of the posterior medial compartment. Evaluate the compartment for meniscal tears, loose bodies, osteochondral injuries, or other intra-articular pathology. Visualization of the posterior medial compartment can be enhanced by externally rotating the foot and extending the knee.

18. Inspect the intercondylar notch (**Fig. 24–4B**). Move the arthroscope laterally into the intercondylar notch while keeping the knee flexed. Maintain the standard arthroscope and camera orientation. Evaluate the intercondylar notch for cruciate ligament tears (**Fig. 24–4D**), loose bodies, or other intra-articular pathology.

19. Inspect the lateral compartment. Place the leg in the "figure four" position by flexing the knee and externally rotating the hip so the operative ankle lays on the anterior portion of the contralateral leg (**Fig. 24–5A**). This position improves visualization by "opening" the lateral compartment. Adjust the arthroscope and camera to maintain the standard orientation with the arthroscope rotated so it parallels the joint line and looks lateral (**Fig. 24–5B**). Orient the camera so the femur is superior and the tibia inferior on the video monitor (**Fig. 24–6A**). The anterior portion of the compartment is inspected by rotating the scope 90 degrees so it looks down toward the tibia. Evaluate the compartment for meniscal tears, loose bodies, popliteus tendon injuries, osteochondral injuries, or other intra-articular pathology.

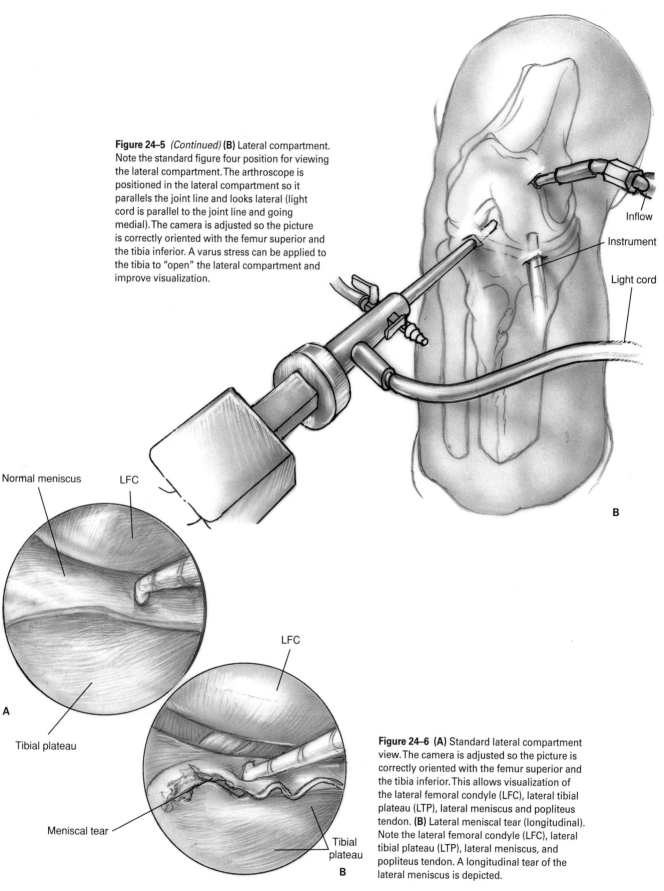

Figure 24–5 *(Continued)* **(B)** Lateral compartment. Note the standard figure four position for viewing the lateral compartment. The arthroscope is positioned in the lateral compartment so it parallels the joint line and looks lateral (light cord is parallel to the joint line and going medial). The camera is adjusted so the picture is correctly oriented with the femur superior and the tibia inferior. A varus stress can be applied to the tibia to "open" the lateral compartment and improve visualization.

Inflow

Instrument

Light cord

B

Normal meniscus

LFC

A

Tibial plateau

LFC

Meniscal tear

Tibial plateau

B

Figure 24–6 (A) Standard lateral compartment view. The camera is adjusted so the picture is correctly oriented with the femur superior and the tibia inferior. This allows visualization of the lateral femoral condyle (LFC), lateral tibial plateau (LTP), lateral meniscus and popliteus tendon. **(B)** Lateral meniscal tear (longitudinal). Note the lateral femoral condyle (LFC), lateral tibial plateau (LTP), lateral meniscus, and popliteus tendon. A longitudinal tear of the lateral meniscus is depicted.

If needed, alter the knee position to improve visualization. In general, increased knee flexion improves posterior structure (i.e., popliteus or posterior lateral meniscus) visualization. However, knee flexion can also restrict the fluid inflow, thereby impairing visualization. If necessary, the inflow can be improved by moving it so the fluid flows into the joint through the arthroscope's cannula.

20. Perform appropriate procedures depending on the intra-articular pathology found.

Partial meniscectomy

➤ Perform a partial meniscectomy if a meniscal tear is felt not appropriate for an attempt at meniscal repair.

➤ In general, attempt to limit the amount of meniscus removed to the degree necessary to leave a stable peripheral meniscal rim.

➤ The exact meniscectomy technique will depend on the type and severity of the tear present. Commonly, a combination of techniques is used depending on the specific meniscal pathology. General guidelines follow.

a. *Bucket handle tears*
Evaluate the extent of the tear with a probe. Use a biting instrument to incise the posterior horn of the meniscus at the level of the posterior extent of the tear. Then incise the meniscus's anterior horn attachments at the level of the anterior extent of the tear. Grasp the torn meniscal fragment with a grabber and remove it through a portal. Use an arthroscopic shaver to contour the meniscal remnant into a stable peripheral meniscal rim. Probe the meniscal remnant to ensure that the remaining peripheral meniscal is stable.

b. *Radial or complex degenerative tears*
Evaluate the extent of the tear with a probe (**Figs. 24–4C and 6B**). Use a biting instrument to morselize the torn portion of the meniscus. Remove only enough meniscal tissue to leave a stable peripheral meniscal rim. Use an arthroscopic shaver to contour the meniscal remnant into a stable peripheral meniscal rim. Probe the meniscal remnant to ensure that the remaining peripheral meniscal is stable.

Meniscal repairs

➤ Perform a partial meniscectomy if a meniscal tear is felt to be appropriate for an attempt at meniscal repair. Various methods can be employed. These include placement of sutures using either inside-out or outside-in techniques or placement of absorbable intra-articular fixation devices ("arrows" or "tacks").

Anterior cruciate ligament (ACL) tears

➤ For treatment of anterior cruciate ligament (ACL) tears (**Fig. 24–4D**), see Chapters 25 and 26.

Loose body removal

➤ Loose bodies can be difficult to find in the knee. Thus, when a loose body is found, it is appropriate (and desirable) to immediately proceed with its removal while it is easily visualized. Standard removal techniques require triangulation with the arthroscope and arthroscopic grabber and removal of the loose body through the appropriate portal. If necessary, make accessory portals to aid in loose body removal.

Arthroscopic debridement

➤ If desired, loose and fibrillated articular cartilage can be debrided arthroscopically. Use an arthroscopic shaver to debride the loose or fibrillated articular cartilage.

➤ In general, attempt to limit the amount of debridement performed to the amount necessary to remove only the severely diseased articular cartilage. If possible, avoid debriding back to subchondral bone as this can be counterproductive.

Closure

21. After the operative arthroscopy is completed, re-evaluate the knee to ensure there is no further pathology amenable to treatment.

22. Copiously irrigate the joint.

23. Inject bupivacaine (0.25%) into the joint to minimize postoperative pain.

24. Close the portals per surgeon's preference. The author prefers a subcuticular suture and steristrips.

25. Dress the wound sterilely in the operating room. Transfer the patient to the recovery room.

Suggested Readings

Boland AL, Southerland SR. Meniscal tear and cyst: arthroscopic menisectomy. In: Craig EV, ed. *Clinical Orthopaedics*. Baltimore, MD: Lippincott Williams & Wilkins, 1999, pp. 741–749.

Cannon WD Jr. Arthroscopic survey of the knee joint. In: Scott WN, ed. *The Knee*. St. Louis, MO: Mosby-Year Book, 1994, pp. 497–514.

CHAPTER 25

Anterior Cruciate Ligament Surgery

Two Incision

Gordon W. Nuber

Indications

1. Active individual with an acute torn anterior cruciate ligament (ACL)
2. Individual with recurrent instability who has failed rehabilitation and bracing
3. A sedentary individual who displays instability related to his or her anterior cruciate ligament—deficient knee with daily activities

Contraindications

1. Active knee infection
2. Lack of neurovascular control
3. A sedentary individual without demonstrable instability
4. Older age (relative)
5. Pediatric patient with open growth plate

Preoperative Preparation

1. Knee radiographs: anteroposterior (AP), lateral, and skyline
2. Magnetic resonance imaging (MRI): not a necessity, but helps to assess other injuries.
3. Wait for knee swelling and active range of motion to normalize prior to surgery (may necessitate preoperative physical therapy).

Special Instruments, Position, and Anesthesia

1. Position the patient supine on the operating room table.
2. The contralateral extremity should be padded to avoid pressure on susceptible areas.
3. Leg holder or post
4. General, epidural, or spinal anesthetic
5. Routine arthroscopic setup and routine orthopaedic surgical instruments
6. Tibial and femoral alignment guides for positioning the tunnel guide pins
7. Interference screws for graft fixation; these can be metal or bioabsorbable. A screw and washer may be used as a "post."
8. A tendon passer (either wire loop, Hewson tendon passer)

Tips and Pearls

1. The anterior knee incision should extend from the lower pole of the patella to a point slightly medial to the tibial tubercle.
2. The lateral incision extends proximal from the lateral epicondyle, approximately 2 to 3 cm.
3. Examine the knee under anesthesia. Assess the stability and document.

4. Document all other intra-articular pathology. Consider meniscal repair when appropriate to aid knee stability.

5. The tibial hole should enter the joint at the posterior insertion of the anterior cruciate ligament's remnant. This is just anterior to the posterior cruciate ligament.

6. The femoral guide pin enters the joint within 5 to 6 mm of the intercondylar notch's back wall. This corresponds to an 11 o'clock position on a right knee and a 1 o'clock position on a left knee.

7. Make an adequate notchplasty to optimize visualization of the drill holes.

8. Rasp the ends of the tunnels to avoid sharp edges.

9. Use a "carrot" to plug the tibial tunnel and avoid fluid extravasation after the tunnel is created.

10. Use a rongeur to contour the end of the bone plug into a bullet; the tip aids graft passage.

11. Minimize tourniquet use if possible.

12. In most cases, aim to harvest 25-mm-long bone plugs from the patella and the tibia.

13. Insert the interference screw with the use of a guide pin.

14. If a meniscal repair is indicated, this should be performed prior to the anterior cruciate ligament reconstruction.

What To Avoid

1. Minimize the chance of patella fracture by avoiding excessively long or deep bone cuts.

2. Lift the femoral guide's handle to avoid breaking out the back wall while creating the femoral tunnel.

3. Take care to minimize the chance of dropping the graft on the floor.

Postoperative Care Issues

1. Consider placing a suction drain in the lateral incision.

2. Place the leg in a compressive dressing with an elastic wrap after surgery. Consider cryotherapy.

3. If a continuous passive motion (CPM) machine is used, it can begin at 0 to 40 degrees on day 1 with daily incremental increases of 5 to 10 degrees.

4. A hinged brace can be used when ambulating the first 4 weeks after surgery. Lock the brace in extension for 2 weeks, then unlock and allow free range of motion for 2 weeks. Alternatively, a knee immobilizer can be used for the first few weeks after surgery (commonly the first 2) and then discontinued when the patient regains adequate quadriceps control.

5. An accelerated rehabilitation protocol begins immediately after surgery. Normally, active and active-assisted flexion exercises and passive extension exercises are instituted.

6. Patients commonly either go home the day of surgery or spend one night in the hospital.

7. Protected weight bearing as tolerated with the immobilizer or hinged-brace is allowed after surgery. Most patients can wean themselves off crutches during the first 2 weeks postsurgery.

Operative Technique

1. Position the patient supine on the operating room table. Apply a thigh tourniquet as proximal as possible on leg. Place the opposite leg on a bolster to flex the hip and avoid stretching the femoral nerve. In addition, loosely tape the opposite leg to the table (the leg of a large athlete may fall off a narrow operating table).

2. Examine the knee and leg after adequate anesthesia is obtained. This examination under anesthesia (EUA) should assess medial, lateral, anterior, and posterior knee stability prior to applying the leg holder. Document the examination.

3. Prepare and drape the surgical leg in the hospital's routine manner. Exanguinate if inflating the tourniquet at this point. Alternatively, exsanguination and tourniquet inflation can be done later in the procedure at the time of graft harvesting. Try to minimize tourniquet time, as increased tourniquet use can increase postoperative leg atrophy.

Arthroscopic evaluation and notchplasty

4. Make routine arthroscopic portals. The inflow portal is made medial and superior to patella into the suprapatellar pouch. The medial and lateral joint line portals are made just to the side of the patellar tendon and are used for instruments and the 30-degree arthroscope (see Chapter 24) (**Fig. 25–1**).

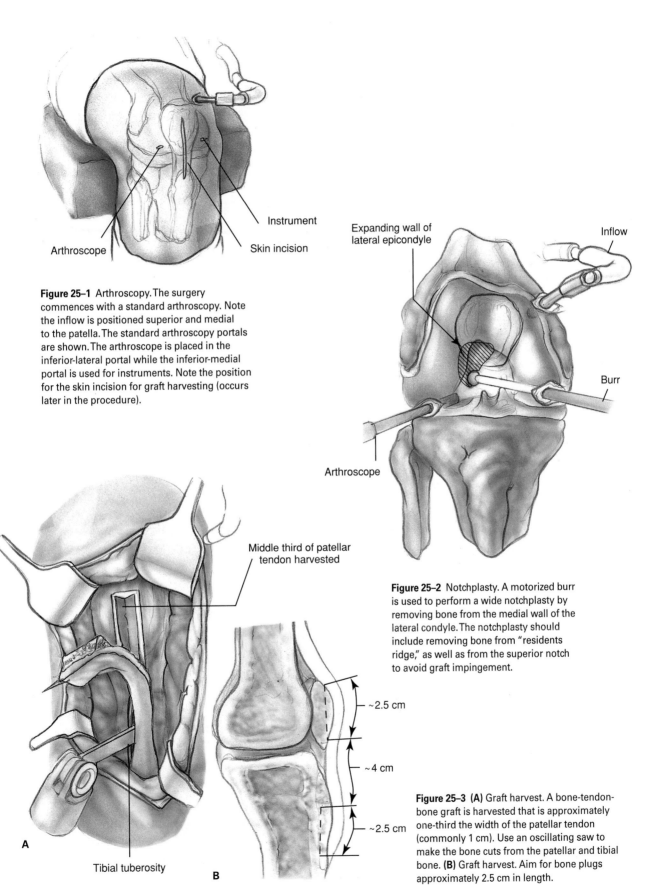

Arthroscope

Instrument

Skin incision

Figure 25–1 Arthroscopy. The surgery commences with a standard arthroscopy. Note the inflow is positioned superior and medial to the patella. The standard arthroscopy portals are shown. The arthroscope is placed in the inferior-lateral portal while the inferior-medial portal is used for instruments. Note the position for the skin incision for graft harvesting (occurs later in the procedure).

Expanding wall of lateral epicondyle

Inflow

Burr

Arthroscope

Figure 25–2 Notchplasty. A motorized burr is used to perform a wide notchplasty by removing bone from the medial wall of the lateral condyle. The notchplasty should include removing bone from "residents ridge," as well as from the superior notch to avoid graft impingement.

Middle third of patellar tendon harvested

~2.5 cm

~4 cm

~2.5 cm

Figure 25–3 (A) Graft harvest. A bone-tendon-bone graft is harvested that is approximately one-third the width of the patellar tendon (commonly 1 cm). Use an oscillating saw to make the bone cuts from the patellar and tibial bone. **(B)** Graft harvest. Aim for bone plugs approximately 2.5 cm in length.

Tibial tuberosity

A

B

Figure 25–4 Rear entry femoral drill guide. Note that the introducer for the rear entry guide has been inserted through the lateral arthroscopy portal and exits the capsule posteriorly. The rear entry guide is attached to the eyelet in the introducer and pulled back into the joint.

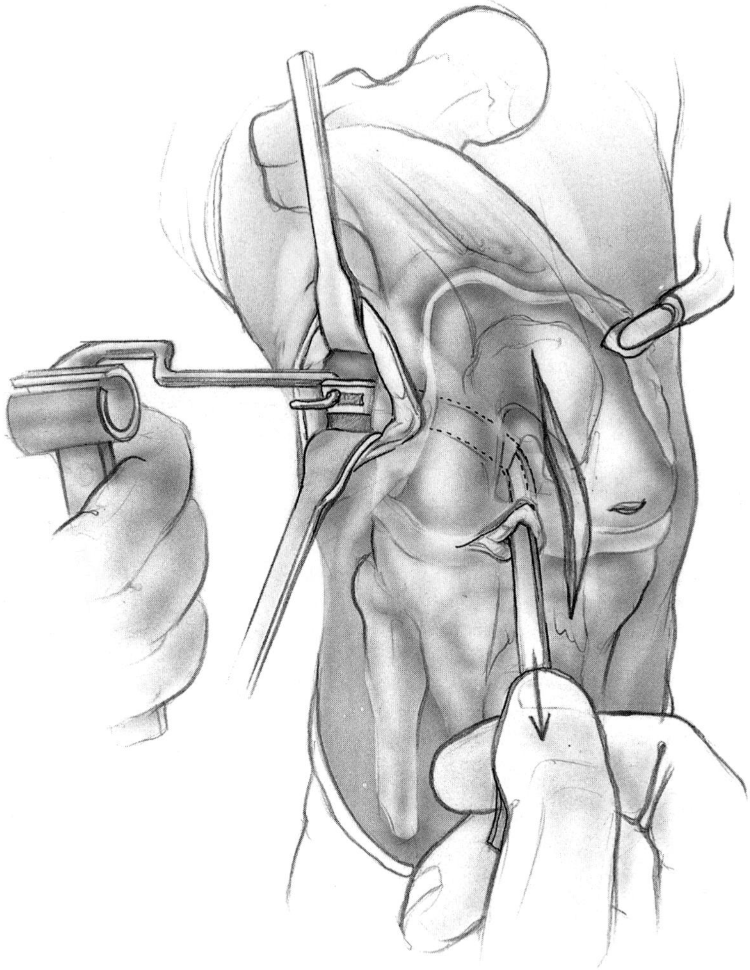

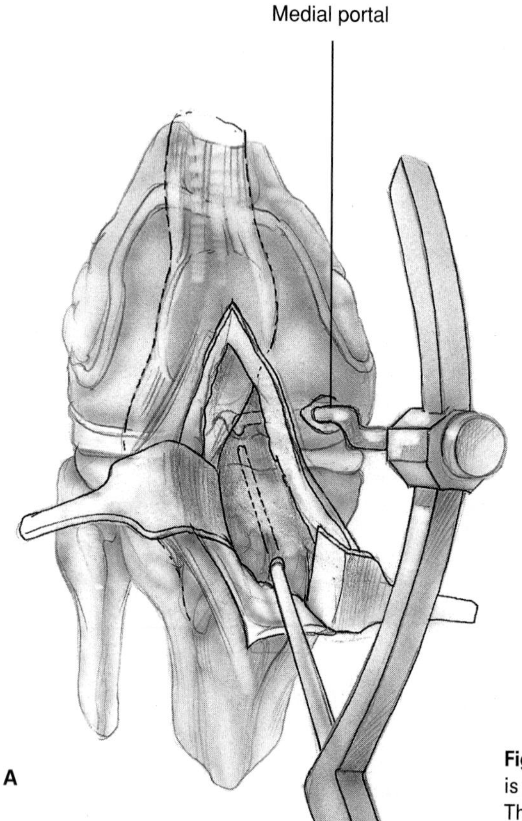

Medial portal

A

Figure 25–5 (A) Tibial guide. Note the arthroscope is positioned in the lateral portal for this step. The tibial guide is inserted through the medial portal. The insertion of the guide pin starts on the anterior surface of the tibial metaphysis. The starting point should be just medial to the tibial tubercle and at least 2 cm distal to the joint line.

5. Perform a standard arthroscopic knee evaluation in a systematic manner. Examine the suprapatellar pouch, patella femoral joint, lateral gutter, medial gutter, medial compartment, intercondylar notch, and lateral compartment. This systematic approach allows an adequate assessment of the menisci, ligaments, and tendons about the knee.

   a. Confirm the anterior cruciate ligament tear.
   b. Repair or resect the menisci as appropriate. Remove any loose bodies.
   c. Evaluate any chondral injuries. Debride and treat them if appropriate (chondral microfracture or chondral transplantation).

6. If a torn anterior cruciate ligament is confirmed, debride the ligament's stump. If the notch is narrow, perform a wide notchplasty. Remove part of the lateral femoral wall along with "residents ridge," as well as the superior notch to avoid graft impingement (Fig. 25–2).

Graft harvest and preparation

7. Remove the arthroscopic instruments from the knee.
8. Make a skin incision from lower pole of the patella to a point just medial to the tibial tubercle (Fig. 25–1).
9. Incise the subcutaneous tissue and peritenon layer directly over the patellar tendon.
10. Measure the patellar tendon's width. Harvest a graft approximately one third the width of the patellar tendon (commonly 1 cm). An oscillating saw is used to make the bone cuts from the patella and tibia. The bone plugs are removed from their donor sites with the help of a curved osteotome. Avoid levering the osteotome against the underlying bone. Aim for bone plugs approximately 2.5 cm long and 1 cm wide from both patella and tibia (Fig. 25–3A and 3B).
11. After graft harvest, use sizing rings to determine the actual size and length of the bone plugs and to determine the exact size of the femoral and tibial tunnels to be created.
12. Trim the bone plugs and contour the ends into a blunt tip with a rongeur to aid in passage through the tunnels.
13. Make two 2.0-mm holes in each bone plug. Place a #5 nonabsorbable suture through each bone hole. Place a #2 nonabsorbable suture at the bone tendon junction.

Tunnel preparation

14. Denude the periosteum over the metaphyseal bone just medial to the tibial tubercle and 2 cm distal to the joint line for the entrance point to the tibial hole. This area should be approximately 1.5 cm in diameter.
15. Make a skin incision extending proximally from the lateral epicondyle 2 to 3 cm.
16. Dissect down through the subcutaneous tissue. Longitudinally split the iliotibial band anterior to the intermuscular septum. Place a "Z" or other type of retractor under the vastus lateralis muscle and retract the muscle medially.
17. Clean the soft tissue from the flair of the lateral epicondyle with a periosteal elevator. Coagulate the lateral geniculate vessels. Make a small split in the intermuscular septum with a hemostat. Leave the "Z" retractor in place.
18. Return the arthroscopic instruments to the operative field. Place the arthroscope through the medial incision to optimize visualization of the rear entry guide. Insert the introducer for the rear entry guide through the lateral arthroscopic portal. It should hug the wall of the lateral intercondylar notch and lateral femoral condyle and exit the capsule posteriorly. The surgeon's finger can guide it through the capsule posteriorly and out the lateral incision.
19. Attach the rear entry guide to the eyelet in the introducer. Bring the internal tip of the rear entry guide back into the joint. Position it in the notch within 5 mm of the back wall at the 11 o'clock position for a right knee or the 1 o'clock position for a left knee. Insert the bullet tip obturator into the hole in the external portion of the rear entry guide. The obturator is pushed against the femoral condyle and locked into position (Fig. 25–4).
20. Insert a guide pin through the obturator directed from the lateral femoral condyle into the intercondylar notch. Use a probe to help ascertain that the guide pin enters the notch in the proper position. The entry point position should prevent the subsequent reamed hole from breaking out the posterior cortex of the femoral condyle.
21. Switch the arthroscope to the lateral portal. Insert the tibial guide so that the intra-articular guide pin enters the joint through the posterior half of the ACL's tibial footprint. This is a point just anterior to

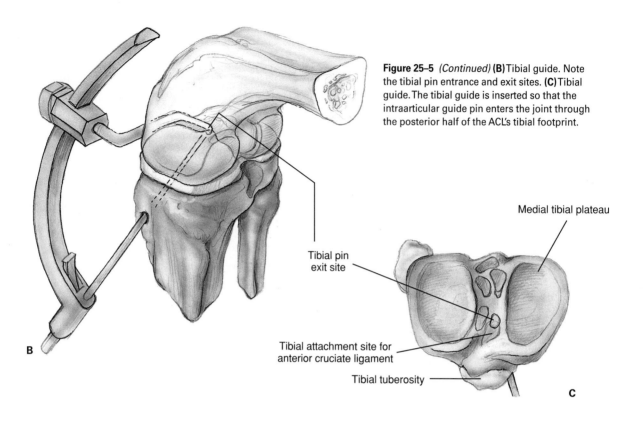

Figure 25–5 *(Continued)* **(B)** Tibial guide. Note the tibial pin entrance and exit sites. **(C)** Tibial guide. The tibial guide is inserted so that the intraarticular guide pin enters the joint through the posterior half of the ACL's tibial footprint.

Medial tibial plateau

Tibial pin exit site

Tibial attachment site for anterior cruciate ligament

Tibial tuberosity

B

C

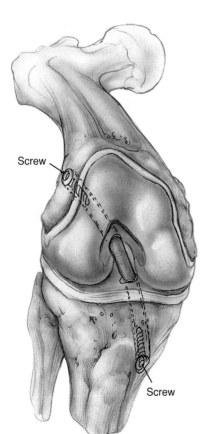

Screw

Screw

Figure 25–6 Graft fixation. For femoral fixation, an interference screw is inserted proximal and anterior to the bone plug. For tibial fixation, either a post or an interference screw (depicted in the picture) can be used.

the posterior cruciate ligament. Start the guide pin on the anterior surface of the tibial metaphysis. The starting point is just medial to the tibia tubercle and at least 2 cm distal to the joint line. This corresponds to the previously denuded area of periosteum (**Fig. 25–5**).

22. Insert the guide pin through the tibia and a few millimeters into the knee joint to ascertain its position. Run the knee through a range of motion. Arthroscopically visualize the guide pin with the knee extended. Ensure that it clears the superior notch and that the graft will not impinge.

23. Over-ream each of the guide pins with disposable reamers (generally 9 to 12 mm diameter). Rasp the edges of each hole to smooth the border. An arthroscopic shaver can be used to clean soft tissue from the intraarticular holes. Use a "carrot" to plug the tibia hole to prevent fluid extravasation.

Graft passage

24. Insert a malleable tendon passer (Hewson or wire loop) into the tibial hole and through the femoral hole so it exits through the lateral incision. Place the patellar tendon graft sutures through the loop in the tendon passer. Pull the sutures back through the femoral and tibial tunnels.

25. Using the sutures, pull the graft into the femoral tunnel and down into the tibial tunnel. Use the probe to assist graft passage into the tibial tunnel. If the femoral and tibial tunnels are different sizes, the lead end of the graft should have the smallest bone plug. Using this technique, the bone plug ends usually sit flush with the tibial and femoral cortex.

26. Arthroscopically visualize the graft to ensure that it does not impinge against either the lateral or superior notch as the knee is run through a range of motion.

Graft fixation

➤ Fix the bone plugs either with interference screws or over a "post" depending on surgeon's preference. A half-turn twist in the graft is felt to strengthen it prior to fixation.

➤ Use a guide wire to assist placement of an interference screw. Slide the guide wire into the tunnel along the side of the bone plug. The wire should slide easily, so it can be removed once the interference screw engages in the hole.

27. Fix the femoral side first. Insert an interference screw proximal and anterior to the bone plug (**Fig. 25–6**).

28. Fix the tibial side.

    a. If using an interference screw, insert it anterior and medial to the bone plug (**Fig. 25–6**).

    b. If using a "post," insert a low-profile screw from anterior to posterior 1 cm distal to the tibial hole. Tie the graft sutures around the screw. Fully seat the screw.

29. Maintain tension on the graft with the knee at 30 degrees of flexion or near full extension while fixing the tibial bone plug.

30. After graft fixation, perform a Lachman test to assess knee stability. Range the knee to assess for graft impingement. If impingement is present, expand the notchplasty.

Closure

31. Pack extra bone removed from the graft bone plugs into the patellar and tibial defects as a bone graft.

32. Close the patellar tendon defect loosely with absorbable sutures.

33. Close the paratenon over the patellar tendon as a separate layer.

34. Close the subcutaneous tissue with absorbable suture. Close the skin and portals per surgeon's preference.

35. A drain may be used in the lateral wound but must be removed prior to the patient's departure from the hospital.

36. Inject intra-articular marcaine into the wounds and the knee joint after closure to diminish postoperative pain.

37. Place a surgical dressing on the wound. Apply a hinge brace or knee immobilizer in the operating room.

Suggested Reading

Nogalski MP, Bach BR Jr. Acute anterior cruciate ligament injuries. In: Fu FH, Harner CD, Vince KG, eds. *Knee Surgery*. Baltimore, MD: Williams & Willkins, 1994, pp. 679–730.

CHAPTER 26

Anterior Cruciate Ligament Surgery

Endoscopic

Steven H. Stern

Indications

1. Active individual with an acute tear of the anterior cruciate ligament
2. Individual with a chronic tear of the anterior cruciate ligament with recurrent instability, who has failed nonoperative treatment
3. A sedentary individual, who displays instability related to his anterior cruciate ligament deficient knee with daily activities

Contraindications

1. Active knee infection
2. Lack of neurovascular control
3. A sedentary individual without demonstrable instability
4. Older age (relative)
5. Pediatric patient with open growth plate
6. Patella alta with extremely long patella tendon (relative); consider two-incision technique

Preoperative Preparation

1. Knee radiographs: anteroposterior (AP), lateral, and skyline
2. Magnetic Resonance Imaging (MRI): not a necessity, but helps to assess other injuries.

3. Wait for knee swelling and active range of motion to normalize prior to surgery (may necessitate preoperative physical therapy).

Special Instruments, Position, and Anesthesia

1. Position the patient supine on the operating room table. The patient's position should allow for knee hyperflexion during the procedure.
2. The contralateral extremity should be padded to avoid pressure on susceptible areas.
3. Leg holder or post
4. General, epidural, or spinal anesthetic
5. Routine arthroscopic setup and routine orthopaedic surgical instruments
6. Tibial and femoral alignment guides for positioning the tunnel guide pins
7. Interference screws for graft fixation; these can be metal or bioabsorbable. A screw and washer may be used as a "post."

Tips and Pearls

1. The anterior knee incision should extend from the lower pole of the patella to a point slightly medial to tibial tubercle.
2. Examine the knee under anesthesia. Assess the stability and document.

3. Document all other intra-articular pathology. Consider meniscal repair when appropriate to aid knee stability.
4. Attempt to make the portals as close to the mid-line as possible without violating the patella tendon. This position optimizes visualization into intercondylar notch.
5. The tibial hole should enter the joint at the posterior insertion of the anterior cruciate ligament's remnant. This is just anterior to the posterior cruciate ligament.
6. The femoral hole needs to be positioned posteriorly, but care should be taken to minimize the chance of "blowout" of the posterior femoral wall.
7. Make an adequate notchplasty to optimize visualization of the drill holes.
8. Rasp the ends of the tunnels to avoid sharp edges.
9. Use a "carrot" to plug the tibial tunnel and avoid fluid extravasation after the tunnel is created.
10. Use a rongeur to contour the end of the bone plug into a bullet; the tip aids graft passage.
11. Minimize tourniquet use if possible.
12. In most cases, aim to harvest 25-mm-long bone plugs from the patella and the tibia.
13. Insert the femoral interference screw with the knee hyperflexed to help optimize its position.
14. Insert the interference screws with the use of a guide pin.
15. If a meniscal repair is indicated, this should be performed prior to the anterior cruciate ligament reconstruction.

What To Avoid

1. Minimize the chance of patella fracture by avoiding excessively long or deep bone cuts.
2. Avoid positioning the patient on the proximal part of the table. The patient must be positioned as distal as possible on the surgical table. This allows for knee hyperflexion, which is essential in optimizing position of the femoral interference screw. Do not overlook this small technical point.
3. Take care to minimize the chance of dropping the graft on the floor.

Postoperative Care Issues

1. Place the leg in a compressive dressing with an elastic wrap after surgery. Consider cryotherapy.
2. If a continuous passive motion machine (CPM) is used, it can begin at 0 to 40 degrees on day one with daily incremental increases of 5 to 10 degrees.
3. A knee immobilizer can be used for the first few weeks after surgery (commonly the first two) and then discontinued when the patient regains adequate quadriceps control. Alternatively, a hinged brace can be used when ambulating during the first four weeks after surgery. Lock the brace in extension for two weeks, then unlock and allow free range of motion for two weeks.
4. An accelerated rehabilitation protocol begins immediately after surgery. Normally active and active-assisted flexion exercises and passive extension exercises are instituted.
5. Patients commonly either go home the day of surgery or spend one night in the hospital.
6. Protected weight bearing as tolerated with the immobilizer or hinged-brace is allowed after surgery. Most patients can wean themselves off crutches during the first two weeks status post surgery.

Operative Technique

1. Position the patient supine and as distally as possible on the operating room table to allow for knee hyperflexion later in the procedure. Apply a thigh tourniquet as proximal as possible on the leg. Pad pressure points and the contralateral Achilles tendon.
2. Examine the knee and leg after adequate anesthesia is obtained. This examination under anesthesia (EUA) should assess medial, lateral, anterior, and posterior knee stability. Document the examination.
3. Prepare and drape the surgical leg in the hospital's routine manner. Exanguinate if inflating the tourniquet at this point. Alternatively, exsanguination and tourniquet inflation can be done later in the procedure at the time of graft harvesting. Try to minimize tourniquet time because increased tourniquet use can increase postoperative leg atrophy.

Arthroscopic evaluation and notchplasty

4. Make routine arthroscopic portals. The inflow portal is made medial and superior to the patella into a supra-patellar pouch. The medial and lateral joint line portals are made just to the side of the patellar tendon, and are used for instruments and the 30-degree arthroscope (see Chapter 24) **(Fig. 26–1)**.

5. Perform a standard arthroscopic knee evaluation in a systematic manner. Examine the supra-patellar pouch, patella femoral joint, lateral gutter, medial gutter, medial compartment, intercondylar notch, and lateral compartment. This systematic approach allows an adequate assessment of the menisci, ligaments, and tendons about the knee.

   a. Confirm the anterior cruciate ligament tear.
   b. Repair or resect the menisci as appropriate. Remove any loose bodies.
   c. Evaluate any chondral injuries. Debride and treat them if appropriate.

6. If a torn anterior cruciate ligament is confirmed, debride the ligament's stump. If the notch is narrow, perform a wide notchplasty. Remove part of the lateral femoral wall along with "residents ridge," as well as the superior notch to avoid graft impingement **(Fig. 26–2)**.

Graft harvest and preparation

➤ In certain cases when the surgeon is convinced that there is a complete anterior cruciate ligament tear, the graft can be harvested prior to performing the initial arthroscopic evaluation.

7. Remove the arthroscopic instruments from the knee. Position the operating room table so the knee is slightly flexed. Exsanguinate the limb and inflate the tourniquet.

8. Make a skin incision from the lower pole of the patella to a point just medial to the tibial tubercle. Use a sharp and blunt dissection to carefully define the borders of the patella tendon. Take care to ensure that the incision is long enough to achieve adequate visualization in both the patella and tibial tubercle region.

9. Incise the subcutaneous tissue and peritenon layer directly over the patella tendon.

10. Measure the patellar tendon's width and mark the desired area for graft harvesting. Aim to harvest a graft approximately one-third the width of the patellar tendon (commonly 10 or 11 mm).

11. Use a knife to longitudinally cut the patella tendon in the desired area for graft harvest. Keep the tendon under tension by maintaining knee flexion. Use a knife or electrocautery to mark the desired areas on the patella and tibial tubercle for the bone plugs. Aim for bone plugs approximately 2.5 cm long and 1 cm wide from both patella and tibia.

12. Use an oscillating saw to make the bone cuts from the patella and tibia. Take care to angle the cuts approximately 45 degrees and limit the resection depth to 10 mm. Avoid over-cutting of the bone, especially in the patella region. Remove the bone plugs from their donor sites with the help of a curved osteotome. Avoid levering the osteotome against the underlying bone **(Figs. 26–3A and 3B)**.

13. After graft harvest, use sizing rings and a ruler to determine the actual size and length of the bone plugs, and to determine the exact size of the femoral and tibial tunnels to be created.

14. Commonly, plan to position the graft in the knee so that the bone plug resected from the tibia will be placed in the femoral tunnel. This is because the patellar tendon's insertion on the tibial tubercle allows for more clearance when inserting the femoral interference screw and thus helps minimize the chance of cutting the graft. Thus, the tibial bone plug (which will be placed within the femur) must be the same or a smaller size than the patella bone plug (which will be placed within the tibia).

15. Trim the bone plugs and contour the ends into a blunt tip with a rongeur to aid in passage through the tunnels.

16. Make the drill holes in the bone plugs. There is significant variation among surgeons in the number of drill holes they make, as well as the type of suture used for graft passage. The author places two 1.6-mm holes in each bone plug. Through the tibial bone plug (which will be placed within the femur), one #2 nonabsorbable suture is placed within each hole. For the patella bone plug (which will be placed within the tibia), two #2 nonabsorbable sutures are placed within each hole (total of four strands).

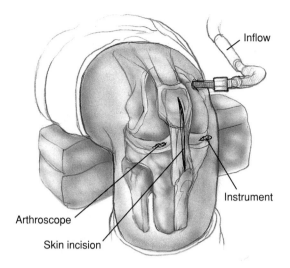

Figure 26–1 Arthroscopy. The surgery commences with a standard arthroscopy. Note the inflow is positioned superior and medial to the patella. The standard arthroscopy portals are shown. The arthroscope is placed in the inferior-lateral portal while the inferior-medial portal is used for instruments. Note the position for the skin incision for graft harvesting (occurs later in the procedure).

Figure 26–2 Notchplasty. A motorized burr is used to perform a wide notchplasty by removing bone from the medial wall of the lateral condyle. The notchplasty should include removing bone from "residents ridge," as well as from the superior notch to avoid graft impingement

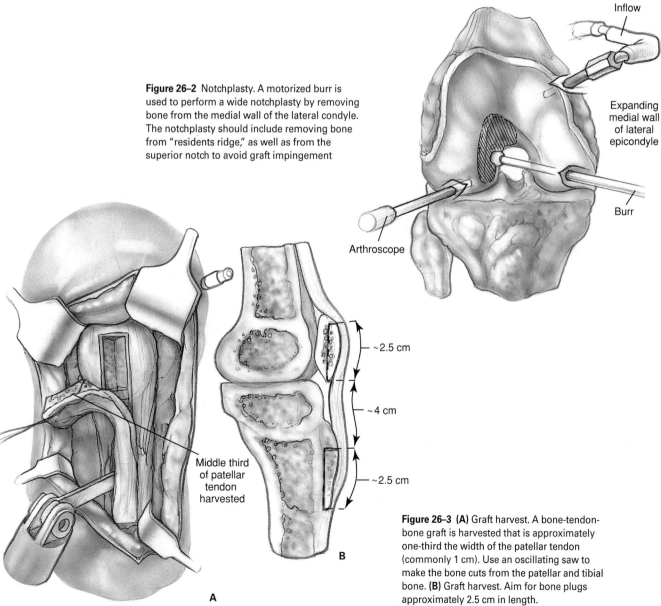

Figure 26–3 (A) Graft harvest. A bone-tendon-bone graft is harvested that is approximately one-third the width of the patellar tendon (commonly 1 cm). Use an oscillating saw to make the bone cuts from the patellar and tibial bone. **(B)** Graft harvest. Aim for bone plugs approximately 2.5 cm in length.

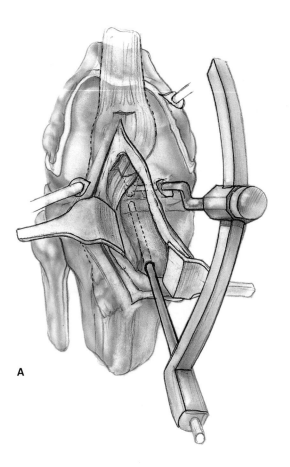

A

Figure 26–4 (A) Tibial guide. The knee should be flexed to approximately 80 degrees. The tibial guide is inserted through the medial portal. The breakaway guide pin is inserted through the anterior surface of the tibial metaphysis and through the tibial bone under arthroscopic visualization. The starting point should be just medial to the tibial tubercle and at least 2 cm distal to the joint line. **(B)** Tibial guide. Note the tibial pin entrance and exit sites. Take care to ensure that the guide is posterior enough within the tibia, since the tendency is to place the guide pin and hence the tibial tunnel too anterior. The tibial guide is normally set at approximately 55 to 60 degrees. Take care to position the starting point as distal as possible on the anterior tibia in order to maximize the length of the tibial tunnel. **(C)** Tibial guide. The tibial guide is inserted so that the intra-articular guide pin enters the joint through the posterior half of the ACL's tibial footprint.

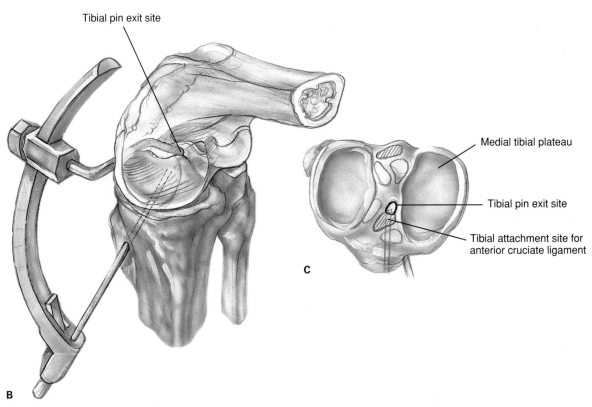

Tibial pin exit site

Medial tibial plateau

Tibial pin exit site

Tibial attachment site for anterior cruciate ligament

B

C

Tunnel preparation

17. Denude the periosteum over the metaphyseal bone just medial to the tibial tubercle and 2 cm distal to the joint line for the entrance point to the tibial hole. This area should be approximately 1.5 cm in diameter.

18. Replace the arthroscopic instruments in the knee. Place the tibial alignment guide through the medial portal and into the intercondylar notch. Flex the knee to approximately 80 degrees. Position the tibial alignment guide so that the intra-articular guide pin enters the joint through the posterior half of the ACL's tibial footprint. This is a point just anterior to the posterior cruciate ligament. Take care to ensure that the guide is posterior enough within the tibia, since the tendency is to place the guide pin and hence the tibial tunnel too anterior **(Figs. 26–4A, 4B, and 4C)**.

19. Drill the break-away guide pin through the anterior surface of the tibial metaphysis and through the tibial bone under arthroscopic visualization. The tibial guide is normally set at approximately 55 to 60 degrees. Take care to position the starting point as distal as possible on the anterior tibia in order to maximize the length of the tibial tunnel. The starting point is just medial to the tibia tubercle and at least 2 cm distal to the joint line. This corresponds to the area previously denuded of periosteum.

20. Insert the guide pin through the tibia and a few millimeters into the knee joint to ascertain its position. Run the knee through a range of motion. Arthroscopically visualize the guide pin with the knee extended. Ensure that it clears the superior notch and that the graft will not impinge. If the position of the guide pin is felt to be unsatisfactory, the pin is removed and reinserted.

21. Over-ream the guide pin with the appropriate size disposable reamers. The reamer normally corresponds to the larger sized bone plug (commonly 10 or 11 mm in diameter). Rasp the edge of the hole to smooth the border. Use an arthroscopic shaver to help clear any soft tissue from the intra-articular tunnel hole. Use a "carrot" to plug the tibial tunnel and prevent fluid extravasation.

22. Flex the knee to approximately 90 degrees. Carefully position the appropriate femoral offset aiming device within the knee. Take care to optimize visualization and fluid inflow at this point in the procedure.

> In general, a 6- or 7-mm femoral offset should be used for a 10-mm femoral tunnel. This helps to ensure a 1 to 2 mm "backwall." If an 11-mm femoral tunnel is desired, consider using a 7-mm femoral offset to help ensure a 1.5-mm "backwall." Similarly for a 9-mm femoral tunnel, consider using a 5- or 6-mm femoral offset to help ensure a 0.5- to 1.5-mm "backwall."

23. While maintaining the knee in the flexed position and aligning the femoral offset guide against the posterior aspect of the intercondylar notch, drill the large beath ("harpoon") guide pin through the femur. The guide pin should exit the anterior lateral femoral cortex and pierce the skin on the anterior lateral thigh. Place a chuck over the tip of the guide pin to minimize injury to the surgical team **(Fig. 26–5)**.

24. Continue to maintain the knee in the same flexed position. Insert the reamer over the guide pin into the knee's intercondylar notch. While maintaining optimal visualization, drill the femoral tunnel. Drill the tunnel to a depth approximately 1 cm greater than the length of the bone plug that will be introduced. Remove the reamer by hand.

25. Use the arthroscopic shaver to debride the intercondylar notch of any small bone fragments or debris that was produced during the reaming. In addition, use the shaver to remove some of the bone along the anterior aspect of the femoral hole. This improves visualization and helps form a starting point for the interference screw to be placed later in the case.

Graft passage

26. Place the tendon graft sutures through the eye of the large beath ("harpoon") guide pin. Pull the guide pin through the knee so the sutures exit the anterior lateral thigh.

27. Pull the leading edge of the graft through the tibial tunnel into the intercondylar notch and then into the femoral tunnel. Visualize the graft as it enters the femoral tunnel to ensure proper rotation (the tendon should be posterior and the cancellous

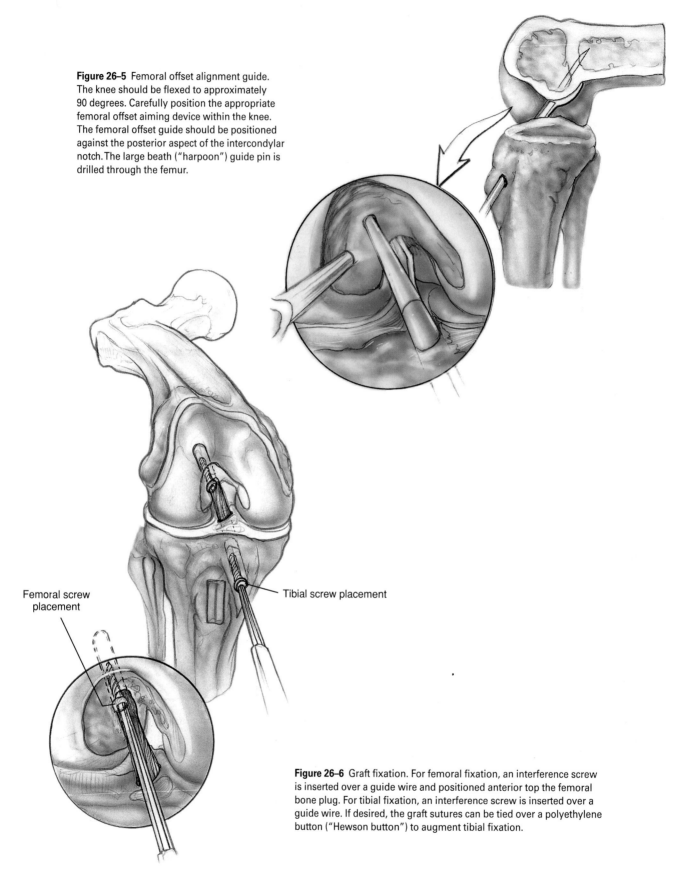

Figure 26–5 Femoral offset alignment guide. The knee should be flexed to approximately 90 degrees. Carefully position the appropriate femoral offset aiming device within the knee. The femoral offset guide should be positioned against the posterior aspect of the intercondylar notch. The large beath ("harpoon") guide pin is drilled through the femur.

Femoral screw placement

Tibial screw placement

Figure 26–6 Graft fixation. For femoral fixation, an interference screw is inserted over a guide wire and positioned anterior top the femoral bone plug. For tibial fixation, an interference screw is inserted over a guide wire. If desired, the graft sutures can be tied over a polyethylene button ("Hewson button") to augment tibial fixation.

portion of the bone plug pointed anterior). If needed, introduce a probe through the medial portal to help align the graft in the proper rotation.

28. Check the position of the graft within the tibial tunnel. If the tibial bone plug is prominent, the graft can be recessed several millimeters into the femoral tunnel.

Graft fixation

29. Fix the femoral side first. Hyperflex the knee. Make a small vertical incision in the medial retinaculum. This should be just medial to the patella tendon and just superior to the top of the tibia.

30. Introduce a guide wire through this rent and position it in the intercondylar notch. It is imperative that visualization is satisfactory at this point in the procedure. In some cases, visualization is improved by turning off the inflow and "going dry."

31. Place the guide wire into the femoral tunnel just anterior to the graft. Insert a 7-mm interference screw over the guide wire. Maintain arthroscopic visualization as the screw is put in place. Recess the screw within the tunnel. Remove the guide wire prior to fully seating the screw (**Fig. 26–6**).

32. Straighten the operative table so the patient lays flat. Insert a guide wire alongside the bone plug within the tibial tunnel. Attempt to place the wire along the side of the bone plug where the sutures do not exit to minimize the risk of cutting the sutures. Use the graft sutures to tension the graft with the knee at 30 degrees of flexion or near full extension, while fixing the tibial bone plug. Remove the guide wire prior to the screw fully seating (**Fig. 26–6**). If desired, the graft sutures can be tied over a polyethylene button ("Hewson button") to augment tibial fixation.

33. After graft fixation, perform a Lachman test to assess knee stability. Range the knee to assess for graft impingement. If impingement is present, expand the notchplasty.

Closure

34. Pack extra bone removed from the graft bone plugs into the patellar and tibial defects as a bone graft.

35. Close the tendon and paratenon with interrupted #1 absorbable sutures. Both can be closed in one layer. Alternatively, the paratenon can be closed as a separate layer with 2-0 absorbable sutures.

36. Close the subcutaneous tissue with absorbable suture. Close the skin and portals per surgeon's preference.

37. Inject intra-articular marcaine into the wounds and the knee joint after closure to diminish postoperative pain.

38. Place a surgical dressing on the wound. Apply a hinge brace or knee immobilizer in the operating room.

Suggested Readings

Bach BR Jr. Endoscopic anterior cruciate ligament reconstruction using autograft patellar tendon substitution. In: Craig EV, ed. *Clinical Orthopaedics.* Baltimore, MD: Lippincott Williams & Willkins, 1999, pp. 750–763.

Kurzweil PR, Jackson DW. Chronic anterior cruciate ligament injuries. In: Fu FH, Harner CD, Vince KG, eds. *Knee Surgery.* Baltimore, MD: Williams & Willkins, 1994, pp. 731–747.

Nogalski MP, Bach BR Jr. Acute anterior cruciate ligament injuries. In: Fu FH, Harner CD, Vince KG, eds. *Knee Surgery.* Baltimore, MD: Williams & Willkins, 1994, pp. 679–730.

CHAPTER 27

Total Knee Arthroplasty

Steven H. Stern

Indications

1. Osteoarthritis knee
2. Rheumatoid arthritis knee
3. Post-traumatic arthritis knee

Contraindications

1. Active knee infection (absolute)
2. Neuropathic joint (relative)
3. Unsatisfactory soft tissue envelope
4. Marked ligamentous insufficiency (requires constrained knee prosthesis)
5. Dysfunctional extensor mechanism

Preoperative Preparation

1. Knee radiographs, including standing anteroposterior (AP), lateral, and skyline views
2. Appropriate medical and anesthetic evaluation
3. Document status of preoperative neurovascular examination
4. Assessment of preoperative mechanical axis (**Fig. 27–1**).

Special Instruments, Position, and Anesthesia

1. The patient is placed supine on the operating room table.
2. All pressure points should be padded.
3. The procedure can be done with general, epidural, or long-acting spinal anesthesia.
4. Routine orthopaedic surgical instrumentation should be available. In addition, the specific instruments and cutting guides unique to the prosthesis to be implanted should be available.

Tips and Pearls

1. If at all possible, prior vertical incision should be incorporated into the current skin incision. Transverse incisions may be crossed at a perpendicular angle.
2. The preoperative arc of motion should be assessed prior to the procedure with special attention to any flexion deformity (inability to fully extend the knee both actively and passively). Extra bone may need to be resected from the distal femur in the event of a fixed flexion deformity.
3. The tourniquet should be placed as proximal as possible on the thigh in order to minimize any infringement on the surgical field. In a patient with significant peripheral vascular disease, or status post bypass surgery, consideration may be given to performing the surgery without tourniquet control.
4. Intravenous antibiotics appropriate for the hospital's bacterial flora should be administered prior to tourniquet inflation.
5. A "quadriceps snip" ("rectus snip") can be used in knees where exposure is difficult and eversion of

the patellar hard to achieve. This is accomplished by making an oblique incision, starting from the most proximal portion of the medial arthrotomy and angled superior and lateral through the quadriceps tendon (**Fig. 27–3**). At the end of the surgery, this incision is closed in a standard fashion; and in most cases, normal postoperative rehabilitation can be instituted.

What To Avoid

1. Because of the problems associated with infection, great care is taken to minimize this complication. Operating room traffic should be minimized, and preoperative antibiotics administered.
2. Ligamentous stability of the knee should be assessed prior to the procedure in order to ascertain the most appropriate prosthesis for implantation.
3. Avoid internal rotation of either the femoral or tibial components.

Postoperative Care Issues

1. A suction-type drain can be used and normally, safely discontinued the morning after surgery.
2. Constant passive motion (CPM) machines can be employed in the postoperative period. These can be started in extension and with gradually increasing flexion, or used with an early motion protocol starting at 50 to 100 degrees the day of surgery, and progressing toward extension.
3. A compressive dressing should be placed at the end of surgery and is normally changed approximately 48 h after the procedure.
4. Assessment of the patient's distal neurovascular examination should be made the evening of surgery. If there is evidence of a peroneal nerve palsy, the dressing should be loosened and the knee placed in a flexed position. Knees with a preoperative valgus alignment or significant preoperative flexion deformities are at particular risk for developing a peroneal nerve palsy (though this complication can occur idiopathically in any knee undergoing an arthroplasty procedure).

Operative Technique

Approach

1. Position the patient supine on the operating room table. Place a thigh tourniquet as proximal as possible on the thigh.
2. Prepare and drape the limb in the hospital's standard sterile fashion. Exsanguinate the limb and inflate the tourniquet.
3. Make an anterior skin incision utilizing either a straight mid-line or a medial parapatellar incision. Dissect directly down to the extensor mechanism while minimizing skin flaps. Adequate exposure of the extensor mechanism with visualization of both the proximal quadriceps tendon and distal patellar tendon should be achieved prior to performing the retinacular arthrotomy (**Fig. 27–2**).
4. Make a medial arthrotomy utilizing either a straight mid-line, medial parapatellar, or mid-vastus retinacular incision. The distal exposure is similar in all of these techniques with the distal limb of the retinacular incision carried along the proximal tibia medial to the tibial tubercle. Extend the retinacular incision as far proximally as necessary to achieve adequate exposure (**Fig. 27–3**).
5. Use a periosteal elevator to subperiosteally strip the periosteum off the proximal medial tibia. Take care to keep this layer in continuity.
6. Evert the patella and flex the knee (**Fig. 27–4**). Take care not to avulse the patellar tendon. If it is not possible to evert the patella, perform a "quadriceps snip" ("rectus snip") (**Fig. 27–3**).
7. Dissect the proximal tibial periosteum.

    a. Varus knees. Continue to subperiosteally strip the proximal medial tibial periosteum and the semimembranosus insertion from the proximal medial tibial brim. Carry this dissection around to the posterior medial corner of the tibia.
    b. Valgus knees. Limit the medial dissection. Strip only enough periosteum to achieve adequate exposure.

8. Remove marginal osteophytes. Resect the anterior cruciate ligament (ACL) or any ACL remnant.

Procedure

The exact technique for performing the bone cuts in total knee arthroplasty are dependent on the specific instruments which are unique to each individual prosthetic knee system. Therefore, the following steps should be used as a general operative guide for total knee arthroplasty; however the exact procedure for implanting specific knee components should be checked with the manufacturer's suggested technique manual. In general, either the femoral or tibial bone cuts can be made first.

9. Proximal tibial cut. Use either an intramedullary or extramedullary alignment guide. In general, the proximal tibia is cut perpendicular to the long axis of the tibia in the frontal plane. Depending on the implant system, the cut should have either a neutral or a posterior slope from front to back. Avoid anterior tilt of the proximal tibia cut (**Fig. 27–5**). Most instrument systems utilize a stylus to help assess the appropriate depth for the tibial resection.

    a. Cruciate retaining (CR) designs. Take care to preserve the PCL. Use retractors, osteotomes, or a posterior bone bridge to preserve the PCL's insertion on the tibia.

    b. Posterior substituting (PS) designs. The tibial cut can be made directly across the proximal tibia without concern for the PCL.

10. Femoral cuts

    a. Use an intramedullary guide for the distal femoral cut. In general, the femur is cut in about 5 to 7 degrees of anatomic valgus. (In knees with a significant preoperative valgus deformity, some surgeons aim for less of a valgus cut.)

    b. Use a drill to make a starting hole in the intercondylar notch for the intramedullary guide. Position the drill so the hole is placed at the intercondylar notch just above the PCL's femoral origin (**Fig. 27–6**).

    c. Widen the starting hole either with a stepdrill or by rotating the regular drill. This helps decompress the intramedullary canal and minimizes fat embolization.

    d. Size the femur. Most surgeons opt to downsize the prosthesis if the femur is between sizes.

    e. Make the anterior and posterior femoral condylar cuts using either anterior or posterior referencing (or a combination of both). Use retractors to protect the medial collateral ligament. Aim for neutral or slight external rotation (~3 degrees) of the femoral component. Avoid internal rotation (**Fig. 27–7**).

11. Excise remnants of the medial and lateral meniscus. Take care on the medial side when dissecting the medial meniscus, since the deep fibers of the MCL are adherent to the periphery of the medial meniscus. Laminar spreaders may be helpful to enhance posterior visualization.

    a. Posterior substituting (PS). Excise the PCL with the knee in flexion. Release the PCL from its insertion on the medial femoral condyle using either a sharp blade or the electrocautery (**Figs. 27–8A and 8B**).

12. Assess both the flexion gap (posterior condyles to proximal tibial) and extension gap (distal femoral to proximal tibial) to ensure optimal knee balance. If needed, release tight ligamentous structures in a sequential fashion to achieve appropriate balance.

    a. Varus knees. Strip the proximal tibial periosteum along the tibial brim around to the posterior medial corner. If needed in knees with a severe preoperative varus deformity, tap an osteotome along the medial tibia with the knee extended to further release fibers of the MCL.

    b. Valgus knees. Release the lateral structures and minimize medial dissection. The structures can be released in various sequences as needed. In general, release the lateral collateral ligament, iliotibial band, popliteus tendon, and lateral capsular structures either sequentially or in a pie-crusting technique.

    c. Tight posterior structures. Resect posterior osteophytes. In CR knees consider conversion to PS design. If needed, release posterior capsule and/or gastrocnemius origin from posterior femur.

13. Resect additional bone if either or both gaps are too tight.

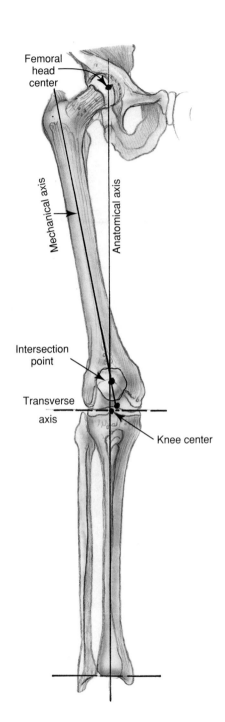

Figure 27-1 Anatomic and mechanical axis. A long radiograph can be utilized to assess the mechanical and anatomic axis of the lower extremity.

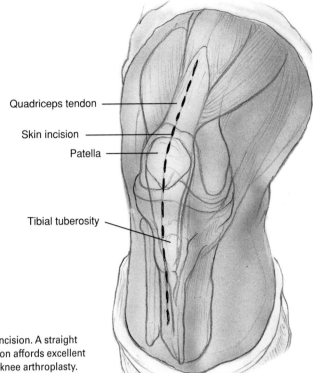

Figure 27-2 Skin incision. A straight anterior skin incision affords excellent exposure for total knee arthroplasty.

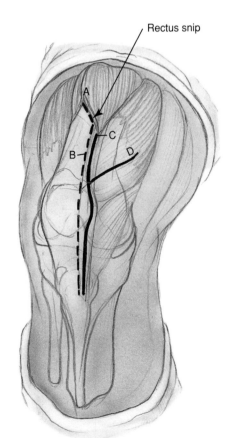

Figure 27-3 Retinacular incisions. Note the varied methods of performing the medial arthrotomy include a straight mid-line (B), medial parapatellar (C), or mid-vastus (D) retinacular incision. The distal exposure is similar in all of these techniques with the distal limb of the retinacular incision carried along the proximal tibia medial to the tibial tubercle. Note the location of the "quadriceps snip" (A), which can be performed to aid exposure in difficult cases.

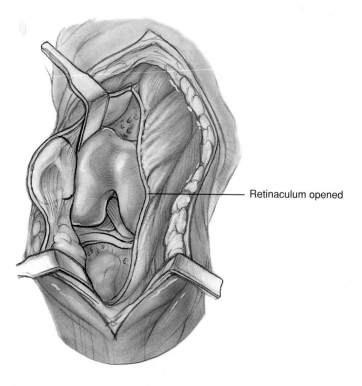

Figure 27–4 Medial arthrotomy. The patella is everted and the knee flexed. This exposes the joint and completes the arthrotomy.

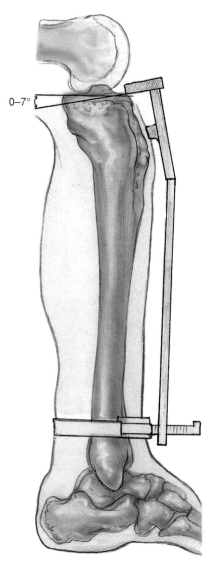

Figure 27–5 Extramedullary tibial alignment guide. In general, the proximal tibia is cut perpendicular to the long axis of the tibia in the frontal plane. Depending on the implant system, the cut should have either a neutral or a slight posterior slope from front to back. Avoid anterior tilt of the proximal tibia cut.

0–7°

Retinaculum opened

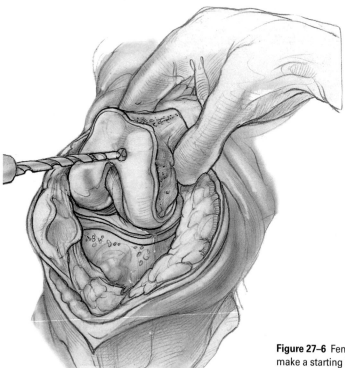

Figure 27–6 Femoral intramedullary starting hole. A drill is used to make a starting hole in the intercondylar notch for the intramedullary guide. The drill is positioned so the hole is placed at the intercondylar notch just above the PCL's femoral origin.

a. Tight extension gap: resect additional bone from the distal femur.

b. Tight flexion gap: angle the proximal tibial cut posteriorly (CR knees) or downsize the femoral component.

c. Tight flexion and extension gaps: resect additional bone from the proximal tibia.

d. Loose flexion and extension gaps: utilize thicker polyethylene.

14. Make the anterior and posterior chamfer cuts and the intercondylar notch cut (PS knees) utilizing the appropriate instrumentation and alignment devices (Fig. 27–9).

15. Prepare the proximal tibia for the tibial base plate utilizing the appropriate instruments. Avoid internal rotation of tibial component.

16. If the patellar is being resurfaced, prepare the patella either with an oscillating saw or with a patellar reamer. Size the patellar component. Drill the fixation holes through a drill guide.

17. Perform a trial reduction with provisional components.

a. Test various size tibial inserts to optimize balance of the flexion and extension gaps.

b. Cruciate retaining (CR). In CR knees special care must be taken to assess the PCL at this stage of the procedure. If the PCL is too tight (commonly manifested by excessive femoral rollback or a tight flexion gap), further balancing is required. The PCL can be "recessed" by sequentially cutting some of the PCL's fibers. Alternately, the proximal tibial cut can be angled posteriorly.

   If the PCL is too loose, consideration should be given to using more constrained components or switching to a PS design.

c. Assess patellar tracking. The patella should easily track within the femoral component's trochlea groove without requiring significant pressure to hold it in place. If the patellar tends to sublux laterally, perform a lateral retinacular release.

i. Perform a lateral retinacular release utilizing an inside-out technique.

ii. Take care to isolate and preserve the superior geniculate vessels.

iii. Dissect through the lateral retinaculum inferior and superior to the preserved vessels. Extend the proximal portion of the retinacular release into the vastus lateralis tendon.

18. Remove the trial components.

19. Depending on surgeon preference and extent of dissection, the tourniquet can be deflated and hemostasis achieved. Reinflate tourniquet.

20. Cleanse the bony surfaces with a pulsatile lavage.

21. Mix the bone cement.

22. Cement the components. In general, the femur is cemented first in posterior cruciate substituting knees. The patellar component can be cemented at any time. Pressurize the cement either with a cement pressurization system or with the implants during implantation. Remove excess cement prior to cement polymerization.

Closure

23. Close the wound.

24. Irrigate the wound with copious antibiotic irrigation.

25. Maintain appropriate hemostasis.

26. If a suction drain is utilized, place it through a separate stab incision beneath the lateral retinaculum. Take care throughout the closure to minimize the risk of inadvertently sewing in the drain.

27. Close the arthrotomy in a meticulous fashion with multiple absorbable sutures (normally zero or #1).

28. Close the subcutaneous tissue in a layered fashion with interrupted absorbable sutures (normally #1, zero and 2-0 sutures).

29. Close the skin with staples, nylon, or prolene.

30. Dress the knee in a sterile fashion with a bulky dressing.

31. Transfer patient to recovery room.

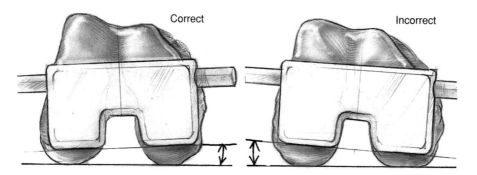

Correct   Incorrect

Figure 27–7 Femoral instrument rotation. Aim to achieve neutral or slight external rotation (~3 degrees) of the femoral component. Avoid internal rotation. This needs to be taken into account when positioning the instrument that sets femoral component rotation rotation.

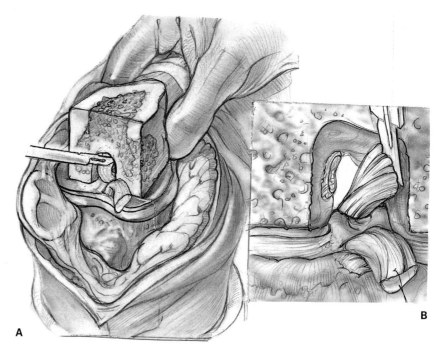

A   B

Figure 27–8 (A) Posterior cruciate excision. In posterior substituting (PS) knees, the PCL is excised from its insertion on the medial femoral condyle with the knee in flexion. This can be done using either a sharp blade or the electrocautery. **(B)** Posterior cruciate excision-close-up. Note the PCL is excised directly off the medial femoral condyle with the knee in flexion.

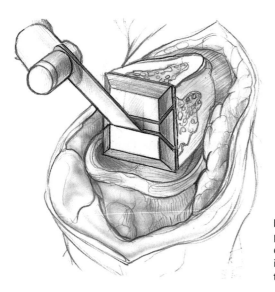

Figure 27–9 Chamfer cuts. The anterior and posterior chamfer cuts are made with an oscillating saw. Commonly, in PS designs this instrument also serves as a guide for making the intercondylar notch cut.

Suggested Readings

Garvin KL, Scuderi G, Insall JN. Evolution of the quadriceps snip. *Clin Orthop* 1995;321:131–137.

Scuderi GR, Insall JN. Fixed varus and valgus deformities. In: Lotke PA, ed. *Master Techniques in Orthopedic Surgery: Knee Arthroplasty*. New York, NY: Raven Press, 1995, pp. 111–127.

Stern SH. Surgical exposure in total knee arthroplasty. In: Fu FH, Harner CD, Vince KG, eds. *Knee Surgery*. Baltimore, MD: Williams & Willkins, 1994, pp. 1289–1302.

Stern SH. Total knee replacement. In: Craig EV, ed. *Clinical Orthopaedics*. Baltimore, MD: Lippincott Williams & Willkins, 1999, pp. 642–649.

Vince KG. Revision knee arthroplasty technique. *Instructional Course Lectures* 1993;42:325–339.

Yashar AA, Venn-Watson E, Welsh T, Colwell CW Jr., Lotke P. Continuous passive motion with accelerated flexion after total knee arthroplasty. *Clin Orthop* 1997; 345:38–43.

Younger AS, Duncan CP, Masri BA. Surgical exposures in revision total knee arthroplasty. *J Am Acad Orthop Surg* 1998;6(1):55–64.

CHAPTER 28

High Tibial Osteotomy

Stephen G. Manifold and Giles R. Scuderi

Indications

1. Unicompartmental medial knee osteoarthritis
2. Age less than 50 years old
3. High activity level (e.g., heavy laborers)
4. Varus deformity 10 degrees or less
5. Flexion arc greater than 90 degrees

Contraindications

1. Rheumatoid arthritis or inflammatory arthritides
2. Flexion contracture greater than 10 degrees
3. Tibiofemoral subluxation (lateral) greater than 1 cm
4. Lateral thrust of knee during gait (high adductor moment)

Preoperative Preparation

1. Knee radiographs, including anteroposterior (AP), lateral, sunrise and standing three-joint films
2. Determine the femoral-tibial angle and the mechanical axis (**Fig. 28–1**).
3. Calculate the size of bone wedge to be removed from the proximal tibia.
4. Consider preoperative physical therapy to increase quadriceps strength and decrease flexion contracture.
5. Patient education to establish reasonable expectations

Special Instruments, Position, and Anesthesia

1. Supine position on a radiolucent operating table with a small padded bolster under the ipsilateral buttock.
2. The surgery can be performed with general, epidural, or long-acting spinal anesthesia.
3. Use basic orthopaedic instrumentation.
4. Use 1/8-in Steinmann pins, sharp straight osteotomes, and a sagittal saw.
5. Consider variable angle proximal tibia cutting guides to make accurate osteotomy cuts.
6. An L buttress plate should be available for fixation of the osteotomy site.
7. Use a fluoroscopic image intensifier for intraoperative imaging.

Tips and Pearls

1. For patients without contraindications (i.e., significant peripheral vascular disease), a tourniquet should be placed as proximal as possible on the thigh to avoid minimizing the surgical exposure.
2. Intravenous antibiotics should be administered prior to inflation of the tourniquet.
3. A vertical skin incision is preferred in order to improve exposure for internal fixation and to facilitate possible total knee arthroplasty in the future.

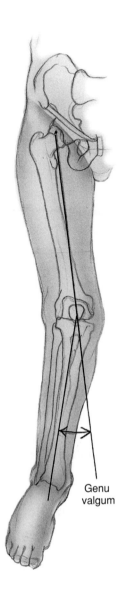

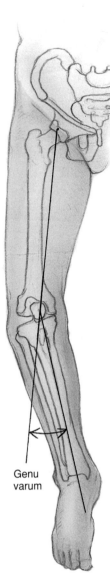

Genu
valgum

Genu
varum

Figure 28–1 Genu valgum. The mechanical axis is defined as the intersection of a line drawn from the femoral head to the center of the knee and a second line drawn from the center of the knee to the center of the ankle. Genu valgum results in a "knock-knee" extremity alignment. Genu varum results in a "bow-legged" extremity alignment.

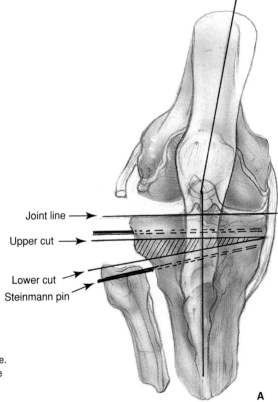

Joint line →

Upper cut →

Lower cut →
Steinmann pin →

A

Figure 28–2 (A) Osteotomy outline. Note the upper osteotomy cut is parallel to the joint line. The lower cut is just above the insertion of the patellar tendon. Note the division of the tibiofibular syndesmosis.

4. The Steinmann pins should be positioned parallel in the lateral plane to avoid rotational problems after the osteotomy.
5. Maintain at least a 2-cm-thick proximal tibial fragment.
6. Obtain stable internal fixation of the osteotomy to allow early aggressive knee rehabilitation.

What To Avoid

1. Do not extend the osteotomy cuts through the medial cortex of the proximal tibia to prevent translation of the osteotomy fragments.
2. Avoid excessive retraction of the soft tissues over the lateral aspect of the knee, which could lead to postoperative peroneal nerve palsy.
3. Avoid undercorrection of the deformity as this can lead to early symptom recurrence.
4. Avoid excessive force during closure of the osteotomy site. If resistance is encountered, verify that the tibio-fibular syndesmosis has been completely disrupted.

Postoperative Care Issues

1. Remove the suction drain from the knee on the first postoperative day. The surgical dressing should be removed on the second postoperative day. Skin sutures or staples are removed approximately 3 weeks from the date of surgery.
2. Place the knee in a continuous passive motion (CPM) machine in the recovery room with initial settings of 0 to 60 degrees. Advance the machine's flexion 10 degrees or more per day as tolerated; 90 degrees of flexion is the goal by the time of hospital discharge.
3. Begin physical therapy on the first postoperative day. Focus on range of motion and isometric exercises. Place the patient in a hinged knee brace. Toe-touch weight bearing is allowed initially; however, progression to full weight bearing status is not allowed for at least 6 weeks.

Operative Technique

1. Place the patient in the supine position on a radiolucent operating table with a bolster under the ipsilateral hip.
2. Prepare and drape the knee in the standard sterile fashion. Elevate the leg and inflate the tourniquet to 350 mm Hg.
3. Make a vertical mid-line skin incision over the anterior aspect of the knee. Carry it down through the subcutaneous tissue. Elevate skin flaps only enough to provide adequate exposure and take care not to violate the extensor mechanism.
4. Incise the fascia over the lateral portion of the proximal tibia. Elevate the overlying muscle and periosteum laterally from the tibial crest using a periosteal elevator. The knee joint should not be entered during this dissection.
5. Disrupt the tibiofibular joint with the elevator during the lateral dissection of the soft tissues. This allows the fibular head to move freely on the tibia. Closure of the tibial osteotomy site requires fibular osteotomy, fibular head resection or tibiofibular joint dissociation. We prefer the latter technique to minimize the risk of injury to the common peroneal nerve (**Fig. 28–2A**).
6. Use the periosteal elevator to continue dissection around the posterior aspect of the proximal tibia. Take care to keep the elevator on the surface of the bone and avoid injury to the posterior neurovascular structures.
7. Measure and mark the level of the proximal tibia 2 cm distal to the joint line using a methylene blue pen or the electrocautery. Identify the joint line either with a needle or by direct inspection.
8. Drill a 1/8-in Steinmann pin at this level parallel to the joint line from a lateral to medial direction. Check the position of the pin in both the AP and lateral planes using the sterile draped C-arm image intensifier. The pin should be parallel to the joint line in both planes.
9. Place a second Steinmann pin distal to the first pin on the lateral aspect of the proximal tibia at a level that will yield the appropriate thickness of bone wedge as determined preoperatively. Consider using templates and cutting guides that incorporate the

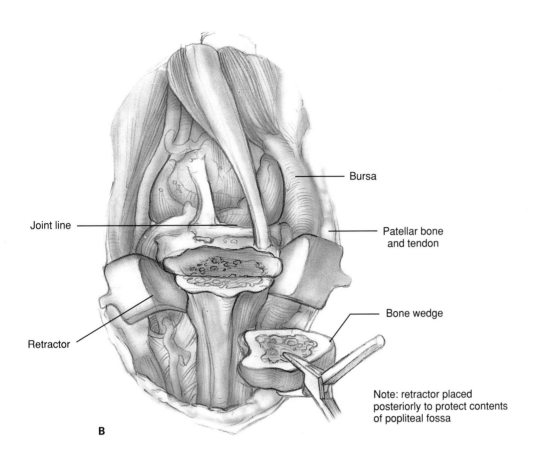

Bursa

Joint line

Patellar bone
and tendon

Bone wedge

Retractor

Note: retractor placed
posteriorly to protect contents
of popliteal fossa

B

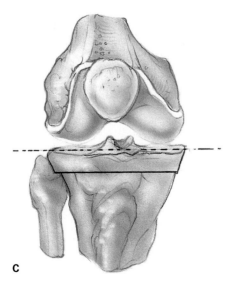

C

Figure 28–2 *(Continued)* **(B)** Lateral osteotomy
view. Note the posterior retractor placement
helps protect the posterior neurovascular
structures. **(C)** Completed osteotomy. After
excision of the bone wedge, the osteotomy is
closed. Note the fibular head slides superiorly.

precise angle of the desired correction to aid in the placement of this second pin. Aim the tip of the second pin so it converges with that of the first pin at the medial tibial cortex.

10. Check the position of the second pin with the C-arm image intensifier. The pins should be parallel to each other in the lateral plane to avoid rotational malalignment during closure of the osteotomy.

11. Place retractors along the posterior surface of the proximal tibia and beneath the patellar tendon to protect the soft tissues from injury during the osteotomy (**Fig. 28–2B**).

12. Start the osteotomy from the lateral side of the proximal tibia. Use a sagittal saw or sharp osteotome to make the initial cut along the axis of the proximal Steinmann pin. Make the second cut along the axis of the more distal Steinmann pin. Extend these osteotomy cuts only approximately three-quarters of the way across the tibia to prevent inadvertent division of the medial tibial cortex.

13. Remove the wedge of bone formed by the osteotomy cuts. Complete the remainder of the osteotomy under direct visualization. Perforate the medial cortex by placing several drill holes through it. However, the periosteal hinge is left intact to prevent translation of the osteotomy fragments (**Fig. 28–2B**).

14. Close the osteotomy site by applying a gentle valgus force to the tibia. Resistance to this maneuver should be minimal. Take care not to close the site with excessive force which could result in fracture of the proximal tibia. Confirm osteotomy closure with the C-arm image intensifier (**Fig. 28–2C**).

15. Use a long alignment rod to assess the overall extremity alignment in a similar manner to a total knee arthroplasty. Align the rod over the center of the ankle joint and the tibial tubercle. This should result in the proximal end of the rod passing at least 2.5 cm medial to the center of the hip joint.

16. Maintain alignment of the fragments with internal fixation. We prefer stable internal fixation with the use of a low-profile L plate secured to the lateral aspect of the proximal tibia. Confirm final alignment and fixation with the image intensifier.

17. Deflate the tourniquet and achieve hemostasis. Copiously irrigate the wound with antibiotic solution.

18. Perform a layered closure over a suction drain. Reapproximate the muscle over the proximal tibia with 0-vicryl sutures. However leave the fascia open to prevent the development of a compartment syndrome.

19. Close the subcutaneous tissue with 00-vicryl sutures. Close the skin with staples.

20. Apply a sterile gauze dressing and secure it with a cotton roll. Wrap an ace bandage loosely around the surgical dressing and connect the collection container for the drain.

21. Take the patient to the recovery room.

Suggested Reading

Insall JN. Osteotomy. In: Insall JN, Windsor RE, Scott WN, Kelly MA, Aglietti P, eds. *Surgery of the Knee*. 2nd ed. New York, NY: Churchill Livingstone, 1993, pp. 635–676.

CHAPTER 29

Supracondylar Femoral Osteotomy

Stephen G. Manifold and Giles R. Scuderi

Indications

1. Unicompartmental lateral knee osteoarthritis
2. Age less than 50 years old
3. High-activity level (heavy laborers)
4. Valgus deformity 15 degrees or less
5. Flexion arc greater than 90 degrees

Contraindications

1. Rheumatoid or inflammatory arthritides
2. Tibiofemoral subluxation (medial) greater than 1 cm

Preoperative Preparation

1. Knee radiographs including anteroposterior, lateral, sunrise, and standing three-joint films
2. Determine the femoral-tibial angle and the mechanical axis (see Chapter 28, **Fig. 28–1**).
3. Calculate the size of bone wedge to be removed from the distal femur.
4. Consider preoperative physical therapy to increase quadriceps strength and decrease flexion contracture.
5. Patient education to establish reasonable expectations

Special Instruments, Position, and Anesthesia

1. Supine position on a radiolucent operating table with a small padded bolster under the ipsilateral buttock

2. Surgery can be performed with general, epidural, or long-acting spinal anesthesia.
3. Use basic orthopedic instrumentation.
4. Use 1/8-in Steinmann pins, sharp straight osteotomes, and a sagittal saw.
5. Consider variable angle proximal tibia cutting guides to make accurate osteotomy cuts.
6. A 90-degree blade plate should be available for fixation of the osteotomy site.
7. Use fluoroscopic image intensifier for intraoperative imaging.

Tips and Pearls

1. Insertion of the 90-degree blade plate-seating chisel should be performed prior to the osteotomy of the distal femur.
2. For patients without contraindications (i.e., significant peripheral vascular disease), a tourniquet should be placed as proximal as possible on the thigh to avoid minimizing the surgical exposure.
3. Intravenous antibiotics should be administered prior to inflation of the tourniquet.
4. A vertical skin incision is preferred in order to improve exposure for internal fixation and to facilitate possible total knee arthroplasty in the future.
5. The Steinmann pins should be positioned parallel in the lateral plane to avoid rotational problems after the osteotomy.
6. Maintain at least a 2-cm thick proximal femoral fragment. Obtain stable internal fixation of the osteotomy to allow early aggressive knee rehabilitation.

What To Avoid

1. Do not violate the lateral cortex of the distal femur during SCFO to prevent translation of the osteotomy fragments.
2. Avoid undercorrection of the deformity as this will lead to early recurrence of symptoms.
3. Avoid excessive force during closure of the osteotomy site to prevent inadvertent fracture.

Postoperative Care Issues

1. Remove the suction drain from the knee on the first postoperative day. The surgical dressing should be removed on the second postoperative day. Skin sutures or staples are removed approximately 3 weeks from the date of surgery.
2. Place the knee in a continuous passive motion (CPM) machine in the recovery room with initial settings of 0 to 60 degrees. Advance the machine's flexion 10 degrees or more per day as tolerated; 90 degrees of flexion is the goal by the time of hospital discharge.
3. Begin physical therapy on the first postoperative day. Focus on range of motion and isometric exercises. Place the patient in a hinged knee brace. Toe-touch weight bearing is allowed initially, however progression to full weight bearing status is not allowed for at least 6 weeks.

Operative Technique

1. Place the patient in a supine position on a radiolucent operating table.
2. Prepare and drape the extremity in the usual sterile fashion. Elevate the leg and inflate the tourniquet to 350 mm Hg.
3. Make a vertical mid-line skin incision over the knee. Dissect down through the subcutaneous tissue to the level of the extensor mechanism.
4. Perform a medial parapatellar arthrotomy. Leave approximately 1 cm of quadriceps tendon medially to provide good tissue for a strong repair during closure. Elevate the periosteum from the anterior, medial, and posterior aspects of the supracondylar femur. Take care not to injure the collateral ligaments at the epicondyles during this dissection.
5. Mark the level and wedge size of the osteotomy site, as calculated from preoperative standing radiographs, on the distal femur with methylene blue. The distal arm of the wedge should be inclined obliquely so that it is parallel to the joint line. The proximal arm is perpendicular to the shaft of the distal femur. This will ensure a transverse osteotomy site following removal of the bone wedge (Fig. 29–1).
6. Insert the blade plate-seating chisel into the lateral femoral condyle at an angle, which is complementary to that of the osteotomy.
7. Insert a 90-degree, 4-hole blade plate until the plate impinges proximally against the lateral cortex of the distal femur. Place the plate laterally because its shape does not fit well on the medial side. In addition, the location of Hunter's canal and its vessels proximally and medially along the distal femur preclude the application of a compressive device in this region.
8. Place retractors on the medial and lateral aspects of the distal femur to protect the surrounding soft tissues during the osteotomy. Maintain the knee in a flexed position during the osteotomy to allow the posterior neurovascular structures to fall away from the bone.
9. Perform the osteotomy of the distal femur in a medial to lateral direction with a power saw. The osteotomy follows the outlined wedge of bone in the distal femur. Extend the cuts only approximately three-quarters of the way through the femur to prevent inadvertent division of the lateral femoral cortex.
10. Remove the wedge of bone formed by the cuts. Complete the remainder of the osteotomy under direct visualization. Perforate the lateral femoral cortex by drilling several holes through it. However, leave the periosteal hinge intact to prevent translation of the osteotomy fragments.
11. Close the osteotomy site by applying a gentle varus force to the distal fragment. Avoid using excessive force to prevent possible fracture of the distal femur. After osteotomy closure, fully seat the lateral plate and secure it with screws to the proximal femur.
12. Evaluate the overall extremity alignment by using a long alignment rod. When the rod is centered over

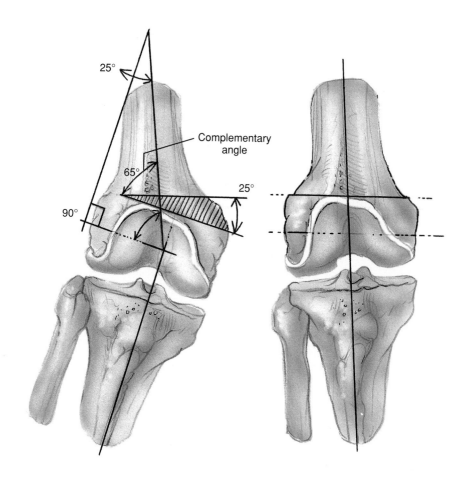

Figure 29–1 Technique distal femoral osteotomy. The angle of the wedge of bone removed is the complement of the femoral–tibial anatomic angle.

the hip and knee, its distal end should align with the lateral malleolus but not be lateral to it. Align the knee in full extension with 2 to 3 degrees of valgus.

13. Deflate the tourniquet and achieve hemostasis. Following hemostasis, copiously irrigate the wound with antibiotic solution.

14. Close the wound in a layered fashion over a suction drain. Close the medial parapatellar arthrotomy using 0-vicryl suture. If patellar tracking is not balanced, a lateral release and, if necessary, proximal realignment of the quadriceps tendon can be performed at this time.

15. Close the subcutaneous tissue with 00-vicryl sutures. Close the skin with staples.

16. Apply a sterile gauze dressing and secure it with a cotton roll. Loosely wrap an ace bandage over the surgical dressing and connect the collection container for the drain.

17. Take the patient to the recovery room.

Suggested Reading

Insall JN. Osteotomy. In: Insall JN, Windsor RE, Scott WN, Kelly MA, Aglietti P, eds. *Surgery of the Knee*. 2nd ed. New York, NY: Churchill Livingstone, 1993, pp. 635–676.

CHAPTER 30

Lateral Tibial Plateau Fracture

Open Reduction and Internal Fixation

Scott D. Cordes

Definitions

There are several classifications for tibial plateau fractures, the most common being the Schatzker classification. Three fracture types involve the lateral condyle: (I) a split fracture of the lateral tibial plateau; (II) a split compression fracture of the lateral tibial plateau; and (III) a compression fracture of the lateral tibial plateau. A type IV fracture involves the medial tibial plateau. Type V is a bicondylar fracture and type VI is a tibial plateau fracture with metaphyseal diaphyseal disassociation. This chapter will address the surgical management of the three fracture patterns involving the lateral tibial plateau.

Indications

1. Knee instability in extension greater than 10 degrees with valgus or varus stress

The following are relative guidelines for consideration of operative treatment.

2. Radiographic lateral tibial plateau tilt greater than 5 degrees (relative)
3. Radiographic depression of the lateral tibial plateau greater than 3 mm (relative)

4. Radiographic evidence of condylar widening of greater than 5 mm (relative)

Contraindications

The following are relative guidelines for consideration of nonoperative treatment.

1. Advanced age (relative)
2. Systemic disease (relative)
3. Severe osteopenia (relative)
4. Pre-existing osteoarthritis (relative)

Preoperative Preparation

1. Standard X-rays anteroposterior (AP), lateral, 45 degree oblique views); consider obtaining a 10 to 15 degree caudad AP view. The X-ray beam in this view matches the posterior slope of the proximal tibia (tibial plateau view).
2. Consider obtaining AP and lateral tomograms at 5-mm intervals or computed tomography (CT). These studies are beneficial in evaluating the extent of the articular injury. CT is felt to be superior in delineating the fracture and is better tolerated by patients. MRI can also be used to assess any cartilage or ligamentous pathology.

Special Instruments, Position, and Anesthesia

1. Place the patient supine on a standard operating table. Positioning a sand bag beneath the ipsilateral buttocks may enhance access to the lateral aspect of the knee.
2. Pad all bony prominences.
3. Use general, epidural, or spinal anesthetic.
4. Use routine orthopedic surgical instrumentation.
5. Use a large fragment bone set (4.5 cortical screws and 6.5 cancellous screws with L or T buttress plates, large bone reduction clamps, and a selection of Kirschner wires for provisional fracture fixation).
6. For limited internal fixation, a large cancellous cannulated screw tray (6.5, 7.0, or 7.3) is required.
7. Autogenous bone graft or synthetic bone filler will be necessary depending on the surgeon's choice. If autogenous iliac bone graft is chosen, the ipsilateral iliac crest should be prepped and draped.

Tips and Pearls

1. Assess the status of the leg compartments. Examine and document the status of the peroneal and tibial nerves and the distal pulses.
2. Perform a careful ligament examination. Assess for any varus–valgus instability with the knee in full extension.

What To Avoid

1. Avoid undermining the soft tissue flaps more than necessary.
2. Avoid further bony devascularization by minimizing soft tissue dissection.
3. Be aware of the peroneal nerve location. Attempt to protect it throughout the procedure to minimize the chance of injury.
4. Avoid injury to the lateral meniscus. Attempt to preserve and protect it throughout the procedure.

Postoperative Care Issues

1. The splint or cast can usually be removed approximately 2 to 6 weeks after surgery and range of motion exercises commenced. The exact timing of removal depends on the complexity of the fracture, the stability of the fixation, and the quality of the bone.
2. Protective weight bearing is continued for approximately 6 to 12 weeks after surgery. This again depends on the complexity of the fracture, the stability of the fixation and the quality of the bone. Radiographic analysis of healing can help guide advancement of weight bearing.

Operative Technique

Type I (split fracture)

In pure type I split fractures where there is no significant comminution or depression, the fracture can often be stabilized with less surgical dissection. Using ligamentotaxis, the type I split fractures can often be reduced anatomically with traction and manipulation, and stabilized using percutaneous cannulated large cancellous screws.

1. Reduce the fracture as described above. Limit the surgical dissection to the amount needed to adequately reduce the fracture if closed techniques are unsuccessful in anatomic restoration.
2. Use fluoroscopy or radiographs to confirm adequate fracture reduction.
3. Make small lateral stab incisions. Insert cannulated guide wires (preferably two or three) 1.5 to 2 cm below and parallel to the joint line. The guide wires should be placed parallel to each other. Use the measuring device to determine screw length.
4. Drill the lateral tibial cortex and metaphysis with the cannulated drill.
5. Insert cancellous screws over the guide wires. When the screw is fully seated, the screw threads should not cross the fracture line. The screw threads should pass beyond the fracture plane and lie within the medial bone fragment (**Fig. 30–5**).

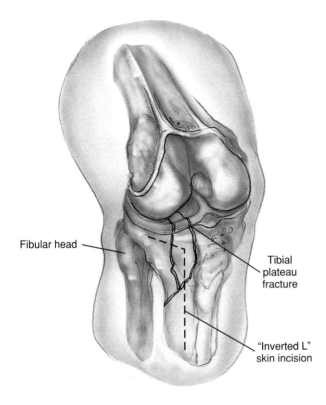

Fibular head

Tibial plateau fracture

"Inverted L" skin incision

Figure 30–1 Skin incision. Expose the lateral condyle in a nonextensile fashion using an inverted L-shaped incision. Place the shorter horizontal segment of the L-shaped incision 5 to 10 mm distal and parallel to the joint line. Do not undermine the soft tissue flaps more than necessary.

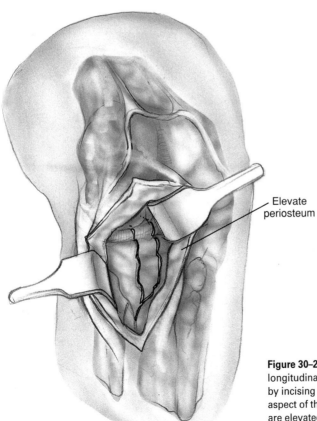

Elevate periosteum

Figure 30–2 Fracture exposure. Expose the longitudinal fracture in the lateral condyle by incising the fascia along the anterolateral aspect of the condyle. The extensor muscles are elevated subperiosteally. The muscle origin is reflected laterally until the fracture line is exposed.

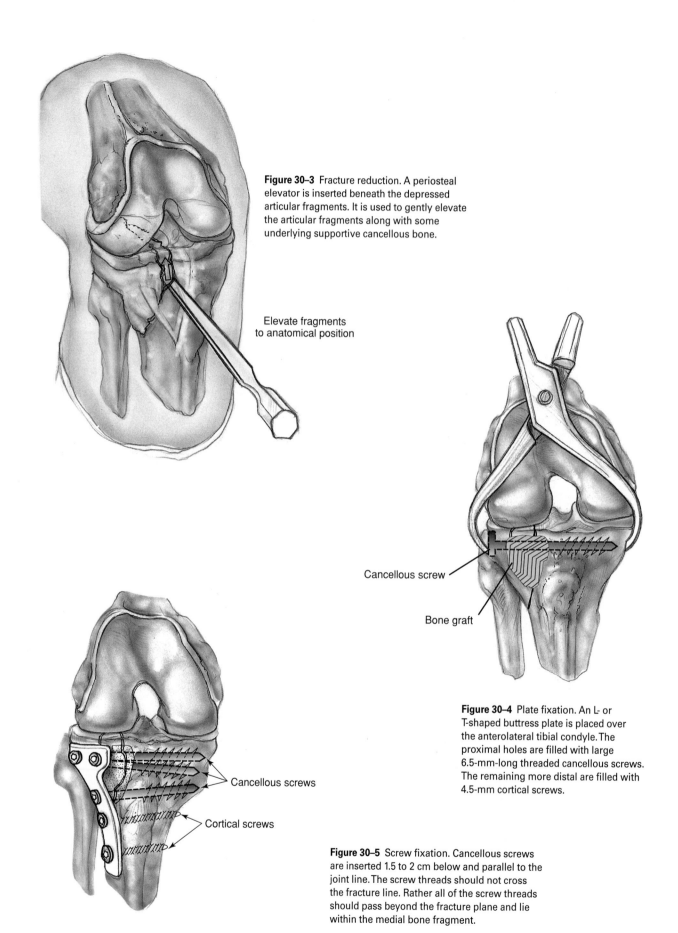

Figure 30–3 Fracture reduction. A periosteal elevator is inserted beneath the depressed articular fragments. It is used to gently elevate the articular fragments along with some underlying supportive cancellous bone.

Elevate fragments
to anatomical position

Cancellous screw

Bone graft

Figure 30–4 Plate fixation. An L- or T-shaped buttress plate is placed over the anterolateral tibial condyle. The proximal holes are filled with large 6.5-mm-long threaded cancellous screws. The remaining more distal are filled with 4.5-mm cortical screws.

Cancellous screws

Cortical screws

Figure 30–5 Screw fixation. Cancellous screws are inserted 1.5 to 2 cm below and parallel to the joint line. The screw threads should not cross the fracture line. Rather all of the screw threads should pass beyond the fracture plane and lie within the medial bone fragment.

6. Use fluoroscopy or radiographs to confirm optimal screw placement.

7. Irrigate and close the stab incisions.

Type II (split compression fracture)

1. Position the patient supine on a translucent operating room table. Place a tourniquet on the ipsilateral thigh.

2. Prepare and drape the limb in the hospital's usual sterile fashion. If the iliac crest is being used for bone graft, prepare and drape this region as well.

3. Exsanguinate the limb and inflate the tourniquet.

4. Use a midline longitudinal extensile skin incision. It should deviate slightly towards the side of the fracture. Alternatively, expose the lateral condyle in a non-extensile fashion using an inverted L-shaped incision (**Fig. 30–1**). This technique minimizes the skin flap that must be raised. However, the disadvantage of this incision occurs if future surgery is required, because there will be a lateral surgical scar that cannot be incorporated into a standard longitudinal midline approach.

    a. Place the shorter horizontal segment of the L-shaped incision 5 to 10 mm distal and parallel to the joint line. Do not undermine the soft tissue flaps more than necessary.

    b. Be aware of the anatomic location of the peroneal nerve and protect it.

    c. Expose the longitudinal fracture of the lateral condyle by incising the fascia along the anterolateral aspect of the condyle. Elevate the extensor muscles subperiosteally. Reflect the muscle origin laterally until the fracture line is exposed (**Fig. 30–2**).

    d. Visualize the joint surface by incising the coronary ligament and elevating the involved meniscus. If at all possible, meniscus preservation is essential. Visualization and exposure of the joint surface is recommended for comminuted split depression fractures where there is extensive comminution of the lateral tibial plateau cortex. Commonly, these fractures require buttressing with an L plate.

5. Once the fracture is adequately visualized, hinge it open to expose the depressed articular surface. Insert a periosteal elevator beneath the depressed articular fragments and use it to gently elevate the articular fragments along with some underlying supportive cancellous bone (**Fig. 30–3**).

6. Fill the metaphyseal cavity with grafting material. Choices for filler material include cancellous autograft, fresh-frozen allograft, or interporous hydroxyapatite.

7. After the articular surface has been elevated and reduced, if necessary insert Kirschner wires to provide temporary provisional fixation. Use fluoroscopy in the AP and lateral planes to help confirm adequate anatomic restoration and hardware placement.

8. Position a T or L buttress plate over the anterolateral tibial condyle. Drill the proximal holes within the plate unicortically approximately 1.5 to 2 cm distal and parallel to the joint line. Insert 6.5-mm-long threaded cancellous screws ("large AO tray") through these plate holes (**Fig. 30–4**).

9. Drill the remaining more distal holes in the plate using standard A-O drilling, tapping, and measuring techniques. Insert 4.5-mm cortical screws in these holes for bicortical fixation.

10. Reconfirm proper hardware placement and optimized fracture restoration (considering nature and severity of fracture) using intraoperative radiographs or fluoroscopy.

Closure

11. Upon completion of fracture reduction and hardware placement, copiously irrigate the wound, and confirm adequate hemostasis.

12. Carefully repair the coronary ligament attachment. Attempt to preserve the meniscus.

13. Re-approximate the fascia with figure eight or vicryl suture.

14. Close subcutaneous tissue with 2-0 vicryl. Close the skin using standard skin closure techniques.

15. Apply a well-padded posterior splint mold, cylinder or long leg cast, per surgeon preference.

Type III (pure central depression fractures)

In these fractures, the articular surface can be elevated through a limited approach using arthroscopy or fluoroscopy to evaluate re-establishment of the joint surface. If the arthroscope is used, it should be used with gravity inflow to prevent over-distension of the knee joint.

1. Make a small longitudinal anterolateral incision 2 to 3 cm distal to the joint over the lateral tibial condyle.
2. Elevate the extensor muscle mass with subperiosteal dissection.
3. Use a 1/4-in osteotome to make a cortical window, just large enough to insert a bone impactor.
4. Elevate the articular surfaces with a periosteal elevator or tamp.
5. Use the arthroscope or fluoroscope to assess adequate reduction of the joint surface.
6. Fill the metaphyseal void with autogenous or synthetic graft or a bone graft substitute such as interporous hydroxyapatite.
7. Insert cannulated guide wires (preferably two) 1.5 to 2 cm below and parallel to the joint line under fluoroscopic control. The guide wires should be placed parallel to each other. Use the measuring device to determine screw length. These screws serve to buttress the previously elevated joint surface and graft material.
8. Drill the lateral tibial cortex with the cannulated drill.
9. Insert large cannulated cancellous screw. Use washers with osteoporotic bone (**Fig. 30–5**).
10. Use fluoroscopy or radiographs to confirm optimal fracture reduction and screw placement.
11. Close the cortical window by lightly impacting the cortex into the cortical window defect.
12. Close the fascia with interrupted vicryl sutures. Close the subcutaneous tissues with interrupted 2-0 vicryl. Close the skin using standard methods.
13. Place the limb in a well-padded brace, posterior splint, cylinder or long leg cast, per surgeon preference.

Suggested Readings

Fractures and Dislocations. In: Canale ST. *Campbell's Operative Orthopaedics*. 9th ed. St. Louis, MO: Mosby-Year Book, 1998, pp. 2094–2111.

Muller ME, Allgower A, Schneider R, Willenegger H. *Manual of Internal Fixation: Techniques Recommended by the AO Group*. New York, NY: Springer-Verlag, 1979, pp. 256–263.

Reid JS. Fractures of the tibial plateau. In: Levine AM, ed. *Orthopaedic Knowledge Update: Trauma*. Rosemont, IL: American Academy of Orthopaedic Surgeons, 1996, pp. 159–169.

Schatzker J, McBroom R, Bruce D. The tibial plateau fracture: the Toronto experience 1968–1975. *Clin Orthop* 1979;138:94–104.

CHAPTER 31

Intramedullary Rodding of Tibial Shaft Fractures

Scott D. Cordes

Indications

1. Closed displaced tibial shaft fractures
2. Open grade 1 tibial shaft fractures (after adequate irrigation and debridement of the open wound)
3. Open grade 2 or 3 tibial shaft fractures (controversial—depends on soft tissue envelope and adequacy of debridement)
4. Nail conversion after external fixator (controversial—can be done acutely 1–2 weeks after fixator application if pin sites are clean and dry without any evidence of drainage or infection)

Contraindications

1. Gross wound contamination
2. Nonviable soft tissues
3. Proximal or distal shaft fractures with significant metaphyseal extension

Preoperative Preparation

1. Appropriate extremity radiographs including knee and ankle joints
2. Template radiographs to ensure that tibial nails of the appropriate length and diameter are available
3. Neurovascular examination with emphasis on assessing arterial blood flow and distal nerve function
4. Assessment of the skin and soft tissues. Evaluate for compartment syndrome.

Special Instruments, Position, and Anesthesia

1. General or regional anesthesia. Avoid long-acting regional anesthesia, as they make assessment of compartment syndrome difficult.
2. Position patient supine on either fracture or radiolucent table. The author prefers a radiolucent table.
3. Check the fluoroscopy prior to draping the patient to ensure that it is in working order and that the C-arm can be positioned to obtain adequate anterioposterior (AP) and lateral images.

Tips and Pearls

1. The more distal the patient is positioned on the radiolucent table, the less likely the table's base will interfere with the C-arm.
2. If a circumferential cast has been previously applied, bivalve it in the preoperative area. This minimizes dust and contamination in the operating room. However, the bivalved cast can be left in place for support and protection until the patient is anesthetized.

3. Make sure the skin over the entry point for the distal screws is not "draped out" of the operative field. The malleoli should be visible after draping has been completed to help optimize rotational alignment of the extremity.

4. Consider "choking up" on the blunt tipped guide rod with the T-handle or vise grip. This will make rod passage easier with less chance of bowing or bending of the guide rod.

What To Avoid

1. Avoid rotational malalignment when impacting the tibial nail. Reconfirm alignment prior to distal locking.

2. Avoid reckless passes with the guide rod. Slow meticulous passage across the fracture site using proprioceptive feel is imperative.

3. Avoid allowing the guide rod to "back out" past the fracture site during reaming.

Postoperative Care Issues

1. If a posterior mold is placed, it can normally be removed within two weeks of the procedure. This is dependent on patient comfort and associated fibular fracture.

2. Initially, most patients are allowed to ambulate either non-weight bearing (NWB) or toe-touch weight bearing (TTWB).

3. Depending on the stability of the fracture, protected weight bearing can be advanced approximately 6 weeks after surgery. This is dependent on radiographic evaluation and clinical symptoms.

Operative Technique

1. Transport the patient to the operating room. Position the patient on a fluoroscopic table. (A fracture table can be used, but the author prefers a standard translucent table.) Care should be taken to ensure that the patient's position allows adequate clearance for the fluoroscopy.

2. After adequate anesthesia is achieved, remove the previously bivalved cast.

3. Place a tourniquet around the proximal thigh. This is not necessarily used during surgery, but is available for use at the discretion of the treating physician.

4. Prepare the entire leg. If possible, hold the extremity using gentle longitudinal traction to minimize further soft tissue trauma. An assistant may be required for prepping.

5. Drape the leg with a standard extremity drape. A sterile adherent dressing can be used for the foot, but it is important to keep the malleoli exposed to allow access for distal locking and to improve visualization of rotational alignment. The drapes should cover both sides of the surgical table.

6. Flex the extremity at the hip and knee. Either have an assistant hold the thigh and leg at the fracture site, or support the extremity with a bolster.

Approach

7. Make a longitudinal incision extending from the inferior pole of the patella to the tibial tubercle (**Fig. 31–1**).

8. Dissect through the soft tissues down to the patellar tendon.

9. Make a longitudinal incision either through the retinaculum just adjacent to the patellar tendon or directly through the patellar tendon. The author prefers to make the longitudinal exposure directly through the tendon.

10. Place a self-retaining retractor in place and expose the proximal tibia. Identify the flattened surface of the anterior proximal tibia. This is roughly 2 cm proximal to the tibial tubercle at the anterior edge of the tibial plateau. This is the standard entry point for the awl (**Fig. 31–2**).

Guide rod insertion

11. Make an entry hole with the awl at the previously identified entry point. Attempt to introduce the awl into the tibia so it parallels the tibia's long axis. Avoid passing the awl's tip posteriorly (**Fig. 31–3**).

12. Pass a blunt tip guide rod down the long axis of the tibia to the fracture site.

13. Based on the fracture pattern, pass the guide rod under fluoroscopic visualization in one of several

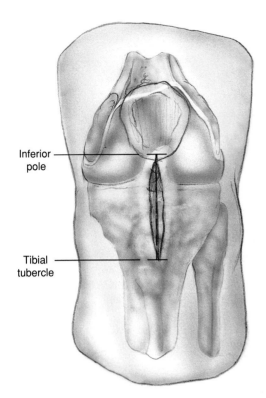

Inferior pole

Tibial tubercle

Figure 31–1 Skin incision. The longitudinal skin incision extends from the inferior pole of the patella to the tibial tubercle.

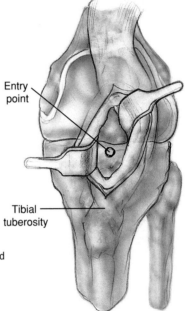

Entry point

Tibial tuberosity

Figure 31–2 Awl entry point. The flattened surface of the anterior proximal tibia is the awl entry point. This is roughly 2 cm proximal to the tibial tubercle at the anterior edge of the tibial plateau.

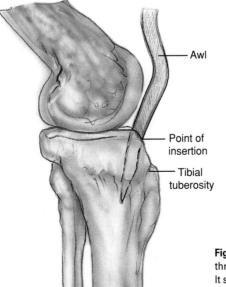

Awl

Point of insertion

Tibial tuberosity

Figure 31–3 Awl introduction. The awl is passed through the previously identified entry point. It should be positioned in the tibia so it parallels the bone's long axis. Do not let the awl's tip pass posteriorly.

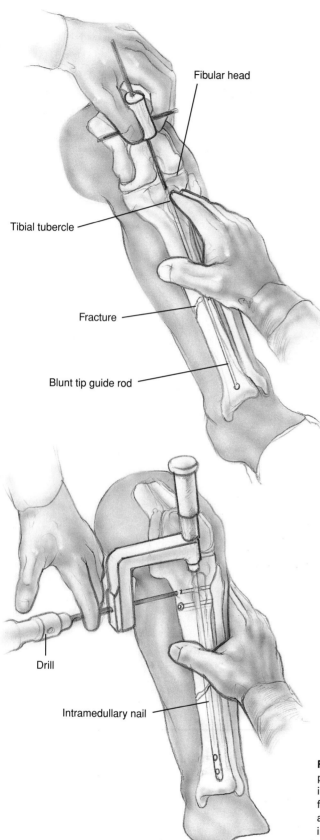

Fibular head

Tibial tubercle

Fracture

Blunt tip guide rod

Figure 31–4 Guide rod passage. The blunt tip guide rod is gently passed down the long axis of the tibia across the fracture site. Use proprioceptive sensation while passing the guide rod across the fracture fragments.

Drill

Intramedullary nail

Figure 31–5 Proximal targeting device. The proximal targeting device allows for accurate introduction of the proximal interlocking screws from medial to lateral. Note: the distal screws are placed from medial to lateral as described in the distal locking screws section.

ways. Passing a guide rod should be as meticulous and gentle a process as possible. This allows for the proprioceptive sensation of passing the guide rod across the fracture fragments, while trying to maintain engagement of the guide rod within the tibial canal (**Fig. 31–4**).

a. With a small bolster beneath the knee and the leg on the table, apply gentle traction to the leg at the ankle, and pass the rod across the fracture site.

b. Drop the leg off the side of the table using gravity for traction and assistance in extremity alignment, and pass the rod across the fracture site. Note, to use this method the sides of the table should be covered with sterile barriers.

14. Depending on the fracture configuration, a very subtle bend can be placed at the end of the blunt tip guide rod to assist in passing it across the fracture site. Remember that the tibial canal has a relatively narrow diameter, so only a slight gentle bend is needed. Fluoroscopy can be used to help rotate the guide rod and fracture fragments to assist in passing the rod across the fracture site.

15. Use fluoroscopy to confirm in both the anteroposterior (AP) and lateral projections that the guide rod is across the fracture site and within the canal of the distal fragment.

16. Impact the guide rod down to the level of the distal epiphyseal scar, which is 1 to 2 cm above the ankle joint line.

17. Place the leg supine and superimpose a standard tibial measuring ruler along the anterior surface of the tibia. Distally, center the end of the ruler over the tibia approximately 1 to 2 cm proximal to the ankle joint. Proximally, align the ruler with the desired entry point for the rod at the proximal tibia. Measure the desired tibial nail length using fluoroscopy. Alternatively, place a second guide rod of identical length against the rod embedded within the tibial canal. Align the second rod with the proximal tibial entry point. Place a clamp on the second rod at the point corresponding to the end of the initial rod. Measure the desired tibial nail length from the clamp to the far end of the second rod.

Reaming (optional)

a. If reaming is desired, start with an 8-mm reamer. Maintain the hip and knee in a flexed position.

b. Use cannulated reamers over the blunt tip guide rod. Increase the reamer size in sequentially 0.5-mm increments.

c. Ream until cortical chatter is noted. Ream 1 to 1.5 mm larger than the diameter of the nail to be used. This step is eliminated when using an unreamed technique.

Unreamed

a. If an unreamed technique is used, determine the tibial nail diameter from the preoperative X-ray. Alternatively, a "sound" or slow velocity reamer can be used to help judge nail diameter.

Guide rod exchange

18. Pass a translucent sleeve over the blunt tip guide rod. Use fluoroscopy to confirm that it is across the fracture site.

19. Exchange the guide rods by removing the blunt tip guide rod and inserting a smooth tip guide rod through the translucent sleeve. Use fluoroscopy to confirm that the smooth tip rod is across the fracture site.

Nail insertion

20. Reconfirm that the proper length and diameter tibial nail has been selected. Mount the proximal targeting device securely to the nail allowing for insertion of locking screws from medial to lateral. Confirm that the anterior bow of the nail corresponds with the anterior bow of the tibia.

21. Impact the tibial nail while maintaining knee flexion. Take care to optimize extremity rotation at this time. In addition, maintain proper rotational control of the implant during insertion. This allows for easier placement of the distal-locking screws later in the procedure.

22. Continue impacting the tibial nail across the fracture site. Periodically check the fluoroscopy to ensure that the nail's length is satisfactory. Ideally, when the nail is fully seated, its proximal tip will be beneath the bony surface, the fracture site will not

be distracted, and the nail's distal tip will be 1 to 2 cm above the ankle joint.

23. Remove the smooth tip guide rod prior to proximal locking.

Proximal locking screws

24. Make medial stab incisions through the proximal targeting device for placement of the proximal locking screws. Maintain the knee in flexion.

25. Utilizing the proximal targeting guide and appropriate drill sleeves, make a bicortical drill hole under fluoroscopic assistance (**Fig. 31–5**).

26. Use a standard depth gauge and insert the appropriate length locking screw. Confirm that the screw heads are flush with the tibial surface with digital palpation and fluoroscopy.

27. If necessary, utilize a similar technique for additional proximal locking screws.

28. Remove the proximal targeting device.

Distal locking screws

29. Bring the leg into full extension. Rest it on a translucent base, elevating it above the uninvolved opposite extremity.

30. Adjust the fluoroscopy so it is exactly perpendicular to the tibia's long axis. Use the fluoroscopy to visualize the distal holes in the nail as perfect circles on the lateral image. If the nail holes appear as ellipses on the image, either internally or externally rotate the involved limb, or airplane the table until perfect circles are obtained. Normally, only small patient position adjustments are necessary to achieve flawless image circles.

31. Make a small longitudinal stab incision in the skin directly over the visualized nail holes seen on the fluoroscopic image. A ring forcep can be used to locate the appropriate spot.

32. Use a sharp tip Steinman pin or disposable trocar pin to make a starting entry point in the bone. A disposable sharp tip pin minimizes sliding away from the hole's epicenter. Center the pin's tip directly in the middle of the perfect circle seen on the fluoroscopy.

33. After this unicortical hole is established, make a bicortical drill hole through the nail. Alternatively, use a radiolucent drill. Align the targeting device of the drill concentrically with the visualized circular hole in the nail. Use the drill to make a bicortical hole.

34. Similarly to the proximal screws, use a standard depth gauge to measure the desired screw length. Insert the appropriate length distal locking screws.

35. If necessary, utilize a similar technique for additional distal locking screws.

36. Use the fluoroscope to confirm proper nail and screw position in both the AP and lateral projections. Appropriate placed locking screws will obliterate the visualized holes in the tibial nail.

Closure

37. Copiously irrigate the wounds.

38. Reapproximate the patellar tendon with interrupted or figure eight 0 Vicryl sutures.

39. Close the peritenon with interrupted or figure eight 2-0 Vicryl sutures. Use a standard closure for the skin and subcutaneous tissue.

40. Apply a soft compression dressing with or without a posterior mold per surgeon discretion.

Suggested Readings

Fractures and Dislocations. In: Canale ST. *Campbell's Operative Orthopaedics*. 9th ed. St. Louis, MO: Mosby-Year Book, 1998, pp. 2067–2094.

Russell TA. Fractures of the tibial diaphysis. In: Levine AM, ed. *Orthopaedic Knowledge Update: Trauma*. Rosemont, IL: American Academy of Orthopaedic Surgeons, 1996, pp. 171–182.

CHAPTER 32

Operative Treatment of Patella Fractures

Mark E. Easley and Giles R. Scuderi

Indications

1. Extensor mechanism insufficiency
2. Articular incongruency
3. Fracture displacement greater than 3 mm (particularly with a transverse fracture pattern)
4. Open fracture

Contraindications

1. Nondisplaced fracture (nonoperative treatment)
2. Minimally displaced fracture with intact extensor mechanism
3. Fracture of the nonarticular surface with intact extensor mechanism

Preoperative Preparation

1. History and physical examination
2. Knee radiographs

   a. Anteroposterior (AP) and lateral to assess fracture pattern
   b. Sunrise view (may be useful to identify osteochondral/marginal fractures)

3. Other imaging studies

   a. Rarely CT
   b. Rarely arthrography
   c. MRI may be useful in identifying osteochondral/marginal fractures.

Special Instruments, Position, and Anesthesia

1. Supine position
2. If extremity tends to externally rotate, place a "bump" under the ipsilateral hip.
3. General, spinal, or epidural anesthesia

   a. Relaxes muscles to facilitate repair
   b. Permits tourniquet use

4. Intravenous antibiotics
5. Standard instrument set
6. Standard small fragment set
7. Large tenaculum clamps
8. Tension band wire (18 gauge)
9. Cannulated screws (4.0 mm)
10. Kirschner wires (2.0 mm)
11. Nonabsorbable suture (#5)
12. Intraoperative fluoroscopy or X-ray

Tips and Pearls

1. Universal vertical midline incision

   a. Allows adequate exposure
   b. Functional incision if future surgery is needed

2. Place a tourniquet as proximal as possible on the thigh.
3. Remember to perform a meticulous retinacular repair.
4. Remove loose, minor fracture fragments—not all of the bone fragments need to be preserved. Preservation of only the major fragments is necessary.

5. Inspect the articular surfaces of the patella and femur because their condition will have a significant effect on the clinical outcome.

6. If necessary, consider lateral release to improve patella tracking.

Tension band principle

a. Converts distraction forces into compressive forces

b. Strongest fixation

c. Wire tension band must be on the anterior aspect of the patella to ensure compression at the articular surface.

Cannulated screws

a. Wire tension band is passed through the cannulated screws.

b. The cannulated screws must be buried within the bone for the tension band principle to act on the bone (otherwise the tension will only be created on the screw ends).

What To Avoid

1. If skin contamination is present secondary to either an open injury or skin abrasion, then delay internal fixation until the wound is clean.

2. Avoid creating multiple layers. Attempt to create two full-thickness tissue flaps medially and laterally.

3. If possible, avoid prolonged operative delay. Aim for surgery within the first 10 to 14 days after injury.

4. Avoid intra-articular step-off. If possible, palpate the patella's articular surface.

5. Avoid improper placement of the wire tension band (otherwise the compressive effect will be forfeited).

6. If possible, avoid performing a patellectomy (only indicated if bone comminution and/or articular surface damage is too extensive for repair).

Postoperative Care Issues

1. Suction drain for 24 hours may avoid hematoma. Compressive dressing for 24 to 48 hours is also useful.

2. Immobilize for 4 to 6 weeks in either a knee immobilizer or cylinder cast. However, earlier mobilization of the knee is permitted for patella fractures when fixation is adequate. This applies particularly to fractures repaired with the tension band principle in which motion results in compression across the fracture.

3. Weight bearing as tolerated with knee immobilized in extension

4. Weight bearing may actually reduce the forces across the quadriceps when compared to forces required to support the limb in non-weight bearing.

Operative Technique

General principles

➤ Debride minor fracture fragments and evacuate hematoma.

➤ Inspect joint.

➤ Remove loose bone fragments.

➤ Identify any osteochondral injuries.

Approach

1. Position patient supine on the operating room table. Place thigh tourniquet as proximal as possible on the thigh.

2. Prepare and drape the limb in the hospital's standard sterile fashion. Exsanguinate the limb and inflate the tourniquet.

3. Make an anterior skin incision utilizing a straight midline incision. Dissect directly down to the extensor mechanism while minimizing skin flaps.

Transverse fracture (tension band technique K-wires)

a. Excise any comminuted fracture fragments from the central portion of the patella.

b. Reduce the major fracture fragments with a tenaculum clamp (**Fig. 32–1A**).

c. Ensure that the articular surface is congruent by palpating the articular surface through the retinacular defects.

d. Place Kirschner wires (2.0 mm) or lag screws across the fracture. A slightly anterior position helps to optimize the tension band principle (**Fig. 32–1A**).

e. Pass the 18-gauge wire through the quadriceps tendon at the patella's superior pole and through the patella tendon at the patella's inferior pole. The wire

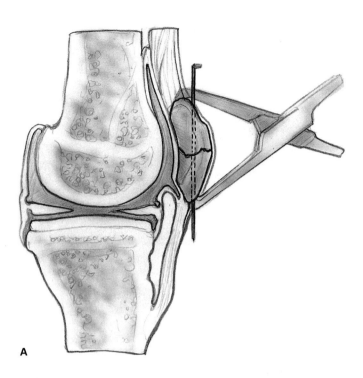

A

Figure 32–1 **(A)** Fracture reduction. Reduce the major fracture fragments with a tenaculum clamp. **(B)** Tension band. Place two longitudinal K-wires (2.0 mm) across the fracture. Pass an 18-gauge wire in a figure eight pattern over the anterior patella. The wire is passed through the quadriceps tendon at the patella's superior pole and through the patella tendon at the patella's inferior pole. The wire should be passed deep to the Kirschner wires or screw heads. **(C)** Final tension band. Loops on both the medial and lateral aspect of the wire are tensioned simultaneously. The pins and wire are cut and the residual wire is buried.

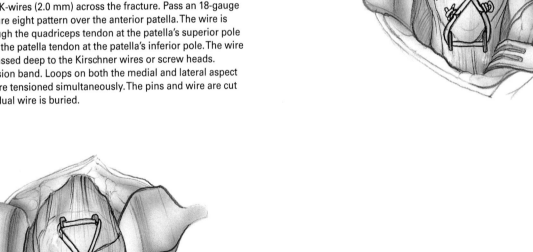

B

C

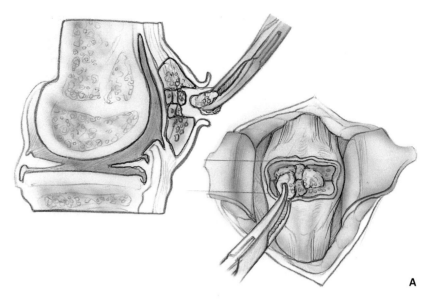

A

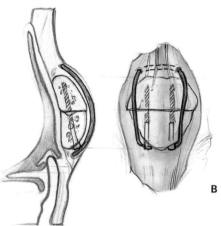

B

Figure 32–2 (A) Fragment excision. Debride and remove small nonviable fracture fragments from the central portion of the patella. (B) Partial patellectomy and repair comminuted patella. Residual fragments are reduced and then secured with compression screws and a cerclage wire.

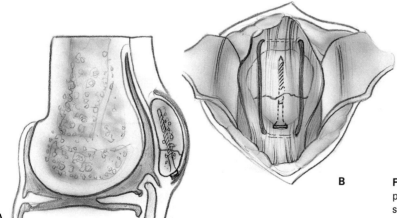

A

B

Figure 32–3 (A) Avulsion fracture inferior pole patella. After reduction, a longitudinal compression screw is placed. (B) Fixation is augmented with a cerclage wire to reinforce the repair.

should be passed deep to the Kirschner wires or screw heads.

f. Remove all "slack" from the wire.

g. Pass the wire in a figure eight pattern over the anterior patella (**Fig. 32–1B**).

h. A single- or two-wire technique may be used. Tighten the wire(s) using a double twist loop with the loops at the medial and lateral margins of the patella.

i. If a single wire is used, create a loop in the continuous portion of the wire opposite the location where the two free ends are tensioned (medial and lateral).

j. Tension both loops simultaneously.

k. Do not overtension the wire. The wire will begin to "double up" when it is tight.

l. Cut any excess wire.

m. Bury the prominent residual wire into the medial and lateral recesses adjacent to the patella (**Fig. 32–1C**).

Transverse fracture

(tension band technique cannulated screws—4.0 mm)

➢ May be used as an alternative to K-wires

a. Recess the screws within the patellar bone.

b. Pass the tension band through the screws. Tension the wire as described above.

c. If the screws are not buried in the bone, the tension band will act on the screws rather than on the patella.

Vertical fracture pattern

a. The tension band principle is not critical, since the fracture is in line with the extensor forces.

b. Transverse screw fixation and/or a simple cerclage wire are typically adequate.

Comminuted fractures

a. Excise comminuted fracture fragments from the central portion of patella (**Fig. 32–2A**).

b. Attempt to reduce the major fragments. If necessary, cut the residual bone to create even surfaces.

c. Ensure that the articular surface is congruent by palpating the articular surface through the retinacular defects.

d. Place a cerclage wire around the patella to approximate the fragments.

e. Place vertical Kirschner wires (2.0 mm) (as described above).

f. Pass a second wire using the figure eight tension band principle (as described above).

g. Further tighten the initial cerclage wire.

h. If necessary, consider using multiple screws and/or Kirschner wires to maintain reduction of major fracture fragments, then pass the initial cerclage wire (**Fig. 32–2B**).

Patella pole fracture

a. Debride minor fracture fragments and evacuate hematoma.

b. Inspect the articular surfaces.

c. Reduce the major fracture fragments.

d. Palpate the articular surfaces to ensure that the surfaces are congruent.

e. Fix the fracture with a single lag screw from the small fragment set (**Fig. 32–3**).

f. Pass a cerclage wire to reinforce the repair (through the quadriceps tendon at the superior pole of the patella and through the patellar tendon at the inferior pole) (**Fig. 32–3**). If the pole fragment is small, nonarticular, or comminuted:

   i. Excise the fragment from the respective tendon while preserving the tendon [i.e., shell out the fragment(s)].

   ii. Reattach the tendon to the patella (see the osseoustendinous repair techniques in Chapter 33).

Patellectomy

➢ If at all possible, preserve the patella as it greatly improves extensor mechanism function and protects the femur.

➢ However, there are instances when the comminution or articular surface damage (on the patella or femur) is so severe that open reduction and internal fixation is not possible; in these cases, patellectomy may be warranted.

a. Shell out fragments.

b. Preserve as much tendon and as much soft tissue as possible.

c. Repair the extensor mechanism.

d. Tensioning is critical.

e. End-to-end repair is rarely ideal.

f. Imbrication is typically indicated to avoid an extensor lag.

g. However, excessive imbrication may result in an extension contracture.

h. The repair should be tight between 45 to 90 degrees of flexion (if it only tightens beyond 90 degrees of flexion, then an extension lag will usually result).

Closure

4. Repair the retinaculum.

a. Begin the retinacular repair with the most posterior defects. Close toward the patella.

b. Use either nonabsorbable or absorbable suture. If nonabsorbable suture is used, attempt to bury the knots.

5. Reinforce the soft-tissue repair anterior to the patella with absorbable sutures.

6. Consider a lateral release if the patella tracking is not satisfactory. This can be performed prior to the lateral retinacular repair.

7. Close the subcutaneous tissue and skin in a standard fashion.

Suggested Reading

Bono JV, Haas SB, Scuderi GR. Traumatic maladies of the extensor mechanism. In: Scuderi GR, ed. *The Patella*. New York, NY: Springer-Verlag, 1995, pp. 253–276.

CHAPTER 33

Extensor Mechanism Injuries

Quadriceps Ruptures and Patella Tendon Ruptures

Mark E. Easley and Giles R. Scuderi

Indications

Extensor mechanism insufficiency with:
1. Complete ruptures
2. Partial ruptures
3. Chronic ruptures

Contraindications

1. Functional extensor mechanism (no extensor "lag")

Preoperative Preparation

1. History and physical examination
2. Knee radiographs

   a. Lateral—to identify patella baja (quadriceps rupture) or patella alta (patella tendon rupture)
   b. Consider obtaining comparison radiographs of the contralateral knee.

3. Other imaging studies

   a. MRI is often useful in identifying discontinuity in tendon substance if diagnosis is in doubt or if partial tear is present.

Special Instruments, Position, and Anesthesia

1. Supine position
2. If extremity tends to externally rotate, place a "bump" under the ipsilateral hip.
3. General, spinal, or epidural anesthesia

   a. Relaxes muscles to facilitate repair
   b. Permits tourniquet use

4. Intravenous antibiotics
5. Standard instrument set
6. Nonabsorbable suture (#5)
7. Drill
8. Keith needle
9. Suture passer
10. Beath needle
11. Pneumatic burr
12. Cerclage wire
13. Nonabsorbable tape (such as mersilene tape)
14. Intraoperative fluoroscopy or X-ray

15. Tendon stripper (if patella tendon repair warrants augmentation with the semitendinosus or gracilis)

Tips and Pearls

1. Universal vertical midline incision

   a. Allows adequate exposure
   b. Functional incision if future surgery is needed

2. Place a tourniquet as proximal as possible on the thigh.
3. Remember to perform a meticulous retinacular repair.
4. Use a Krakow suture technique (interlocking stitch) to ensure adequate purchase of the suture in the tendon.
5. Beath needle

   a. Use to pass suture through patellar tunnels (in lieu of drilling) and then passing a Keith needle or suture passer
   b. Saves a step and minimizes the difficulty of finding the tunnel after drilling

6. Tendon stripper (in the event that patella tendon repair requires augmentation with the semitendinosus or gracilis)
7. If necessary, consider a lateral release to improve patella tracking.

What To Avoid

General principles:

1. If skin contamination is present secondary to either an open injury or skin abrasion, then delay internal fixation until the wound is clean.
2. Avoid creating multiple layers. Attempt to create two full-thickness tissue flaps medially and laterally.
3. If possible, avoid prolonged operative delay. Aim for surgery within the first 10 to 14 days after injury.
4. Avoid reattaching the tendon on the anterior aspect of the patella (this leads to tilt of the patella with tension).
5. Avoid overtightening the patella tendon repair (will create a patella infera). Check intraoperative fluoroscopy or knee X-ray at 45 degrees of flexion; the

inferior pole of the patella should be superior to the roof of the intercondylar notch.

Postoperative Care Issues

1. A suction drain for 24 hours may avoid hematoma. Compressive dressing for 24 to 48 hours is also useful.
2. Immobilize for 4 to 6 weeks in either a knee immobilizer or cylinder cast.
3. Weight bearing as tolerated with knee immobilized in extension
4. Weight bearing may actually reduce the forces across the quadriceps when compared to forces required to support the limb in non-weight bearing.

Operative Technique

Approach

1. Position patient supine on the operating room table. Place thigh tourniquet as proximal as possible on the thigh.
2. Prepare and drape the limb in the hospital's standard sterile fashion. Exsanguinate the limb and inflate the tourniquet.
3. Make an anterior skin incision utilizing a straight midline incision. Dissect directly down to the extensor mechanism while minimizing skin flaps.

I.   Quadricep Tendon

Acute ruptures quadricep tendon (mid-substance)

a. Debride damaged tissue back to normal-appearing tendon. However, avoid excising too much tissue.
b. Repair end-to-end using #2 or #5 nonabsorbable sutures (interrupted).
c. Repair the retinaculum with a nonabsorbable or absorbable #0 suture.
d. If necessary, perform a lateral release to improve patellar tracking.
e. If repair is tenuous, reinforce repair with a cerclage wire or nonabsorbable tape (such as mersilene tape).
f. Proximally, pass the reinforcing wire or tape transversely through the quadriceps tendon.
g. Distally, pass the reinforcing wire or tape transversely through a drill hole in the patella.

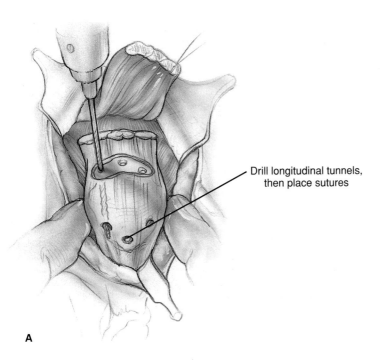

A

Drill longitudinal tunnels,
then place sutures

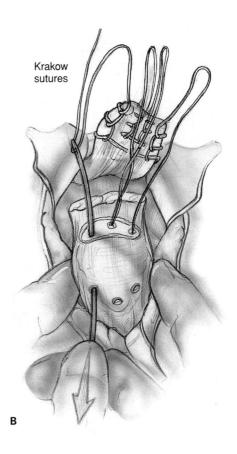

Krakow
sutures

B

Figure 33–1 (A) Drill longitudinal tunnels. A transverse bony trough
is made in the proximal pole of the patella. A drill is used to create
3 (or 4) longitudinal tunnels in the patella. **(B)** Suture passage. Parallel
Krakow (interlocking) sutures are placed in the quadriceps tendon. These
sutures are passed through tunnels using a (straight) Keith needle,
a Hughston suture passer, or a Beath needle. **(C)** Suture tensioning.
The sutures are tensioned and tied over an osseous-tendinous bridge
at the patella's distal pole.

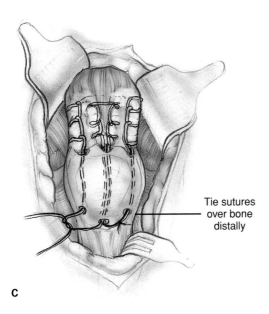

Tie sutures
over bone
distally

C

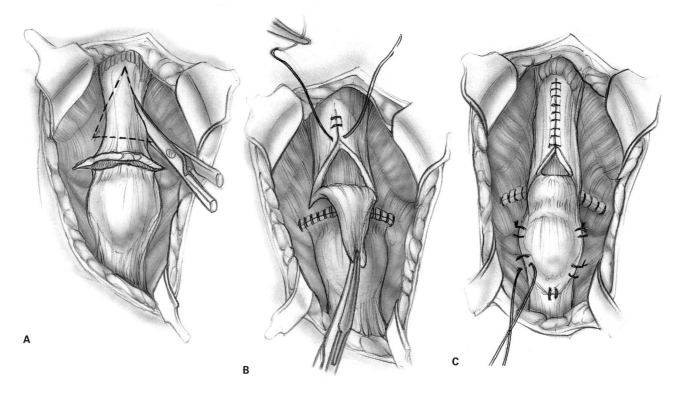

Figure 33–2 (A) Chronic rupture. A full-thickness inverted "V" is cut through the tendon proximal to the rupture. **(B)** Chronic rupture. The chronically ruptured tendon ends are repaired with nonabsorbable #5 suture. The inverted "V" flap is folded distally over the repair to augment the reconstruction. **(C)** Chronic rupture. The inverted "V" flap is sutured over the patella using nonabsorbable sutures.

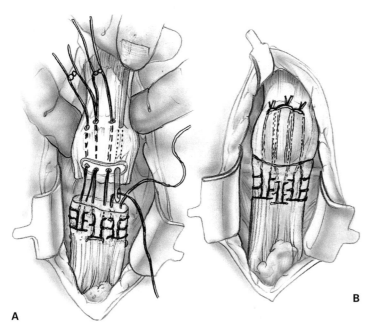

Figure 33–3 (A) Suture passage. Parallel Krakow (interlocking) sutures are placed in the patellar tendon. These sutures are passed through tunnels using a (straight) Keith needle, a Hughston suture passer, or a Beath needle. **(B)** Suture tensioning. The sutures are tensioned and tied over an osseous-tendinous bridge at the patella's proximal pole.

Acute ruptures quadricep tendon (osteotendinous junction)

a. Debride back to healthy tendon and evacuate hematoma.

b. Create a transverse bony trough in the proximal pole of the patella (**Fig. 33–1A**).

c. To avoid patella tilting after the repair, place the trough near the patella's anterior cortex, but not at the patella's articular surface.

d. Place 2 (or 3) parallel Krakow (interlocking) sutures in the tendon (#5 nonabsorbable suture).

e. Create 3 (or 4) vertical tunnels in the patella (**Fig. 33–1A**).

f. Pass the lateral suture through the lateral tunnel, the two central sutures through the central tunnel(s), and the medial suture through the medial tunnel (**Fig. 33–1B**).

g. Traditionally, the suture is passed using either a (straight) Keith needle or a Hughston suture passer (**Fig. 33–1B**).

➤ Alternatively, the tunnels may be drilled using a Beath needle.

   i. The Beath needle has an eye so that the sutures can be passed using the same "needle" that was used to drill the tunnels.

h. Tension the sutures and tie them over an osseous-tendinous bridge at the distal pole of the patella (**Fig. 33–1C**).

Chronic ruptures quadricep tendon

➤ If the tendon ends cannot be opposed, use the Cordivilla technique.

a. Create a full-thickness inverted "V" cut through the tendon proximal to the rupture (**Fig. 33–2A**).

b. Extend the inverted "V" approximately 1 to 2 cm proximal to the rupture (**Fig. 33–2A**). The inverted "V" allows for tissue advancement to reapproximate the ruptured tendon ends (**Fig. 33–2B**).

c. Freshen the chronically ruptured tendon ends and repair them with nonabsorbable #5 suture (**Fig. 33–2B**).

d. Repair the retinaculum.

e. Fold the inverted "V" flap distally over the repair to augment the reconstruction (**Fig. 33–2B**). Suture the extensor mechanism over the patella using non-absorbable suture (if possible bury the sutures) (**Fig. 33–2C**).

f. Close the proximal gap using absorbable or non-absorbable suture in a side-to-side fashion (**Fig. 33–2C**).

II. Patella Tendon Ruptures

Acute ruptures patella tendon (osteotendinous junction)

a. Debride back to healthy tendon and evacuate hematoma.

b. Create a transverse trough in the inferior pole of the patella.

c. Place 2 (or 3) parallel Krakow (interlocking) sutures in the patellar tendon (#2 or #5 nonabsorbable sutures) (**Fig. 33–3A**).

d. Make 3 (or 4) longitudinal tunnels in the patella (**Fig. 33–3A**).

e. Pass the lateral suture through the lateral tunnel, the two central sutures through the central tunnel(s), and the medial sutures through the medial tunnel (**Fig. 33–3A**).

f. Traditionally, the suture is passed using either a (straight) Keith needle or a Hughston suture passer (**Fig. 33–3A**).

➤ Alternatively, the tunnels may be drilled using a Beath needle.

   i. The Beath needle has an eye so that the sutures can be passed using the same "needle" that was used to drill the tunnels.

g. Tension the sutures. Use a smooth clamp to provisionally hold the sutures at the proximal pole of the patella.

h. Move the knee through a range-of-motion to assess tension and tracking.

i. Avoid overtightening the patella tendon repair (this will create a patella infera). Check intraoperative fluoroscopy or knee X-ray at 45 degrees of flexion: inferior pole of patella should be superior to the roof of the intercondylar notch.

j. If the patella is maltracking, perform a lateral release.

k. Tension the sutures. Tie them over an osseous-tendinous bridge at the proximal pole of the patella (**Fig. 33–3B**).

l.   Repair the retinaculum using absorbable or nonabsorbable suture.

➤ If the repair is tenuous, reinforce it with mersilene tape or a cerclage wire.

   i. Pass the reinforcing wire or tape through a transverse drill hole in the patella and a transverse drill hole in the tibial tubercle. It is prudent to place the transverse drill hole in the patella at a different level than the longitudinal tunnels to avoid compromise of the sutures. Ideally, create both tunnels prior to passing the sutures (requires early assessment of the patellar tendon).
   ii. The repair can also be reinforced using a semitendinosus/gracilis autograft (see below).

Acute ruptures patella tendon (mid–substance)

a. Debride back to healthy tendon and evacuate hematoma.
b. Repair the patellar tendon with running interlocking sutures (#2 nonabsorbable sutures) (**Fig. 33–4B**).
c. Reinforce the proximally based tendon with interlocking sutures in the tendon passed through a transverse drill hole in the tibial tubercle (**Fig. 33–4A,B**).
d. Reinforce the distally based tendon with interlocking sutures in the tendon passed through longitudinal drill holes in the patella (described above) (**Fig. 33–4A,B**).
e. Repair the medial and lateral retinaculum with absorbable or nonabsorbable suture.

Acute ruptures patella tendon (tenuous repair)

➤ Augment the repair with mersilene tape or a cerclage wire (described above).
➤ Alternatively, augment with the semitendinous (ST) +/– gracilis (G).

a. Identify the pes anserinus insertion of the ST and G through the same incision.
b. Preserve the distal tendon insertions of the ST and G.
c. Use a tendon stripper to harvest the ST +/– G (similar to the technique utilized for ACL reconstructions).
d. Create an oblique tunnel in the tibial tubercle from medial to lateral (**Fig. 33–5A**).
e. Pull the tendon(s) through the tibial tubercle tunnel so they exit superiorly (**Fig. 33–5A**).

f. Create a transverse tunnel in the inferior patella from lateral to medial (**Fig. 33–5A**).
g. Pull the tendon(s) through the patella so they exit medially (**Fig. 33–5A**).
h. Suture the free ends of tendon to their insertion site at the pes anserinus (**Fig. 33–5B**).
i. This creates a "box" around the patellar tendon to reinforce the repair (**Fig. 33–5B**).
j. Use intraoperative X-rays or fluoroscopy to ensure that the augmentation is not overtightened (see above).

Chronic rupture patella tendon

➤ If the proximal extensor mechanism is contracted and scarred, mobilize it.

a. Clear medial and lateral gutters up to the suprapatellar pouch.
b. Superiorly, elevate the vastus intermedius from the anterior femur.
c. If necessary, perform a lateral retinacular release.
d. As noted above, the key is to reposition the inferior pole of the patella just proximal to the roof of the intercondylar notch with the knee in 45 degrees of flexion (check intraoperative X-ray or fluoroscopy). Consider comparing with either preoperative contralateral knee X-rays or with preoperative X-rays of the affected knee.

Chronic rupture patella tendon (reconstruction)

➤ Reconstruct with allograft (Achilles) or autograft (quadriceps with patellar bone block) tissue transfer. The quadriceps autograft and Achilles allograft techniques are particularly useful when the patellar tendon rupture is associated with compromise of the tibial tubercle.

a. Create a trough in the tibial tubercle (approximately 2.5-cm long x 1.5-cm wide x 1.5-cm deep).

Achilles allograft

   i. Match the calcaneal bone block to the tibial tubercle trough. However, it should be slightly oversized to create an interference fit.
   ii. Insert bone block into the trough and secure with 2 screws (4.0-mm cancellous screws).

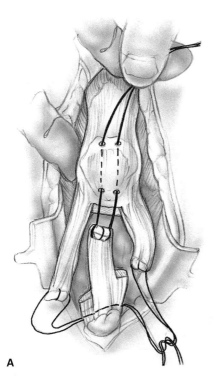
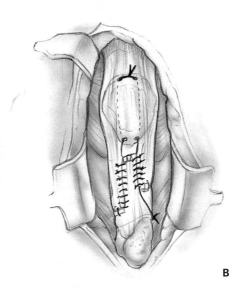

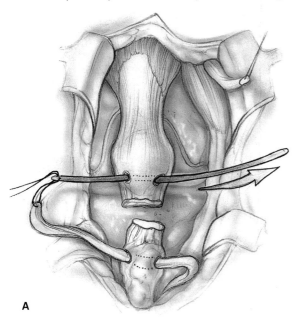
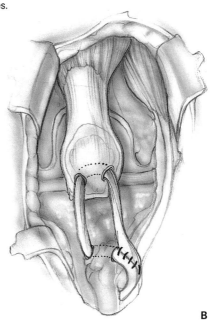

Figure 33–4 **(A)** Patellar tendon rupture. The proximally based tendon is reinforced with interlocking sutures passed through a transverse drill hole in the tibial tubercle. The distally based tendon is reinforced with interlocking sutures in the tendon and passed through longitudinal drill holes in the patella. **(B)** Suture tensioning. The sutures are tensioned and tied over an osseous-tendinous bridge at the patella's proximal pole. The patellar tendon is repaired with running interlocking sutures.

Figure 33–5 **(A)** Semitendinous augmentation. The tendon(s) are passed through the tibial tubercle tunnel so they exit superiorly. The tendon(s) are passed through the patella so they exit medially. **(B)** Suture tensioning. The free suture ends of tendon are tensioned and then sutured to their insertion site at the pes anserinus. This creates a "box" around the patellar tendon to reinforce the repair.

iii. Split the Achilles tendon longitudinally into thirds.

iv. Place interlocking sutures into each third with excess tendon at the free ends.

v. Create a longitudinal tunnel in the patella from the inferior pole to the superior pole.

vi. Pass the central third of the Achilles tendon through the longitudinal patellar tunnel.

vii. Use intraoperative fluoroscopy or X-ray to set the proper tension in the reconstruction.

viii. Secure the central third of the tendon to the quadriceps proximally and the inferior pole of the patella distally (using a nonabsorbable suture).

ix. Use nonabsorbable suture to secure the medial and lateral thirds to the medial and lateral retinaculi.

Suggested Readings

Bono JV, Haas SB, Scuderi GR. Traumatic maladies of the extensor mechanism. In: Scuderi GR, ed. *The Patella*. New York, NY: Springer Verlag, 1995, pp. 253–276.

CHAPTER 34

Tibial Fasciotomy

Bradley R. Merk

Indications

1. Acute compartment syndrome of the leg
2. Major arterial disruption of the lower extremity with ischemia times greater than 4 to 6 hours prior to revascularization
3. Full thickness extremity burns at initial presentation
4. Chronic exertional compartment syndrome

Contraindications

1. None

Preoperative Preparation

1. Initial stabilization by ATLS protocols
2. Anteroposterior (AP) and lateral radiographs of the knee, tibial shaft, and ankle
3. Careful documentation of preoperative neurovascular status
4. Careful assessment of soft tissue injuries (obvious or occult); administer appropriate antibiotics and tetanus prophylaxis in the event of an open fracture.
5. Noncircumferential splinting of fractures allows extremity access for serial examinations.
6. If the compartment syndrome diagnosis is equivocal, measure intracompartmental pressure in all four compartments (pressures greater than 30 mm Hg or within 20 mm Hg of diastolic blood pressure is suggestive of compartment syndrome).

Special Instruments, Position, and Anesthesia

1. Supine position on the operating room table
2. Consider using a radiolucent table in fracture cases.
3. General anesthesia or regional techniques are acceptable. However, regional anesthesia may cloud postoperative neurologic evaluation.
4. Basic orthopedic surgical tray
5. Concomitant soft tissue or skeletal injury dictates additional instruments.

Tips and Pearls

1. In patients at risk for compartment syndrome, constant vigilance with regard to diagnosis and treatment must be maintained.
2. The earliest and most reliable signs of compartment syndrome is pain out of proportion to the injury, firm or tense swelling of the involved compartment, and pain with passive stretch of the involved musculotendinous units.
3. Paresthesias are a later finding. Unreliable signs of compartment syndrome are skin color and pedal pulses. Commonly, the foot remains pink with intact pulses during a compartment syndrome.
4. Avoid circumferential casts and tight dressings in patients with high-risk injuries.
5. There is no such thing as a mini-open fasciotomy and the skin as well as the fascia should be divided adequately.

6. If necessary, consider consulting the plastic surgery service early in the course of treatment to facilitate early wound closure via split thickness skin grafts or flaps.

What To Avoid

1. Avoid misdiagnosing a compartment syndrome.
2. Avoid incomplete dermofascial release.
3. Attempt to protect the superficial peroneal nerve and the saphenous vein and nerve to minimize the risk of operative injury.
4. If possible, avoid excessive delays in second look procedures because difficulty with skin closure, which is always present, can increase over time.

Postoperative Care Issues

1. The wounds should be packed open.
2. The leg is immobilized in a posterior mold splint with a bulky loose circumferential dressing.
3. If possible, the patient is returned to the operating room several days later for wound inspection and repeat debridement.
4. If the wounds are clean at this point, consider secondary closure with supplemental split thickness skin graft as needed.
5. If the muscle or wound margins are necrotic, delay skin closure and proceed with serial inspection and debridements. These serial procedures are commonly done every 2 to 3 days until the wound is felt to be satisfactory for skin closure or grafting.
6. In the setting of repeat debridements, some institutions employ sequential quantitative wound cultures to aid in the timing of wound closure.
7. In the event of significant soft tissue defects, rotational or free flaps may be required.

Operative Technique

➤ In general, a two-incision technique is preferred to adequately release all four compartments, although others have advocated a perifibular single-incision technique or partial fibulectomy (**Figs. 34–1 and 34–2**).

1. Place the patient supine on the operating room table.
2. Avoid use of a tourniquet since it will hinder accurate assessment of tissue viability.
3. Prepare and drape the extremity in the usual sterile fashion.

Anterolateral incision (Fig. 34–3A)

4. Make a 20- to 25-cm incision. Place the incision at the midpoint between the tibial crest and the fibular shaft and extend it along the long axis of the limb.
5. Raise subcutaneous flaps to expose the anterior fascial compartment, the anterior intermuscular septum, the superficial peroneal nerve (running just posterior to the septum), and the lateral fascial compartment.
6. Make a transverse fascial incision at the midpoint of the wound to allow for clear definition of the intermuscular septum and the superficial peroneal nerve.
7. Use Metzenbaum scissors to divide the anterior and lateral fascia proximally and distally. This completes the release of the anterior and lateral compartments.

Posteromedial incision (Fig. 34–3B)

8. Make a second longitudinal incision 2 cm posterior to the posterior margin of the tibia. It should extend a similar distance along the leg's long axis as the lateral incision.
9. Protect the saphenous vein and nerve throughout the procedure. They run parallel to the incision.
10. Make a transverse fascial incision at the midpoint of the wound to allow for identification of the septum separating the superficial and deep posterior compartments.
11. Completely release each of these compartments using Metzenbaum scissors.
12. If a fracture is present, operative stabilization is undertaken as indicated.

Closure

13. Copiously irrigate and pack open the wounds.
14. Apply a sterile bulky nonadherent dressing.
15. Transfer the patient to the recovery room.

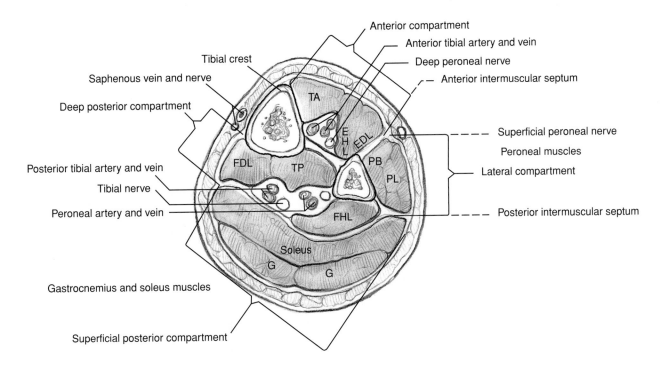

Figure 34–1 Cross sectional anatomy of the leg.

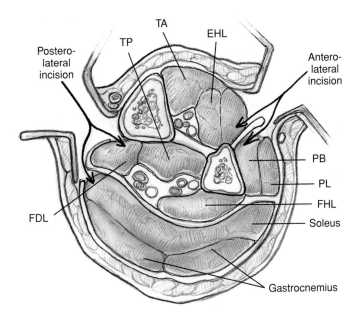

Figure 34–2 Cross sectional path of two-incision technique. Note the path of the anterolateral and posteromedial incisions. The anterolateral incision allows release of both the anterior and lateral compartments on both sides of the anterior intermuscular septum. The posteromedial incision allows release of both the deep and superficial posterior compartments on both sides of the posterior intermuscular septum.

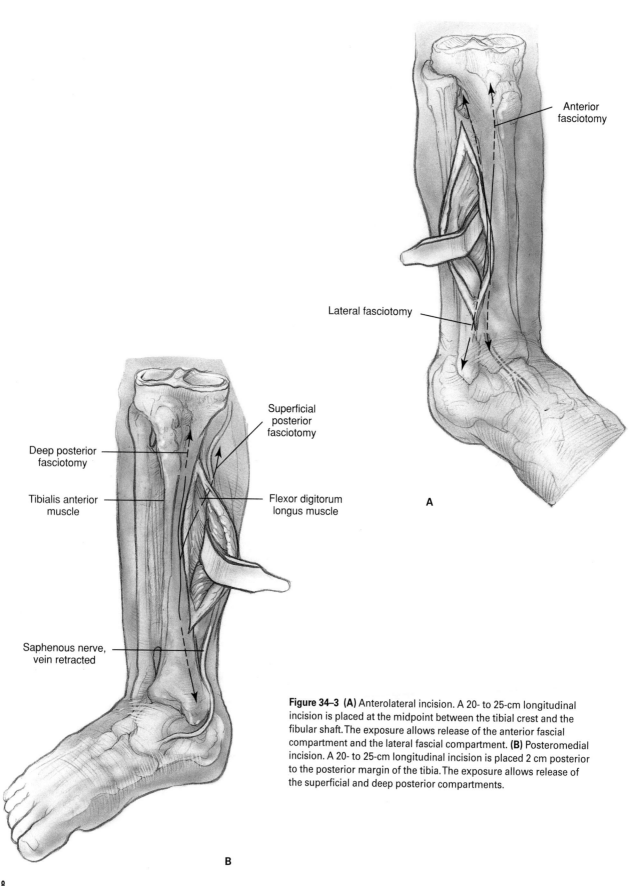

Anterior
fasciotomy

Lateral fasciotomy

A

Superficial
posterior
fasciotomy

Deep posterior
fasciotomy

Tibialis anterior
muscle

Flexor digitorum
longus muscle

Saphenous nerve,
vein retracted

Figure 34–3 **(A)** Anterolateral incision. A 20- to 25-cm longitudinal
incision is placed at the midpoint between the tibial crest and the
fibular shaft. The exposure allows release of the anterior fascial
compartment and the lateral fascial compartment. **(B)** Posteromedial
incision. A 20- to 25-cm longitudinal incision is placed 2 cm posterior
to the posterior margin of the tibia. The exposure allows release of
the superficial and deep posterior compartments.

B

Suggested Readings

Hoppenfeld S, deBoer, MA. *Surgical Exposures in Orthopaedics: The Anatomic Approach*. 2nd ed. Philadelphia, PA: J.B. Lippincott, 1994.

Mubarak SJ, Owen CA. Double-incision fasciotomy of the leg for decompression in compartment syndrome. *J Bone Joint Surg* 1977; 59A:184.

Section Six

Ankle and Foot

CHAPTER 35

Ankle Arthroscopy

Armen S. Kelikian

Indications

1. Loose bodies
2. Anterior tibiotalar osteophytes
3. Soft tissue impingement
4. Osteochondritis dessicans
5. Synovectomy
6. Arthritis

Contraindications

1. Soft tissue infection (cellulitis)
2. End stage arthritis
3. Peripheral vascular disease
4. Marked limitation of motion
5. Sympathetic dystrophy

Preoperative Preparation

1. Thorough history and physical examination
2. Check for instability patterns
3. Examine subtalar joint
4. Weight-bearing anteroposterior/lateral radiographs of ankle
5. Optional views include mortise, Broden's, and stress X-rays
6. CT/MRI for osteochondral lesion staging

Special Instruments, Position, and Anesthesia

1. Regional/general anesthesia
2. Place the patient supine on a standard operating room table. Secure the opposite limb.
3. Flex the hip and knee 45 degrees with a soft bump or use a thigh holder proximal to the popliteal fossa (**Fig. 35–1**).
4. 4.0- and 2.7-mm (short) arthroscopes with 30- and 70-degree obliquity
5. Small arthroscopy instruments: probes, basket forceps, graspers, awls, and curettes
6. Motorized 3.5- and 2.9-mm shaver tips
7. High flow-inflow system
8. Noninvasive soft tissue distraction system

Tips and Pearls

1. Mark and identify anatomical landmarks such as the dorsalis pedis artery, superficial and deep peroneal nerves, peroneus tertius and anterior tibial tendons, and both malleoli (**Fig. 35–2**).
2. The patient should be as far cephalad on the operating room table as possible to allow for optimal utilization of the distal distraction device.
3. Invert the foot to visualize the superficial peroneal nerve.

4. The foot and ankle should be freely suspended.

5. Manually attach the foot strap and then pull the distraction lever bar out to length and clamp it. Now begin distraction.

6. Suck all air bubbles out of the high-inflow line.

What To Avoid

1. Attempt to minimize the risk of neurological complications from injuries to the peroneal, saphenous or sural nerves at the portal sites. The key to limiting neurological complications is preoperative anatomical markings and the safe use of portals. Avoid the posteromedial and central portals. With noninvasive distraction, there are fewer complications than with invasive techniques with distraction pins.

Postoperative Care Issues

1. Close the portals with 4-0 interrupted nylon to minimize risk of sinus tract formation.

2. Splint the ankle in a bulky dressing and posterior mold for 5 to 7 days at zero degrees dorsiflexion.

3. May begin weight-bearing as tolerated and rehabilitation when posterior mold is removed.

4. If microfracture or fixation was used for osteochondral lesions, weight-bearing is delayed 4 to 6 weeks.

Operative Technique

1. Prepare and drape the ankle in the hospital's standard sterile fashion ensuring adequate exposure.

2. At the joint line, usually 1 cm above the tip of the medial malleolus and just medial to the anterior tibial tendon, introduce a #18 gauge spinal needle angled obliquely from anteromedial to posterolateral.

3. Insufflate the joint with 10 to 20 ccs of fluid.

4. Cut the skin with a #15 scalpel. Use a hemostat to spread the incision in a vertical direction. Penetrate the joint capsule with the hemostat to establish the anteromedial portal.

5. Introduce the arthroscope/cannula into the ankle. Begin inflow and visualize the joint (**Fig. 35–3**).

6. Establish the anterolateral portal by way of a needle just lateral to the peroneus tertius. Avoid the peroneal nerve. Cut the skin as in Step 3 and bluntly dissect with a hemostat.

7. If necessary, an optional posterolateral portal can be created by passing the arthroscope from anteromedial to posterolateral through the notch of Harty. Palpate the fibular tip and introduce a spinal needle 1.5 cm above the fibular tip and just lateral to the Achilles. Introduce a #18 gauge needle angling obliquely 45 degrees from posterolateral to anteromedial. The needle should pass between the posteroinferior tibial/fibular ligament. This portal can be used for inflow, visualization, or instrumentation by utilizing interchangeable cannulas.

8. Examine the ankle systematically. Start from anteromedial to anterolateral, then centrally and finally posteriorly using the 21 point reference examination of Ferkel.

Specific pathologies

a. *Loose bodies.* Distraction and patience are prerequisites for removal of loose bodies. Anterior loose bodies are easily removed while visualized from the opposite portal. When posterior, they can be manipulated anteriorly and removed or viewed from anterior and removed through a posterior portal.

b. *Tibiotalar osteophytes.* These usually occur anterolaterally, but may occur on the medial or posterior malleoli. Expose the osteophyte by shaving the synovium or the anterior capsule. A 4.0-mm high-speed burr can then facilitate a thorough removal. Optionally, a lateral radiograph or fluoroscopy can be utilized to assess the degree of bone removed.

c. *Soft tissue impingement.* The fascicle of the anteroinferior tibial/fibular ligament can impinge on the talus anterolaterally. Impingement may also occur in the lateral gutter (evaluate with the 70-degrees arthroscope introduced from the anteromedial portal), syndesmosis, or posteriorly. Begin debridement with a basket forceps then a motorized shaver.

d. *Osteochondritis dessicans.* These lesions usually occur anterolaterally or posteromedially. At first glance, prior to limited synovectomy and probing,

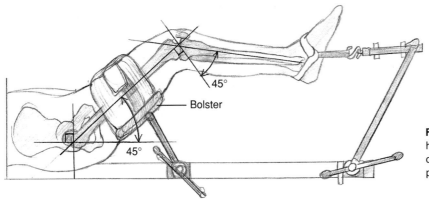

45°

Bolster

45°

Figure 35–1 Extremity position. Flex the hip and knee 45 degrees with a soft bump or use a thigh holder proximal to the popliteal fossa.

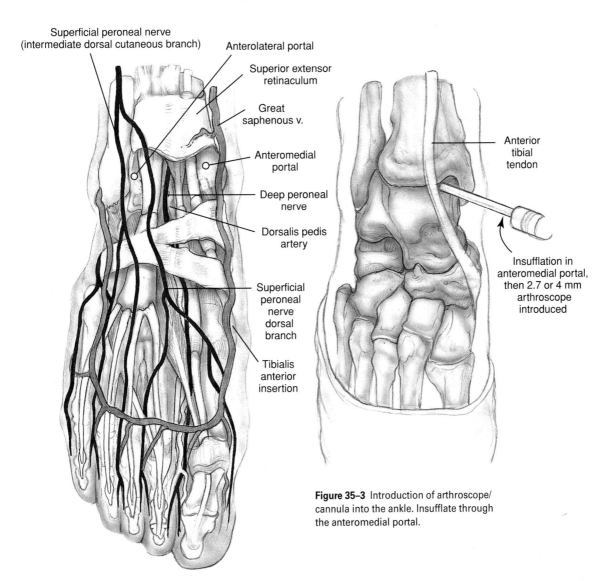

Superficial peroneal nerve (intermediate dorsal cutaneous branch)

Anterolateral portal

Superior extensor retinaculum

Great saphenous v.

Anteromedial portal

Deep peroneal nerve

Dorsalis pedis artery

Superficial peroneal nerve dorsal branch

Tibialis anterior insertion

Figure 35–2 Anatomical landmarks.

Anterior tibial tendon

Insufflation in anteromedial portal, then 2.7 or 4 mm arthroscope introduced

Figure 35–3 Introduction of arthroscope/cannula into the ankle. Insufflate through the anteromedial portal.

235

they may seem miniscule. Acute lesions may be pinned with polylactic acid (PLLA) absorbable pins. Chronic lesions can be debrided and drilled either with a 0.062-in K-wire or with right-angled awls. A transmalleolar drilling guide or free-hand technique can be used (microvector). Ideally, the holes should be drilled to a depth of 10 mm with interval separation of 5 mm. By flexing and extending the ankle, multiple talar holes can be drilled through 1 or 2 tibial entry sites. Alternatively, for large lesions or failed debridement, the OATS procedure has shown promise.

e. *Synovectomy.* Limited or extensive synovectomy can be performed for inflammatory or infectious arthritis. The full radius 3.5 or 2.9 shavers can be used.

9. After the arthroscopy is complete, close the portals with 4-0 interrupted nylon to minimize risk of sinus tract formation.

Suggested Readings

Ferkel RD, Scranton PE Jr. Arthoscopy of the ankle and foot. *J Bone Joint Surg* 1993;75A:1233–1242.

Ferkel RD, Cheng JC. Ankle and subtalar arthroscopy. In: Kelikian AS, ed. *Operative Treatment of the Foot and Ankle.* Stamford, CT: Appleton & Lange, 1999, pp. 321–350.

Hangody L, Kish G, Karpatiz Z, Szerb I, Eberhardt R. Treatment of osteochondritis dessicans of the talus: use of mosaicplasty technique—a preliminary report. *Foot Ankle Int* 1997;18:628–634.

CHAPTER 36

Ankle Fractures

Open Reduction and Internal Fixation

Scott D. Cordes

Classification

Danis-Weber AO classification is based on the level of the fibula fracture: Type A, infrasyndesmotic; Type B, transsyndesmotic; Type C, suprasyndesmotic.

Indications

1. Displaced lateral malleolus fracture associated with deltoid ligament disruption resulting in medial joint space widening
2. Unstable trimalleolar fractures
3. Any combination of bony and/or ligamentous injury that disrupts the integrity of the ankle mortise

Contraindications

1. Nonviable soft tissue envelope
2. Anatomic reduction and the ability to maintain that reduction
3. Although best results can be seen with open reduction and internal fixation in all age groups, clinical judgment must be used in the face of advanced age, systemic disease, and severe osteopenia.
4. Acute surgical management of open grade III B ankle fractures remains controversial. However, lesser grade open fractures can be stabilized acutely after satisfactory thorough irrigation and debridement.

5. Fracture blisters are associated with increased complication rates, presumably related to significant underlying soft tissue damage. The exact timing of surgery in patients with fracture blisters remains controversial.

Preoperative Preparation

1. Perform a systemic evaluation that includes examination of both malleoli, fibular shaft, proximal fibula, deltoid ligament, and syndesmosis.
2. Obtain appropriate extremity radiographs including anteroposterior (AP), lateral and mortise views of the ankle joint. Any shift of the talus within the mortise implies instability and must be recognized.
3. Assess the skin, soft tissues and neurovascular status of the extremity.

Special Instruments, Position, and Anesthesia

1. The procedure can be done with general, epidural, or spinal anesthesia.
2. Position patient supine on either a standard operating room table (if intraoperative plain radiographs are planned) or a radiolucent table (if intraoperative fluoroscopy is planned).
3. Pad all bony prominences.

4. A sand bag placed under the ipsilateral buttocks aids in internal rotation of the leg. Internal rotation enhances exposure of the distal lateral fibula.

5. A tourniquet should be placed on the upper thigh.

6. Instruments: complete small screw fragment set (3.5-mm cortical screws, 4.0-mm cancellous screws and 1/3 semitubular plates). Optional: cannulated 3.5- to 4-0-mm screws are useful for medial malleolus fracture fixation.

Tips and Pearls

1. If a circumferential cast has been previously applied, bivalve it in the preoperative area. This minimizes dust contamination in the operating room. The bivalved cast can be left in place for support and protection until the patient is anesthetized. However, if the condition of the skin needs to be inspected, the anterior half of the cast can be removed.

2. If both the lateral and medial malleolus require open reduction and internal fixation, stabilize the fibula first.

3. Whenever possible, use an interfragmentary screw to enhance fixation in oblique fibula fractures (Fig. 36-3).

4. Carefully review an intraoperative radiograph obtained after completion of the open reduction and internal fixation. Check for proper hardware placement, satisfactory fracture reduction, proper ankle mortise spacing, and syndesmotic ligament integrity. Make necessary changes or proceed with wound closure once these findings have been reviewed.

What To Avoid

1. While bone reduction clamps are useful in holding a fracture in anatomic alignment prior to internal fixation, avoid using excessive force with these instruments which could cause further fracture comminution.

2. Avoid excessive soft tissue stripping. Limit soft tissue dissection to what is needed to assist reduction and obtain adequate visualization.

3. Avoid missing syndesmotic ligament disruptions. The more proximal the fibular fracture extension, the higher the index of suspicion should be.

4. Respect the articular confines of the ankle mortise. Avoid screw penetration into the ankle joint especially during fixation of distal fibular or medial malleolus fractures.

5. Avoid missing a "Maisonneuve" fracture (proximal fibular fracture associated with ankle instability). Tenderness anywhere along the fibular shaft on examination warrants radiographs of the entire fibula.

Postoperative Care Issues

1. After surgery, the extremity is placed in either a posterior mold or a formal cast. The mold or cast is normally removed 2 to 6 weeks after surgery depending on the quality of the internal fixation and bone.

2. Commonly, the extremity is placed in a short leg brace after the mold or cast is discontinued. The brace can be intermittently removed to allow commencement of ankle range-of-motion exercises.

3. Initially, most patients are allowed to ambulate non-weight-bearing (NWB).

4. Depending on the stability of the fixation and quality of the bone, protected weight bearing can be advanced approximately 6 weeks after surgery. This is dependent on radiographic evaluation and clinical symptoms.

Operative Technique

1. Transport the patient to the operating room. Position the patient on a radiolucent table. (A standard operating table can be used if plain radiographs are planned for later in the case to evaluate hardware position; however, the author prefers using a radiolucent table in conjunction with fluoroscopy.) Care should be taken to ensure that the patient's position allows adequate clearance for the fluoroscopy.

2. After adequate anesthesia is achieved, remove the previously bivalved cast.

3. Place a tourniquet around the proximal thigh.

4. Prepare and drape the foot, ankle, and distal leg. The drapes should cover both sides of the surgical table.

Approach (distal fibula)

5. Make a longitudinal incision along the distal fibula in a line parallel to its axis. Center the incision over the fracture site by checking the radiographic location of the fracture and by palpating the fracture site (**Fig. 36–1**).

6. Dissect down through the soft tissues. Split the fascia in a longitudinal line parallel to the skin incision. Remember that sural nerve is more vulnerable to injury, the more proximal the fibula fracture. Identify and protect it in higher-level fibular fractures.

7. Identify the fibular fracture. Visualize the entire fracture including the most superior and inferior extensions of the fracture. Ensure that the dissection is carried over the anterior aspect of the fibula just proximal to the fracture site.

8. Use a periosteal elevator to elevate the periosteum approximately 2 mm from either side of the fracture. This enhances visualization of the ensuing fracture reduction and prevents soft tissue interposition (**Fig. 36–2**).

9. Irrigate the fracture site to help remove any debris or hematoma.

Fibular fixation (spiral or oblique displaced fibular fractures)

a. Reduce the fracture fragments. Commonly, fracture reduction is optimized with a combination of longitudinal traction and internal rotation of the distal fragment. This helps bring the fibula out to its anatomic resting length and enhances alignment of the fracture fragments.

b. Use a bone reduction clamp to maintain fracture reduction. Ensure that adequate dissection has been performed over the anterior aspect of the fibula just proximal to the fracture site.

c. If possible, insert an interfragmentary screw perpendicular to the fracture site angled from anterior to posterior. Use the 2.5-mm drill to make a bicortical hole for the screw. Start the drill on the anterior aspect of the proximal fibular fracture fragment. Aim the drill posterior and inferior so the hole is perpendicular to the fracture site and exits through the posterior aspect of the distal fibular fracture fragment (**Fig. 36–3**).

d. Measure the length of the drill hole with a depth gauge.

e. Use a 3.5-mm drill bit to over drill the proximal portion of the drill hole. This allows the cortical screw to function as a "lag" screw.

f. Tap the distal portion of the drill hole.

g. Insert a 3.5-mm cortical screw across the fracture site. This screw should help compress the fracture and augment the provisional clamp fixation.

h. Place a 5- or 6-hole 1/3 semitubular plate over the distal lateral fibula. Contour the plate to the shape of the distal fibula as needed. If possible, position the plate superior-inferior to avoid placing a screw hole at either the level of the fracture site or the interfragmentary screw. This is not always possible.

i. Insert the screws (**Fig. 36–4**).

   i. For screws proximal to the ankle mortise, make a bicortical drill hole with a 2.5-mm bit; measure the hole length with a depth gauge, and tap the hole with the 3.5-mm cortical tap. Insert the appropriate 3.5-mm cortical screws.

   ii. For screws at or below the ankle mortise, make a unicortical drill hole with a 2.5-mm bit and measure the hole length with a depth gauge. Tapping is rarely required. Insert the appropriate 4.0-mm cancellous screws.

   iii. Do not fill holes in the plate, if the screw hole is at the level of the fracture site, or if inserting a screw would interfere with the pre-positioned interfragmentary screw.

Syndesmosis assessment

➤ Assess the anterior tibiofibular syndesmotic ligament complex. If radiographic evaluation or physical examination confirms disruption of the syndesmotic ligament complex, a syndesmotic screw will be required.

➤ Either a 3.5- or 4.5-mm cortical screw is inserted through the fibula into the lateral cortex of the tibia.

➤ The syndesmotic screw is not a lag screw. It is designed to maintain the correct reduced position of the fibula during healing of the syndesmotic ligaments.

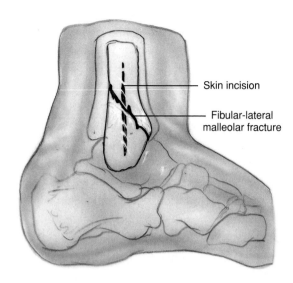

Figure 36–1 Skin incision. The longitudinal incision is made along the distal fibula in a line parallel to its axis. Center the incision over the fracture site by checking the radiographic location of the fracture and by palpating the fracture site.

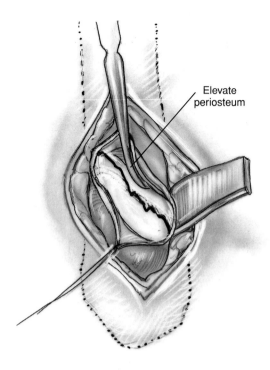

Figure 36–2 Elevate periosteum. The periosteum is elevated approximately 2 mm from either side of the fracture with a periosteal elevator. This enhances visualization of the ensuing fracture reduction and prevents soft tissue interposition.

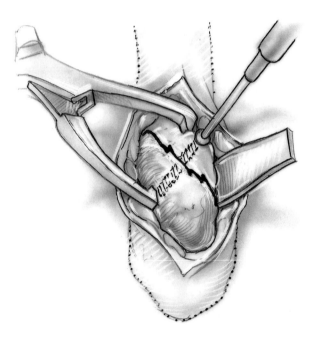

Figure 36–3 Interfragmentary screw. The interfragmentary screw is inserted using a "lag" screw technique. The screw is placed perpendicular to the fracture site angled from anterior to posterior. The 2.5-mm drill is used to make a bicortical hole. Subsequently, the proximal portion of the drill hole is over drilled with the 3.5-mm drill bit. This allows the cortical screw to function as a "lag" screw.

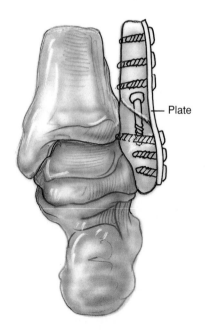

Figure 36–4 Fibular fixation (spiral or oblique displaced fibular fractures). Note the common method of fixation for these fractures with a 1/3 semitubular plate. The proximal cortical screws are placed through both cortices. The distal cancellous screws are placed only through the lateral cortex so they do not enter the ankle mortise. Note the position of the interfragmentary screw.

➤ The syndesmotic screw is positioned 2 to 3 cm above the ankle joint. Typically, this position allows the syndesmotic screw to be placed through a hole in the semitubular plate. In high-fibular fractures (type C), the proximal location of the fracture requires the syndesmotic screw to be placed distal to the plate.

a. Position the drill bit along the lateral fibular cortex 2 to 3 cm proximal to the ankle joint. Aim the drill slightly anteriorly, since the tibia lies anterior to the fibula. Keep the ankle dorsiflexed during drilling for, and inserting of, the syndesmotic screw.

b. Drill through the fibula and through the medial tibial cortex, preferably under fluoroscopic visualization. Keep the drill bit parallel to the ankle joint.

c. Measure the length of the drill hole with a depth gauge.

d. Tap the three cortices.

e. Insert either a 3.5- or 4.5-mm cortical screw.

Proximal transverse or short oblique fibular fractures (type C)

➤ Proximal fibula fractures (type C) are associated with syndesmotic ligament disruption. These fractures should be stabilized and commonly require a syndesmotic screw.

➤ Because of the short oblique or transverse fibula fracture, typically it is not feasible to place an interfragmentary screw across the shortened fracture pattern. Consider using a six-hole low-profile compression plate for the fixation of these fractures.

a. Position the middle of the plate directly over the fracture site. Clamp the plate to the bone with a bone reduction clamp.

b. Generally, it is easier to first stabilize the plate to the proximal bone fragment prior to reducing the fracture fragments. Use 3.5-mm cortical screws to fix the plate to the proximal bone fragment. Insert the screws using standard drilling, measuring and tapping techniques.

c. Reduce the unstable distal fibula fragment to the proximal construct (proximal fibula fracture fragment and plate). Attempt to achieve an anatomic reduction by allowing the fracture fragments to interdigitate at the fracture site. The lateral plate provides a buttress.

d. Clamp the plate to the distal fracture fragment with a bone reduction clamp.

e. Make an eccentric drill hole, using the offset drill guide, through any hole in the plate. This provides 1 mm of compression across the fracture site. Insert a 3.5-mm cortical screw after using standard measuring and tapping techniques.

f. Insert 3.5-mm cortical screws through the remaining holes in the plate using standard (neutral hole) drilling, measuring, and tapping techniques.

g. Insert a syndesmotic screw 2 to 3 centimeters above the ankle joint as described above.

Approach (medial malleolar fracture)

➤ Consider using a cannulated screw system to fix the medial malleollar fracture.

➤ Commonly, two 4.0-mm-long threaded cannulated screws are used to fix the fracture.

➤ On occasion, a small medial malleolar fragment necessitates using only a single screw or a screw and K-wire construct.

10. Identify the inferior aspect of the medial malleolus by palpation. Make an anteromedial "hockey stick" incision around the medial malleolus. Extend the incision proximally in a curvilinear direction over the anterior aspect of the ankle joint (**Fig. 36–5**).

11. Identify and protect the saphenous vein.

12. Remove any interposed soft tissues from the fracture site. Reflect the periosteum 2 mm from either side of the fracture site.

13. Inspect the ankle joint anteriorly. Irrigate the ankle joint and remove any hematoma or cartilaginous debris.

14. Use a towel clip or bone reduction clamp to reduce and then temporarily hold the medial malleolar fragment. Place a "bump" beneath the calf. This acts to take pressure off the heel and assist in optimizing reduction of the medial malleolar fragment.

15. Retract the skin with a narrow ribbon retractor to visualize the tip of the medial malleolus.

16. Advance two guide wires from the tip of the medial malleolus, across the fracture site, and into the tibial metaphysis. If possible, use fluoroscopy to assess the reduction and guide wire placement. Specific fluoroscopic assessment of the mortise view ensures

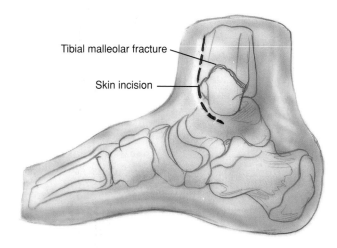

Tibial malleolar fracture

Skin incision

Figure 36–5 Skin incision. The curvilinear "hockey stick" incision is made anteromedial and curves around the medial malleolus.

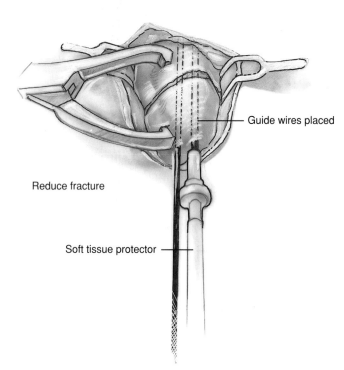

Guide wires placed

Reduce fracture

Soft tissue protector

Figure 36–6 Guide wire placement. Two guide wires are placed across the fracture site tibial metaphysis. If possible, use fluoroscopy to assess the reduction and guide wire placement. Specific fluoroscopic assessment of the mortise view ensures that the guide wires have not inadvertently been inserted into the ankle joint.

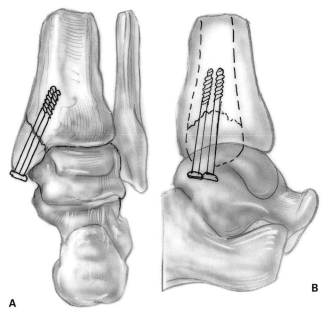

A

B

Figure 36–7 Tibial fixation (medial malleolar fracture). **(A)** AP view. **(B)** Lateral view. Note the common method of fixation for these fractures with two 4.0-mm cannulated screws. The screw threads are placed so they are in the tibial metaphysis and do not lie across the fracture site.

that the guide wires have not inadvertently been inserted into the ankle joint (**Fig. 36–6**).

17. After adequate guide wire position is confirmed, insert two 4.0-mm cannulated screws over the guide pins if the fracture is of satisfactory size. This is accomplished by drilling the outer cortex with the cannulated drill and using a standard depth gauge. If necessary, tap the outer cortex. Occasionally, in small medial malleolar fragments, only a single screw and/or screw and K-wire fixation can be used (**Figs. 36–7A and 7B**).

Intraoperative assessment

18. Use intra-operative fluoroscopy or standard radiographs to assess hardware placement and fracture alignment.

   a. Confirm proper hardware placement. Ensure that the screws do not penetrate into the ankle mortise and their lengths are satisfactory.

   b. Confirm anatomic restoration of the ankle mortise and the fibula. If there was evidence of deltoid ligament disruption, ensure closure of the medial joint space.

   c. If there was an associated syndesmotic disruption, confirm proper syndesmotic screw placement and an anatomic restoration of the ankle mortise.

   d. If a posterior malleolar fracture was present, confirm that it has satisfactorily been reduced with restoration of appropriate fibular length.

Closure

19. Irrigate both wounds.

20. Reapproximate the periosteum over the medial malleolus and the subcutaneous tissues with interrupted 2-0 vicryl.

21. Laterally, close the fascia with figure eight or interrupted 0-vicryl sutures. Close the subcutaneous tissues with interrupted 2-0 vicryl. Optionally, a drain can be used per surgeon preference.

22. Close the skin using standard skin closure techniques, preferably staples or interrupted nylon suture.

23. Place the leg in a well padded posterior mold or short leg cast, with the ankle immobilized at 90 degrees.

Suggested Readings

Gregory PR, Sanders RW. Ankle and foot injuries. In: Levine AM, ed. *Orthopaedic Knowledge Update: Trauma*. Rosemont, IL: American Academy of Orthopaedic Surgeons, 1996, pp. 191–209.

Muller ME, Allgower A, Schneider R, Willenegger H. *Manual of Internal Fixation: Techniques Recommended by the AO Group*. 2nd ed. New York, NY: Springer-Verlag, 1979, pp. 282–299.

Whittle AP. Fractures of lower extremities. In: Canale ST, ed. *Campbell's Operative Orthopaedics*. 9th ed. St. Louis, MO: Mosby-Year Book, 1998, pp. 2043–2066.

CHAPTER 37

Achilles Tendon Repair

Steven Kodros

Indications

1. Acute rupture of the Achilles tendon in a competitive or high-level athlete
2. Acute ruptures of the Achilles tendon in which treatment has been delayed: the exact length of delay that "requires" operative intervention is debatable, but treatment delays beyond approximately 2 weeks generally increase the benefits of surgery. In the event that treatment has been extensively delayed (e.g., greater than 6 to 8 weeks), surgical repair of the ruptured Achilles tendon may require additional augmentation with fascial turndown flaps or flexor hallucis longus tendon transfer.

Contraindications

1. Poor skin or soft tissue condition in the area of desired surgical repair
2. Patients with conditions that may increase the risk of wound-healing problems (e.g., peripheral vascular disease, diabetes mellitus, heavy tobacco use) (relative)

Preoperative Preparation

1. Evaluate the patient to assess the benefits of surgical versus nonoperative treatment.
2. Discuss both surgical and nonsurgical treatment (and their respective pros and cons) options with the patient.

3. If a calcaneal avulsion fracture is suspected, radiographs of the ankle and foot may be beneficial.
4. While an appropriate history and physical examination can reliably identify most Achilles tendon ruptures, consider obtaining a MRI if diagnosis is in doubt.

Special Instruments, Position, and Anesthesia

1. If augmentation with the plantaris tendon or other additional procedures is being considered, tendon strippers and weavers may be beneficial.
2. The procedure is usually done with the patient in the prone position. However, if desired, the procedure can be done with the patient supine by placing a rolled blanket beneath the contralateral buttock to externally rotate the affected limb.
3. A thigh tourniquet is utilized.
4. The procedure is done with either general or spinal anesthesia.

Tips and Pearls

1. Preoperatively, pay close attention to the normal plantarflexion resting position and tone of the contralateral foot and ankle in order to reproduce this as best as possible when repairing the ruptured side. If necessary, both lower extremities can be prepped and draped to allow this comparison intraoperatively.

2. Use great care in handling the skin and soft tissues during the procedure to minimize the incidence of postoperative wound-healing problems. However, since postoperative wound-healing problems remains a risk even with meticulous technique, this possibility should be reviewed with patients preoperatively.

3. Use a medial incision. This avoids the sural nerve laterally and allows better access to the plantaris, flexor hallucis longus, and flexor digitorum longus tendons that are occasionally required for augmentation of the repair.

4. Make sure all suture knots in the repair are deeply buried and do not lie superficial under the wound closure.

5. Carefully close the paratenon in order to relieve tension on the skin closure and minimize wound complications. If this closure is tight or difficult to perform, consider making a longitudinal relaxing incision in fascia of the deep posterior compartment immediately anterior to the Achilles tendon.

What To Avoid

1. Avoid excessive undermining or subcutaneous tissue dissection superficial to the paratenon layer.

2. Attempt to avoid making the reconstructed tendon either too long or too short. The goal is to repair the tendon so it returns as close to its normal length as possible.

Postoperative Care Issues

1. After surgery the foot and ankle are placed in either a well-padded posterior splint or a plaster reinforced Jones-type dressing. The foot and ankle are maintained in a neutral to slightly plantar flexed position. If a stable repair has been achieved, it is not necessary to immobilize the foot and ankle in extreme equinus.

2. At 1 week postsurgery, the splint is removed and the wound inspected. If a stable repair was achieved at surgery, early active range-of-motion may be begun at this time. The patient is encouraged to perform active dorsiflexion and plantarflexion exercises with as much force as possible, using only the affected extremity's muscle groups. No resistance exercise or passive range-of-motion or stretching is allowed. When not exercising, the patient is protected in a removable short-leg brace with a heel lift. Strict non-weight-bearing ambulation is continued.

3. At 3 weeks postsurgery, the sutures are removed and the patient begins scar mobilization with manual massage to prevent adherence to the underlying tendon.

4. At 6 weeks postsurgery, full weight-bearing is allowed with the use of the removable short-leg brace with a heel lift. Water exercises, swimming, and stationary cycling (with minimal resistance) may be instituted. Otherwise, the rehabilitation program remains unchanged.

5. At 10 to 12 weeks postsurgery, the removable short-leg brace is discontinued and use of a regular shoe with a heel lift commences. At this time more aggressive progressive resistance-strengthening exercises, including double-limb toe raises, can be gradually implemented. In addition, light jogging on level ground or a treadmill and proprioception training exercises can be commenced. If necessary, knee-high compression stockings can help limit dependent swelling.

6. As strength and motion improve, activity and athletic participation can progress. A good benchmark to aid in timing a safe return to competitive sports is the patient's ability to successfully perform a single-limb toe rise on the involved side.

Operative Technique

1. After successful induction of anesthesia, position the patient prone on the operating room table. Use padded chest rolls to allow the abdomen to hang freely. Prevent injury to the brachial plexus by avoiding hyperextension of the shoulders. Pad all bony prominences.

2. Evaluate the normal plantarflexion resting position and tone of the contralateral foot and ankle. In addition, assess its normal passive plantarflexion response to a manual squeeze of the calf musculature (i.e., normal Thompson test response). Alternatively prepare and drape the normal side in addition to the affected side to allow these comparisons to be made during the procedure.

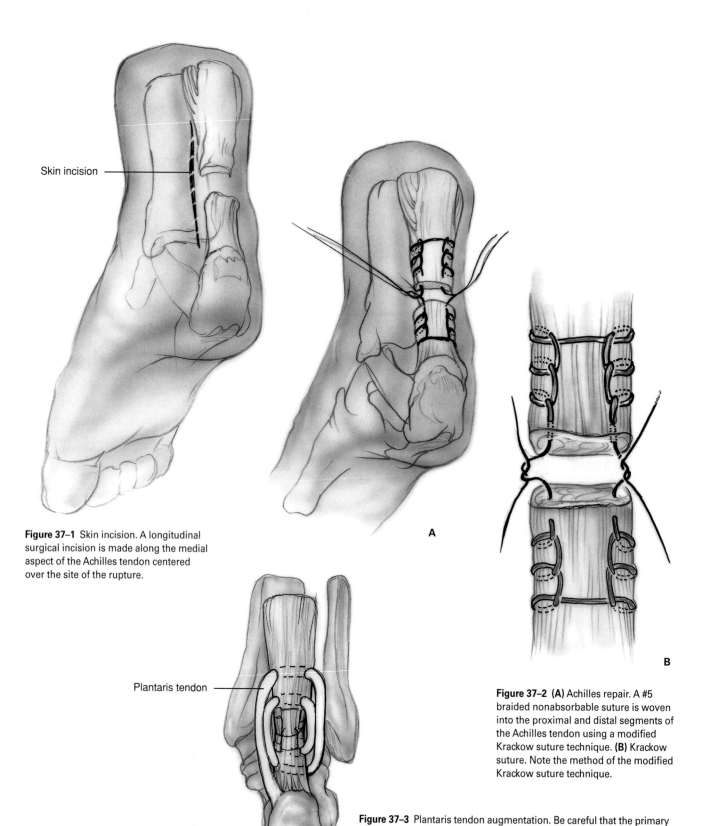

Figure 37–1 Skin incision. A longitudinal surgical incision is made along the medial aspect of the Achilles tendon centered over the site of the rupture.

A

B

Plantaris tendon

Calcaneus

Figure 37–2 **(A)** Achilles repair. A #5 braided nonabsorbable suture is woven into the proximal and distal segments of the Achilles tendon using a modified Krackow suture technique. **(B)** Krackow suture. Note the method of the modified Krackow suture technique.

Figure 37–3 Plantaris tendon augmentation. Be careful that the primary repair suture is not inadvertently cut or damaged when passing the plantaris through the Achilles tendon. Tack the plantaris tendon with absorbable suture at several points on the lateral side of the Achilles to keep the knots deep to the wound.

3. Place a tourniquet on the thigh. Prepare and drape the limb in a sterile fashion. Exsanguinate the limb and inflate the tourniquet to 300 to 350 mm Hg.

4. Make a longitudinal incision along the medial aspect of the Achilles tendon centered over the site of the rupture (**Fig. 37–1**). Commonly, the rupture site can be identified by the presence of a palpable subcutaneous defect. The incision should be at least 10 cm in length. It is better to lengthen the incision than to use aggressive skin and soft tissue retraction because excessive retraction may increase the risk of wound complications.

5. Sharply dissect straight down through the subcutaneous tissue and identify the underlying paratenon layer. Take care to avoid undermining the subcutaneous tissue superficial to the paratenon. Utilize an atraumatic or "no touch" technique when handling the skin edges and soft tissues. These efforts help to minimize the risk of wound complications.

6. Longitudinally incise the paratenon.

7. Identify the ruptured Achilles tendon and its associated hematoma. If present, the plantaris tendon is also identified. Irrigate the hematoma. Debride any hemorrhagic or hypertrophied tenosynovium. If necessary, debride excessively frayed ends of the ruptured tendon.

8. If augmentation of the Achilles tendon repair with a plantaris tendon weave is desired, harvest the plantaris tendon at this time. Pass a "cork screw"-type tendon stripper over the plantaris subcutaneously and detach it proximally within the calf. Alternatively, detach the plantaris as proximal as possible with a scissors while pulling distally on the visible tendon. Leave the distal insertion of the plantaris tendon on the medial aspect of the calcaneous intact.

9. Weave a #5 braided nonabsorbable suture into the proximal and distal segments of the Achilles tendon using a modified Krackow suture technique (**Figs. 37–2A and 37–2B**). Confirm sturdy purchase within each segment by firmly pulling on the suture ends.

10. Securely tie the suture ends while positioning the ruptured tendon as close as possible to its normal length. Tie the sutures so the knots are deeply buried and do not lie in the subcutaneous tissue directly beneath the skin.

11. Passively dorsiflex the foot and ankle to at least neutral (90 degrees), thereby confirming the repair's stability. Ensure that proper tendon length has been restored by evaluating the plantarflexion resting position of the foot and the response to a Thompson test. Compare these findings with those obtained preoperatively in the contralateral limb (or intraoperatively if it has been prepped and draped).

12. Place a running "baseball"-type stitch circumferentially around the repair site using a 3-0 monofilament absorbable suture. This helps to both smoothly contour the repair and strengthen it.

13. If desired, augment the repair with a plantaris tendon weave (**Fig. 37–3**). Take care to avoid inadvertently cutting or damaging the primary repair suture when passing the plantaris tendon through the torn ends of the Achilles. Use absorbable suture to tack the plantaris tendon down to the Achilles tendon at several points on the lateral side of the Achilles. Keep the knots deeply buried.

14. Extensively irrigate the wound.

15. Close the paratenon layer with interrupted inverted (buried) 2-0 absorbable sutures. Be careful not to catch the underlying Achilles tendon in this layer of closure.

16. Close the skin with interrupted 3-0 nylon sutures.

17. Apply sterile dressings to the wound. Place the extremity in a well-padded posterior splint or plaster reinforced Jones dressing. Maintain the foot and ankle in a neutral to slightly plantarflexed position.

18. Deflate the tourniquet and transfer the patient to the recovery room.

Suggested Readings

Maffuli N. Current concepts review: rupture of the Achilles tendon. *J Bone Joint Surg Am* 1999;81A: 1019–1036.

Mandelbaum BR, Myerson MS, Forster R. Achilles tendon ruptures. A new method of repair, early range of motion, and functional rehabilitation. *Am J Sports Med* 1995;23:392–395.

Wapner KL. Achilles tendon ruptures and posterior heel pain. In: Kelikian AS, ed. *Operative Treatment of the Foot and Ankle*. Stamford, CT: Appleton & Lange, 1999, pp. 369–387.

CHAPTER 38

Bunions and Hallux Valgus

Armen S. Kelikian

Definition

1. Hallux valgus: metatarsus primus varus represents a complex of deformities and deficiencies that require relative versatility and adaptability in treatment.

Indications (Chevron Osteotomy)

1. Painful hallux
2. Intermetatarsal angle (IMA) <15 degrees **(Fig. 38–1)**
3. Distal metatarsal articular angle (DMAA) >10 degrees (bidirectional chevron) **(Fig. 38–1)**

Contraindications

1. Hypermobility of the first tarso-metatarsal joint
2. Revision (relative)
3. Arthritis of the metatarsophalangeal (MTP)
4. Peripheral vascular disease
5. Narcissism

Preoperative Preparation

1. Hallux valgus foot scores <70
2. Anteroposterior (AP) weight-bearing X-rays of the forefoot
3. Harris floor reaction imprints

Special Instruments, Position, and Anesthesia

1. Ankle block and ankle tourniquet (250 mm)
2. Patient positioned supine on standard operating room table
3. Microsagittal saw (medium blades)
4. 0.062- and 0.054-in K-wires with wire driver
5. Tenotomy scissors
6. Banana #67 Beaver blade
7. Ragnell, Davis, and Hohman retractors

Tips and Pearls

1. The Ragnell retractor is used to pull the proximal fragment medially to allow lateral translation of the capital or distal fragments.
2. An intra-articular adductor tenotomy is performed from medial to lateral using a banana blade.

What To Avoid

1. Avoid excessive lateral stripping of head/neck fragments.
2. Avoid crossing the osteotomy ends.
3. Avoid notching the first metatarsal cortex during the exostectomy.

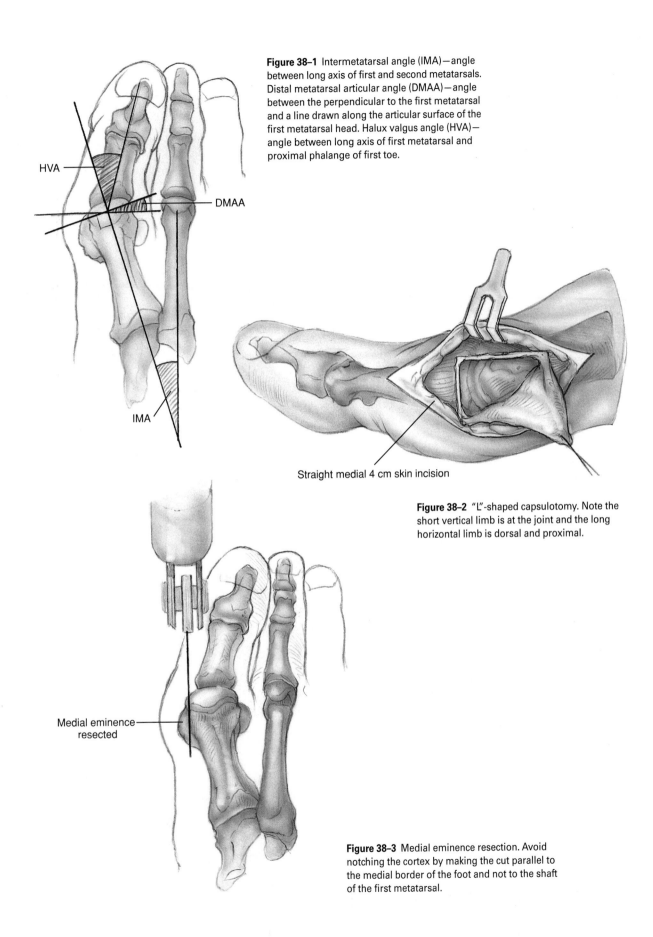

Figure 38–1 Intermetatarsal angle (IMA)—angle between long axis of first and second metatarsals. Distal metatarsal articular angle (DMAA)—angle between the perpendicular to the first metatarsal and a line drawn along the articular surface of the first metatarsal head. Halux valgus angle (HVA)—angle between long axis of first metatarsal and proximal phalange of first toe.

HVA

DMAA

IMA

Straight medial 4 cm skin incision

Figure 38–2 "L"-shaped capsulotomy. Note the short vertical limb is at the joint and the long horizontal limb is dorsal and proximal.

Medial eminence resected

Figure 38–3 Medial eminence resection. Avoid notching the cortex by making the cut parallel to the medial border of the foot and not to the shaft of the first metatarsal.

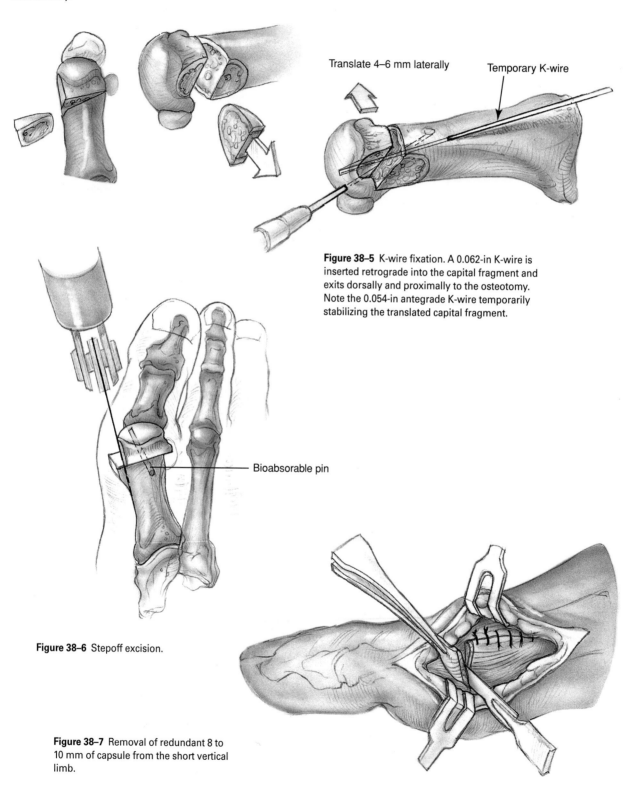

Figure 38–4 Bidirectional chevron osteotomy. Make a 70-degree apex distal cut. The horizontal limb is parallel to the floor. The oblique limb exits dorsally.

Translate 4–6 mm laterally

Temporary K-wire

Figure 38–5 K-wire fixation. A 0.062-in K-wire is inserted retrograde into the capital fragment and exits dorsally and proximally to the osteotomy. Note the 0.054-in antegrade K-wire temporarily stabilizing the translated capital fragment.

Bioabsorbable pin

Figure 38–6 Stepoff excision.

Figure 38–7 Removal of redundant 8 to 10 mm of capsule from the short vertical limb.

Postoperative Care Issues

1. Apply a bulky, bunion compression dressing after surgery. This is removed 5 to 7 days after surgery and a commercial bunion splint is applied.
2. The postoperative shoe is used for 4 weeks. A bunion splint is used at night for an additional 4 weeks. Gym shoes are allowed at this stage using toe spacers.
3. Toe extension exercises are encouraged after the first postoperative visit.

Operative Technique

Approach

1. Prepare and drape the ankle in the hospital's standard sterile fashion ensuring adequate exposure.
2. If a tourniquet is to be utilized, the foot should be exsanguinated and the ankle tourniquet inflated.
3. Make a straight 4-cm medial skin incision centered over the metatarsophalangeal (MTP) joint. Place a retraction skin suture to improve exposure. Elevate dorsal and plantar flaps subfascially with a tenotomy scissors. Identify the dorsal cutaneous nerve.
4. Make an inverted "L"-shaped capsulotomy. The short vertical limb is at the joint and the long horizontal limb is dorsal and proximal (**Fig. 38–2**).

Procedure

5. Expose the metatarsal neck. Remove the exostosis (1 to 2 mm). Caution, one should not be parallel to the shaft of the first metatarsal, but to the medial border of the foot to avoid notching the cortex (**Fig. 38–3**).

6. Make a 70-degree apex distal cut. The horizontal limb is parallel to the floor. The oblique limb exits dorsally. Caution: do not cross the limbs at the center (**Fig. 38–4**).
7. Complete the cuts with thin Mannerfelt osteotomes.
8. Displace the head fibularward by pulling the shaft medially with a Ragnell retractor.
9. If the DMAA is high, make a second dorsal oblique osteotomy. Initially, leave a 1- to 2-mm sliver of bone medially which is subsequently removed.
10. After translation and correction, use a 0.054-in K-wire antegrade to stabilize the head.
11. Insert either an antegrade or retrograde 0.062-in K-wire. The author prefers the retrograde technique beginning in the capital fragment and exiting dorsally and proximally to the osteotomy (**Fig. 38–5**).
12. Measure the length of the pin. Insert a 1.5-mm by either a 20- or 30-mm Bionix (PLLA) pin.
13. If the construct is unstable, add a second pin.
14. Excise the stepoff (**Fig. 38–6**).
15. Perform an adductor tenotomy if needed.
16. Balance the medial capsular tissue. Remove the redundant 8 to 10 mm of capsule from the short vertical limb (**Fig. 38–7**).

Closure

17. Use 2-0 Vicryl suture to perform the capsulorrhaphy.
18. Close the skin with 5-0 Nylon suture. Apply a bulky compression dressing.

Suggested Readings

Kelikian AS. Hallux valgus. In: Kelikian AS, ed. *Operative Treatment of the Foot and Ankle*. Stamford, CT: Appleton & Lange, 1999, pp. 61–94.

CHAPTER 39

Hammer Toe Correction

Armen S. Kelikian

Definitions

1. Mallet toe: flexion deformity at the distal interphalangeal (DIP) joint
2. Hammer toe: flexion deformity at the proximal interphalangeal (PIP) joint and mild extension at the metatarsophalangeal? (MTP) and DIP joints
3. Claw toe: flexion deformity at the PIP joint and hyperextension at the MTP joint
4. Deviated toe: MTP joint in either varus or valgus
5. Crossover toe: medial deviation of the second toe crossing over the first toe with an associated hammer toe deformity
6. Curly toe: the fourth or fifth toes may appear curved, but they are not angulated

Indications

1. Fixed deformity
2. Nonresponsive to conservative measures such as wide toe box shoes and pads, toe crescents

Contraindications

1. Peripheral vascular disease
2. Narcissism

Preoperative Preparation

1. Physical examination
   a. Cock-up test (hyperextension at the MTP joint with plantar pressure)
   b. Lachman test (instability of the second MTP joint)
   c. Assess position of the hallux and first ray.
   d. Examine the foot for associated hard corns, keratoses, and soft corns (clavus).

Special Instruments, Position, and Anesthesia

1. Patient positioned supine on standard operating room table
2. This procedure can de done under local anesthesia.
3. An ankle tourniquet (at 250 mm) is optional.
4. #15 blade
5. Freer elevator
6. Meyerding retractors
7. Double skin hooks
8. Microsagittal saw blade
9. 0.045-, 0.054-, 0.062-in smooth K-wire
10. 3-0 Vicryl sutures
11. 5-0 Nylon sutures

Tips and Pearls

1. A pulse oximeter placed on the toe is an excellent method of checking oxygen delivery to the foot.

What To Avoid

1. If toe circulation is compromised after K-wire instrumentation, it should be removed.

2. If necessary, more of the proximal phalanx may be resected to relax the soft tissue envelope.

Postoperative Care Issues

1. Apply a standard well-padded foot dressing.
2. Remove the K-wires at 3 weeks for PIP joint and DIP arthroplasty, and at 4 weeks when the MTP joint has been crossed.
3. Ambulation should be in stiff-soled postoperative shoes.
4. When the pins are removed, tape the adjacent digits together.

Operative Technique

Approach

1. Prepare and drape the foot in the hospital's standard sterile fashion ensuring adequate exposure available.
2. If a tourniquet is to be utilized, the foot should be exsanguinated and the ankle tourniquet inflated.

Procedure

a. Flexible mallet toes

  i. Make a percutaneous flexor digitorum longus tenotomy through a transverse stab incision at the distal plantarflexion crease.

b. Rigid mallet toes

  i. Make an elliptical incision over the DIP joint (**Fig. 39–1A**).
  ii. Excise skin, tendon and capsule.
  iii. Cut the collateral ligaments and remove the distal 4 to 5 mm of the head of the middle phalanx with an oscillating saw (**Fig. 39–1B**).
  iv. Place a smooth, 0.054-in, K-wire across all three phalanges for about 3 to 4 weeks (**Fig. 39–2**).

c. Flexible hammer toe or a second intermetarsal (IM) space syndrome

  i. A Girdlestone-Taylor flexor to extensor transfer with a dorsal capsular release is appropriate. If there is a fixed hammer toe deformity, this is treated by resection of the distal portion of the proximal phalanx (see below).

  ii. The flexor digitorum longus tendon is harvested through two transverse incisions at the MP and IP creases. The distal portion of the flexor digitorum longus is transected last after being identified with blunt dissection. Alternatively, a longitudinal incision may be made on the volar aspect to harvest the tendon.

  iii. Pass the tendon proximally through the transverse incision at the MTP crease where it lies between the flexor digitorum brevis tendon.

  iv. The two slips of the FDL are split on their raphei. Tie each with a 3-0 Mersilene suture.

  v. The slips of the FDL are passed subperiosteally around the proximal phalanx. They are brought out through a separate dorsal incision over the extensor mechanism centered over the proximal phalanx. With the ankle in neutral position and the toe in 20 degrees of flexion, tie these on to each other and into the extensor hood after step vi.

  vi. Place a 0.062-in K-wire through all the joints. All the joints should be in neutral extension except for the MTP joint which is in 20 degrees of flexion with the ankle at neutral. The wire is left in for 4 weeks.

d. Fixed hammer toe deformities

  i. Make an elliptical incision over the PIP joint (**Fig. 39–1A**).
  ii. Excise the skin and cut the extensor tendon cut. Cut the collateral ligaments from plantar to dorsal, turning the blade at 90 degrees.
  iii. Remove an additional 5 mm of the distal portion of the proximal phalanx (**Fig. 39–1B**).
  iv. Place a 0.054-in K-wire antegrade and retrograde to stabilize the toe and crossing all three phalanges. Check the MTP joint with a cock-up test to ensure that there is no hyperextension. If hyperextension is present, then an extensor tenotomy and dorsal capsular release are necessary. These can be performed through a separate vertical incision over the MTP joint (**Fig. 39–2**).

e. Clawtoe correction (**Fig. 39–3**)

  i. For clawtoe correction, the same procedure is performed at the PIP joint (see section d above).

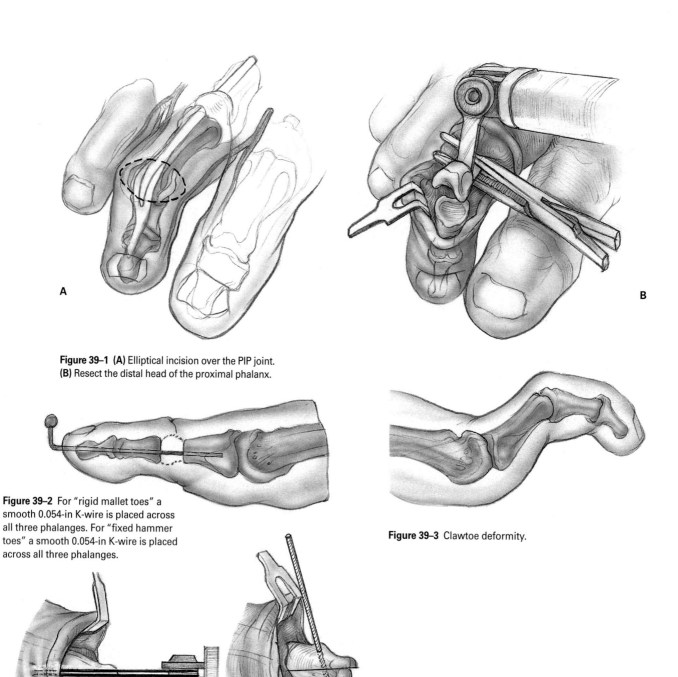

Figure 39–1 (A) Elliptical incision over the PIP joint. **(B)** Resect the distal head of the proximal phalanx.

Figure 39–2 For "rigid mallet toes" a smooth 0.054-in K-wire is placed across all three phalanges. For "fixed hammer toes" a smooth 0.054-in K-wire is placed across all three phalanges.

Figure 39–3 Clawtoe deformity.

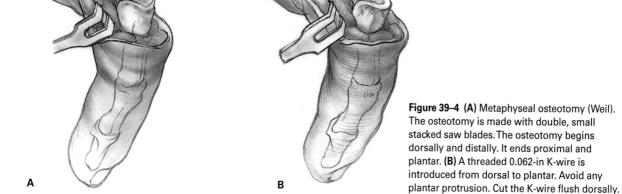

Figure 39–4 (A) Metaphyseal osteotomy (Weil). The osteotomy is made with double, small stacked saw blades. The osteotomy begins dorsally and distally. It ends proximal and plantar. **(B)** A threaded 0.062-in K-wire is introduced from dorsal to plantar. Avoid any plantar protrusion. Cut the K-wire flush dorsally.

For mild deformities, a separate incision may be made over the MTP joint in order to release the dorsal capsule. For moderate claw toe deformities, the author prefers the Sarrafian extensor tenodesis.

ii.   Make a T-incision with the short limb at the PIP joint and the long limb proximal to the MTP joint.

iii. Incise the extensor mechanism at the MTP joint level with the dorsal capsule.

iv.   Free the periosteum, capsule, and extensor mechanism from the lateral band from proximal to distal.

v.   Fold the extensor tendon and retract it distally. Resect the distal 5 to 6 mm of the proximal phalanx after incising the collateral ligaments.

vi.   Make two transverse 0.045-in drill holes 1 cm apart through the proximal phalanx. Pass 3-0 nonabsorbable suture through each pilot hole.

vii. Place an antegrade/retrograde 0.062-in K-wire across the toe and all the joints.

viii. Hold the toe in zero degrees of extension at the DIP and PIP joints and the MTP in 20 degrees of flexion, while the ankle is held in neutral position. The 3-0 nonabsorbable sutures, which were previously passed through the proximal phalanx, are sutured to the extensor tendon which is pulled proximally and then tied.

ix.   The lateral bands are brought dorsally and sutured to the extensor tendon on both sides, both proximal and distal.

Closure

3. The skin is then closed.

Optional (for transfer lesion of the metatarsal)

Always check the adjacent metatarsals for transfer lesions and treat as needed.

a.   If the patient has a transfer lesion of the metatarsal, a plantar DuVries procedure may be performed prior to stabilizing the MTP joint. This is done by removing 25% of the plantar portion of the metatarsal head.

b.   Alternatively, a shortening elevating, oblique, metaphyseal osteotomy (Weil) will achieve the same end as the DuVries condylectomy. If the patient has a relatively long second metatarsal with a transfer lesion, this additional step provides an excellent correction.

i.   Double small saw blades are used stacked on one another. The osteotomy begins dorsally and distally. It ends proximal and plantar (**Fig. 39–4A**).

ii.   The head is shifted dorsally 2 to 3 mm and proximally 6 to 12 mm depending on the correction.

iii. A threaded 0.062-in K-wire is introduced from dorsal to plantar. This should not protrude plantarly. It should be cut flush dorsally (**Fig. 39–4B**).

Suggested Readings

Sarrafian SK. Correction of fixed hammer toe deformities with resection of the heads of the proximal phalanx and extensor tendon tenodesis. *Foot Ankle Int* 1995;16:449–451.

Watson AD, Anderson RB, Davis WH. Toe deformities. In: Kelikian AS, ed. *Operative Treatment of the Foot and Ankle*. Stamford, CT: Appleton & Lange, 1999, pp. 99–115.

CHAPTER 40

Morton's Neuroma Excision

Steven Kodros

➤ Morton's neuromas are felt to be secondary to perineural fibrosis that develops around the interdigital nerve. About 90% of Morton's neuromas occur in the third interspace.

➤ Only about 10% of Morton's neuromas occur in the second interspace. Therefore, remember to consider other possible causes for metatarsalgia symptoms in this area.

Indications

1. Patients with Morton's neuromas who have failed nonoperative treatment (e.g., accommodative shoes, metatarsal pad, cortisone injection)

Contraindications

1. Dysvascular disease
2. Patients with conditions that may increase the risk of wound healing problems (e.g., peripheral vascular disease, diabetes mellitus, heavy tobacco use) (relative)

Preoperative Preparation

1. If circulatory status is questionable (e.g., elderly patients, diabetics, etc.), consider obtaining noninvasive arterial blood flow studies (with absolute toe pressures).
2. Inform patients about permanent numbness of affected toes that results from successful neuroma excision.

Special Instruments, Position, and Anesthesia

1. The procedure can be done under an ankle block with the use of monitored anesthesia care and intravenous sedation. Alternatively, general or other methods of regional anesthesia can be employed.
2. An ankle tourniquet (just above the malleoli) is utilized and set at 250 mm Hg.
3. A small laminar spreader, which can be placed between the respective metatarsals, facilitates exposure.

Tips and Pearls

1. Perform the ankle block prior to prepping and draping the extremity. This helps ensure that there is an adequate amount of time for the block to achieve optimal effectiveness after it has been performed.
2. Elevating the limb for a couple of minutes before tourniquet inflation can exsanguinate the foot.
3. When the proximal portion of the nerve is excised, be sure that a hemostat clamp is used to apply distally directed longitudinal traction on the nerve. A Freer elevator can be used retract the soft tissues proximally and then the nerve should be transected sharply as proximal as possible within the wound. These efforts allow the proximal end of the cut nerve to retract proximally within the midfoot and thereby minimize the risk of developing a symptomatic stump neuroma.

4. The tourniquet should be deflated after the neuroma is excised and before the closure. This helps confirm both that hemostasis has been obtained and that good capillary refill and viability of the respective toes are present.

What To Avoid

1. Avoid attempting to excise neuromas in adjacent interspaces at the same operative sitting. There is always a chance that the digital artery can be injured during the excision of a neuroma. If this were to happen on both sides of a toe, the viability of that toe could be compromised.

Postoperative Care Issues

1. Place the foot in a gentle compression dressing.
2. The patient is allowed to be full weight bearing in a postoperative or wooden shoe. However, weight bearing should be kept to an absolute minimum during the first 12 hours.
3. The dressing is removed 1 week after surgery. However, the sutures should not be removed until 3 weeks after surgery to ensure that complete healing of the wound has occurred.
4. The postoperative shoe should be used for 3 weeks after surgery. After this period of time the patient may progress to an accommodative tennis shoe.

Operative Technique

Approach

1. Position the patient supine on the operating room table. Place a rolled blanket beneath the ipsilateral buttock to internally rotate the limb. Place the ankle tourniquet just above the malleoli.
2. Perform an ankle block with a 1:1 mixture of 1% lidocaine and 0.5% bupivicaine solution (without epinephrine).
3. Prepare and drape the limb in a sterile fashion. Exsanguinate the foot and inflate the tourniquet to 250 mm Hg.

4. Make a longitudinal incision over the dorsum of the involved interspace. This should start at the distal most extent of the web space and extend proximally for about 3 to 4 cm (**Fig. 40–1**).
5. Use careful blunt dissection to deepen the exposure down through the subcutaneous tissue. Cauterize small veins to maintain hemostasis.
6. Identify the transverse intermetatarsal ligament. Place a small laminar spreader between the metatarsals proximal to this structure (**Fig. 40–2**).
7. Bluntly dissect below (plantar) to the transverse intermetatarsal ligament. Isolate the transverse intermetatarsal ligament and then divide it (**Fig. 40–3**).
8. Add additional distraction to the laminar spreader to separate the metatarsals. This will expose the nerve and neuroma.

Neuroma excision

9. Gently free up the nerve and neuroma from the adjacent digital vessels with blunt dissection.
10. Follow the terminal digital branches of the nerve into their respective toes. Transect these terminal branches sharply in the distal most extent of the wound.
11. Proceeding in a distal to proximal direction, dissect and free up the nerve and neuroma.
12. Sharply transect the nerve as far proximal as possible. This is done by maintaining distally directed longitudinal traction on the nerve with hemostat clamp and by retracting the proximal soft tissues with a Freer elevator (**Fig. 40–4**).
13. Remove the nerve and neuroma. Inspect the interspace to confirm that you have excised all abnormal-appearing neural tissue.
14. Remove the laminar spreader and deflate the tourniquet. Confirm adequate hemostasis and good capillary refill of the toes.

Closure

15. Irrigate the wound.
16. Close only the skin using interrupted 4-0 nylon sutures.
17. Apply a sterile dressing to the wound. Place the foot into a gentle compression dressing.
18. Transfer the patient to the recovery room.

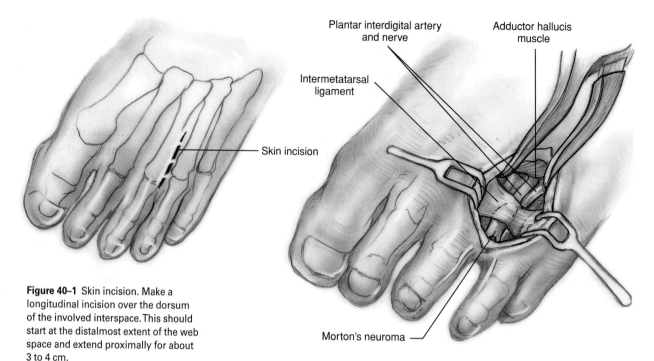

Figure 40–1 Skin incision. Make a longitudinal incision over the dorsum of the involved interspace. This should start at the distalmost extent of the web space and extend proximally for about 3 to 4 cm.

Figure 40–2 Superficial dissection. A small laminar spreader is placed between the metatarsals allowing visualization of the transverse intermetatarsal ligament and the underlying neurovascular structures.

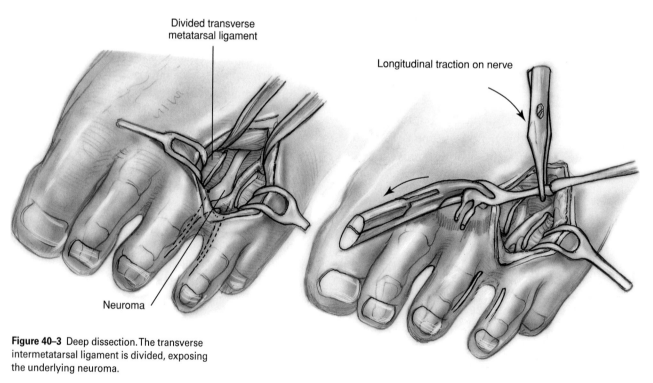

Figure 40–3 Deep dissection. The transverse intermetatarsal ligament is divided, exposing the underlying neuroma.

Figure 40–4 Nerve excision. The nerve is sharply transected as far proximal as possible. This is done by maintaining distally directed longitudinal traction on the nerve with hemostat clamp and by retracting the proximal soft tissues with a Freer elevator.

Suggested Readings

Kodros SA. Armamentarium and implants. In: Kelikian AS, ed. *Operative Treatment of the Foot and Ankle*. Stamford, CT: Appleton & Lange, 1999, pp. 53–60.

Kodros SA. Nerve entrapment. In: Kelikian AS, ed. *Operative Treatment of the Foot and Ankle*. Stamford, CT: Appleton & Lange, 1999, pp. 201–210.

CHAPTER 41

Proximal Fifth Metatarsal Jones Fractures

Internal Fixation

Steven Kodros

➤ Jones fractures are transverse fractures located at the proximal metaphyseal-diaphyseal junction of the fifth metatarsal.

➤ Jones fractures have a much higher incidence of developing a symptomatic nonunion or fibrous union than simple avulsion fractures of the fifth metatarsal tuberosity (located more proximally) **(Fig. 41–1)**.

➤ Commonly, nonoperative treatment includes a short leg cast and non-weight-bearing for 6 to 8 weeks. After this period, patients can be converted to either a short leg brace or walking cast which is maintained until fracture union has occurred (usually another 6 to 8 weeks).

Indications

1. Proximal fifth metatarsal (Jones) fractures that fail to show progression toward bony union after treatment in a non-weight-bearing short-leg cast for 6 to 8 weeks

2. Acute proximal fifth metatarsal (Jones) fractures in young athletic individuals who wish to shorten the time to return to sport and minimize the prolonged course of immobilization and rehabilitation that is associated with nonoperative treatment

3. Proximal fifth metatarsal (Jones) fractures in patients who desire surgical management, as opposed to nonoperative treatment

4. Stress fractures, delayed unions, or nonunions of the proximal fifth metatarsal

Contraindications

1. Medullary canal diameter that is too small to accommodate an adequate-sized screw

2. Patients with conditions that may increase the risk of wound healing problems (e.g., peripheral vascular disease, diabetes mellitus, heavy tobacco use) (relative)

Preoperative Preparation

1. Determine the appropriate screw size by measuring the width of the fifth metatarsal's medullary canal on the preoperative radiographs. Commonly, a screw that is between 4.5 and 6.5 mm in size will usually provide appropriate canal fill and purchase and have adequate strength for internal fixation.

Special Instruments, Position, and Anesthesia

1. A cannulated screw system will facilitate intramedullary screw placement when using a "relatively" percutaneous technique.
2. Intraoperative fluoroscopy and a radiolucent operating table are necessary for accurate screw placement.
3. The patient is positioned supine on the operating table with a large padded roll placed beneath the ipsilateral buttock. This helps to internally rotate the affected extremity.
4. The procedure can be done under an ankle block with the use of monitored anesthesia care and intravenous sedation. Alternatively, general or other methods of regional anesthesia can be employed.
5. An ankle tourniquet (just above the malleoli) is utilized and set at 250 mm Hg.

Tips and Pearls

1. Prior to the procedure, ensure that adequate fluoroscopic images of the fifth metatarsal can be obtained in multiple projections, including anteroposterior, lateral, and oblique views.
2. Prior to the skin incision, place a guide wire directly over the shaft of the fifth metatarsal. Assess its position with fluoroscopic images in the anteroposterior and lateral planes. Use a marking pen to draw lines along the guide wire. These lines will help you to achieve proper placement of the intraoperative intramedullary guide wire.
3. If the initial position of the intraoperative intramedullary guide wire is undesirable, try to reposition it while spinning the drill in reverse (counterclockwise). This helps to prevent the threaded tip of the guide wire from engaging the previous track.
4. If a solid intramedullary screw is desired, the guide wire and cannulated drill bit from a cannulated screw system can be used (if the cannulated drill bit is of the appropriate diameter) to facilitate accurate intramedullary placement of the hole.
5. If a fully threaded screw is used, the near (proximal) segment of the fifth metatarsal should be over drilled to the diameter of the screw. This creates a gliding hole and allows for interfragmentary compression across the fracture site.

What To Avoid

1. Avoid using a screw with a diameter that is too large for the medullary canal of the fifth metatarsal. This can result in an iatrogenic fracture of the fifth metatarsal.
2. Attempt to avoid injuring branches of the sural nerve and developing an incisional neuroma by bluntly dissecting through the subcutaneous tissue.

Postoperative Care Issues

1. The extremity should be placed in a short-leg splint or cast immediately after surgery. Strict non-weight bearing is maintained for the affected foot.
2. At 2 weeks postsurgery, the sutures are removed and the extremity placed in a short leg brace. Early functional rehabilitation exercises for the foot and ankle can be started.
3. For acute fractures at 2 weeks postsurgery, weight bearing can be advanced as tolerated in the short leg brace. At 6 weeks postsurgery, the short leg brace may be discontinued if early fracture healing is apparent radiographically.
4. For nonunions and for some stress fractures, weight bearing should be deferred for approximately 4 to 6 weeks postsurgery and the short leg brace continued until follow-up radiographs show clear signs of fracture healing.

Operative Technique

1. Position the patient supine on the operating room table. Place a rolled blanket beneath the ipsilateral buttock to internally rotate the limb. Place the ankle tourniquet just above the malleoli.
2. Perform an ankle block with a 1:1 mixture of 1% lidocaine and 0.5% bupivicaine solution (without epinephrine).
3. Prepare and drape the limb in a sterile fashion. Exsanguinate the foot and inflate the tourniquet to 250 mm Hg.

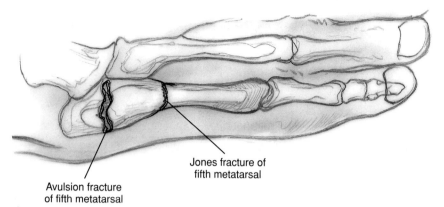

Figure 41–1 Fifth metatarsal fractures. Fifth metatarsal showing location of a tuberosity avulsion fracture and a transverse Jones fracture located at the proximal metaphyseal-diaphyseal junction.

Jones fracture of
fifth metatarsal

Avulsion fracture
of fifth metatarsal

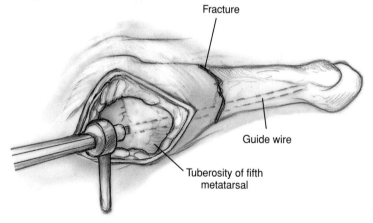

Figure 41–2 Skin incision. A longitudinal incision is made along the lateral aspect of the midfoot. It extends proximally from the tip of the fifth metatarsal tuberosity for about 3 cm.

Skin incision

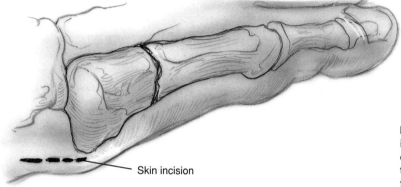

Fracture

Guide wire

Tuberosity of fifth
metatarsal

Figure 41–3 Guide wire placement. Position the guide wire's soft tissue sleeve so that it is directly on the tip of the fifth metatarsal tuberosity. Confirm its location with anteroposterior and lateral fluoroscopic images.

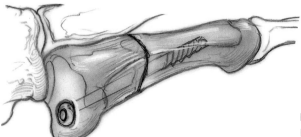

Figure 41–4 Screw position. The final position of the screw is confirmed with the fluoroscopic images.

4. Make a longitudinal incision along the lateral aspect of the midfoot. It should start at the tip of the fifth metatarsal tuberosity and extend proximally about 3 cm (**Fig. 41–2**).

5. Use careful blunt dissection to deepen the exposure down to the tip of the fifth metatarsal tuberosity.

6. Position the guide wire's soft tissue sleeve so that it is directly on the tip of the fifth metatarsal tuberosity. Confirm its location with anteroposterior and lateral fluoroscopic images (**Fig. 41–3**).

7. Orient the shaft of the soft tissue sleeve so it is in line with the shaft of the fifth metatarsal.

8. Drill the guide wire through the soft tissue sleeve and into the fifth metatarsal.

9. Confirm accurate intramedullary placement of the guide wire with fluoroscopy. Multiple projections should be assessed including anteroposterior, lateral, and oblique views.

10. Use the depth gauge to determine the appropriate length for the screw.

11. Drill over the guide wire with the appropriate cannulated drill bit inserted through the soft tissue protector. Periodically stop and remove the drill bit to clean bone debris from its flutes to prevent clogging.

12. Insert the screw over the guide wire. Advance it into the fifth metatarsal.

13. Once the screw has entered the metatarsal's medullary canal, withdraw the guide wire back into the screw. This minimizes the chance of it breaking or becoming incarcerated in the bone. However, do not completely remove the guide wire from the screw until the screw's final position is confirmed as satisfactory with the image intensifier.

14. Assess the screw's final position with fluoroscopic images in the anteroposterior and lateral planes (**Fig. 41–4**).

15. Deflate the tourniquet, confirm hemostasis, and irrigate the wound.

16. Close only the skin using interrupted 4-0 nylon sutures.

17. Apply a sterile dressing to the wound. Place the foot in a well-padded short-leg splint or cast.

Suggested Readings

Kodros SA. Armamentarium and implants. In: Kelikian AS, ed. *Operative Treatment of the Foot and Ankle.* Stamford, CT: Appleton & Lange, 1999, pp. 53–60.

Lawrence SJ, Botte MJ. Jones fractures and related fractures of the proximal fifth metatarsal. *Foot Ankle* 1993;14:358–365.

Trevino SG, Williams RL, Siff TE. Lisfranc and proximal fifth metatarsal injuries. In: Kelikian AS, ed: *Operative Treatment of the Foot and Ankle.* Stamford, CT: Appleton & Lange, 1999, pp. 455–493.

Section Seven

Spine

CHAPTER 42

Lumbar Discectomy

Srdjan Mirkovic

Indications

1. Bowel and bladder dysfunction (absolute)
2. Failure of conservative management (relative)
3. Recurrent sciatica (relative)
4. Duration of symptoms greater than three months (relative)

Contraindications

1. Painless herniated nucleus propulsus (HNP)
2. Ongoing infection
3. Significant nonorganic findings
4. Lack of concordance between clinical presentation, anatomic level, physical examination, and imaging study
5. Low back pain only

Preoperative Preparation

1. Anteroposterior (AP) lateral radiographs of the lumbar spine
2. Imaging studies (MRI, CT, CT myelogram)
3. Neurological evaluation, psychological assessment, and sciatic tension signs
4. Medical and anesthetic evaluation
5. Intravenous antibiotics prior to surgery

Special Instruments, Position, and Anesthesia

1. The patient is placed either prone on chest rolls with hips and knees extended or in the 90-degree knee chest position.
2. Antiembolic stockings and/or compression boots are used.
3. Consider inserting a Foley catheter in older individuals.
4. The arms are placed in a 90/90 position to avoid brachial plexus traction.
5. All pressure points are padded, specifically the chest, elbows, and knees.
6. In males, the groin is checked to ensure no compression.
7. The procedure can be done under general, spinal, or local anesthesia. If not medically contraindicated, consider hypotensive anesthesia with a mean pressure of less than 70 mm Hg which helps minimize epidural bleeding.
8. The procedure is performed under microscope or loop magnification and light augmentation. If using loops, a fiber optic head light is used.
9. Basic lumbar spinal instruments: rongeurs, pituitaries, kerrosens, bipolar cautery, Penfield retractors, gelfoam, thrombin, Cobb elevators, special self-retaining retractors, and either a microscope or loops
10. Consider using spinal cord monitoring.

Tips and Pearls

1. Ensure that the abdomen hangs free in order to diminish venous compression and help control epidural bleeding.
2. The patient should be completely paralyzed in order to facilitate paravertebral muscle retraction.
3. Only approach paracentral disc herniations on the affected side, thereby leaving the contralateral musculature intact. Central disc herniations represent an exception to this rule and should be approached bilaterally.
4. During the procedure, the nerve root should be retracted intermittently while instrumentation is within the discs. This avoids battering the nerve root.
5. Review the patient's history and imaging studies preoperatively in order to ensure that the surgery is performed at the right level and on the appropriate side. Preoperatively ask the patient to indicate the side of his lower extremity symptoms. Mentally, re-check the level and side prior to making the incision and ensure that you are standing on the appropriate side.
6. In males, the top of the iliac crest approximates the L4-L5 level. Avoid rolling your fingers over the iliac crest, which would place the incision at a higher level. The posterosuperior iliac spines approximate the L5-S1 level.
7. To palpate the midline in obese patients, start at a higher level until the spinous processes are felt and line these up with the intergluteal fold.
8. Check the level intraoperatively by placing a radiopaque marker at the surgical site and obtaining lateral X-rays.
9. Assess the presence of spinal anomalies such as spina bifida or abnormal lumbosacral segmentation.

What To Avoid

1. Avoid operating at the wrong level. The tendency is to be too high, particularly in the presence of marked lumbar lordosis.
2. Avoid ignoring a lack of correlation between intraoperative findings and preoperative imaging and physical examination.
3. Avoid missing extruded disc fragments.

Postoperative Care Issues

1. The majority of patients are discharged within 24 to 48 hours.
2. Patients are discharged once they are ambulating; their preoperative symptoms have resolved or are markedly diminished; they have normal bowel and bladder function, are tolerating oral intake, and are not nauseated.
3. Patients are seen in follow-up at two weeks, at which time a cardiovascular conditioning program is instituted. Low back strengthening and conditioning programs are instituted at four weeks postoperatively. Patients involved in heavy labor may require a more prolonged course of physical therapy and possible work hardening.
4. Individuals with sedentary jobs can return to work within 10 to 20 days. Those involved in heavier labor return to work between 3 and 5 months.
5. Postoperative analgesia includes nonsteroidal anti-inflammatories and limited narcotic medication.

Operative Technique

1. Position the patient prone on chest rolls or a Jackson table. Ensure that the abdomen hangs free. Inspect the eyes, ulnar nerves, male genitalia, and the breasts in females to ensure that there are no areas of excessive pressure on the skin.
2. Prepare and drape the back in the hospital's normal sterile fashion.
3. Place an 18-gauge spinal needle at the presumed pathologic level. Use anatomic landmarks to assist in placement. The tip of the iliac crest approximates the L4-L5 level and posterosuperior iliac spine approximates the L5-S1 level. Orient the needle laterally to avoid puncture of the dura. Use either lateral X-ray or lateral fluoroscopy to confirm appropriate needle level.
4. Make a 3- to 4-cm midline incision. Carry this down through the underlying subcutaneous tissues to the level of the lumbodorsal fascia.
5. Coagulate all bleeding vessels using electrocautery. Attempt to maintain a dry field at all times.
6. Retract the soft tissues with a Cobb elevator, while an assistant uses Army-Navy retractors.

7. Use electrocautery to incise the tip of the spinous processes at the desired level.

8. Dissect the paravertebral muscles from the lateral aspect of the spinous processes on the affected side. Dissect down to the lamina. Take care to minimize damage to the intraspinous-supraspinous ligaments. Limit periosteal muscle dissection to the interlaminar level being exposed.

9. Place a self-retaining McCullough retractor.

10. Cauterize all over-hanging soft tissue. If necessary, remove the bulbous facet joints with a burr to optimize visualization. Limit exposure for a one level disc excision to the affected interlaminar level with partial visualization of the superior and inferior laminae (**Fig. 42–1**). If the disc fragment is extruded, additional laminotomy or hemilaminectomy, either cephalad or caudally depending on the level of disc herniation, may be necessary. If a more extensive exposure is required, identification of the parts should be performed to prevent iatrogenic fracture during decompression.

11. Identify the fat pad which commonly overlies the superolateral laminae at the base of the superior facet. Dissect the soft tissues overlying the ligamentum flavum in the interlaminar space. Excise the soft tissues with a pituitary using the fat pad as a safe landmark. Use intermittent bipolar cautery to control all bleeding.

12. Visualize the ligament flavum. It is bordered by the lamina superiorly and inferiorly and the facet joint laterally.

13. Debulk the ligamentum flavum. Scrape it in a distal to proximal direction, starting from its distal insertion at the superior aspect of the caudal lamina. This thins down the ligamentum flavum and facilitates subsequent removal or reflection.

14. Use a kerrosen rongeur to perform a hemilaminotomy or laminectomy. Remove the inferior edge of the superior laminae and the superior aspect of the inferior laminae (**Fig. 42–2**). If additional exposure is needed, perform a medial facetectomy by removing the most medial aspect of the superior facet. This allows excellent visualization of the underlying ligamentum flavum.

15. Use a 2-0 angled Epstein curette to reflect the insertion of the inferior aspect of the ligamentum flavum into the superior aspect of the caudal lamina. This allows visualization into the spinal canal. Do this in a gentle and controlled manner to avoid injury to the dura.

16. Dissect the ligamentum flavum with a 3-P Epstein curette. Initially, dissect laterally under the facet and then extend the dissection superiorly.

17. Insert a short ball-ended probe underneath the ligamentum flavum to free-up the residual attachment of the ligament inferiorly, laterally, and superiorly.

If the interlaminar defect is congenitally large:

 a. Preserve the medial insertion of the ligamentum flavum along its medial raphae.
 b. Reflect the ligamentum flavum medially.
 c. At the procedure's completion, drape it over the dura to minimize scarring.

If the interlaminar defect is not congenitally large:

 a. Excise the ligamentum flavum in its entirety.
 b. Grasp the ligament with fine forceps with teeth. Excise it using kerrosens or a #15 blade. Curettes may also be used (**Fig. 42–3**).

18. Once in the spinal canal, identify the lateral edge of the nerve root using a #4 Penfield or a blunt freer. If the lateral aspect of the nerve root cannot be identified, search for the corresponding pedicle. The distal medial aspect of the nerve root courses around the pedicle. If identification remains difficult, consider several factors. Failure to recognize lateral recess stenosis can lead to persistent nerve root compression and unsatisfactory postoperative result.

➤ Lateral recess stenosis caused by degenerative osteophytes from the medial aspect of the superior facet can obscure the nerve root. Excise the osteophytes using a 2-mm Kerrosen. This allows safe visualization of the lateral aspect of the nerve root.

➤ A disc fragment in the axilla may displace the nerve root medially.

➤ Fibrovascular inflammatory changes may encase the nerve root, obliterating visualization.

➤ Congenital nerve root anomalies may hinder dissection.

19. Once the nerve root is identified, handle it gently. Apply only the force necessary to retract the nerve root. Avoid stretching it. Use the nerve root retractor

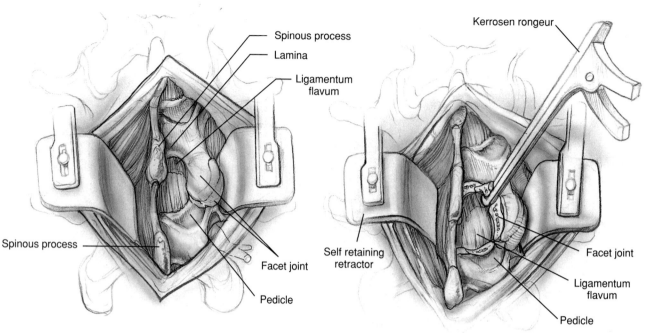

Figure 42–1 Lumbar musculature. The paravertebral muscles are dissected from the lateral aspect of the spinous processes on the affected side down to the lamina. The muscle dissection is limited to the interlaminar level being exposed.

Figure 42–2 Unilateral laminotomy. A kerrosen rongeur can be used to perform a hemilaminotomy or laminectomy. This is done by removing the inferior edge of the superior laminae and the superior aspect of the inferior laminae.

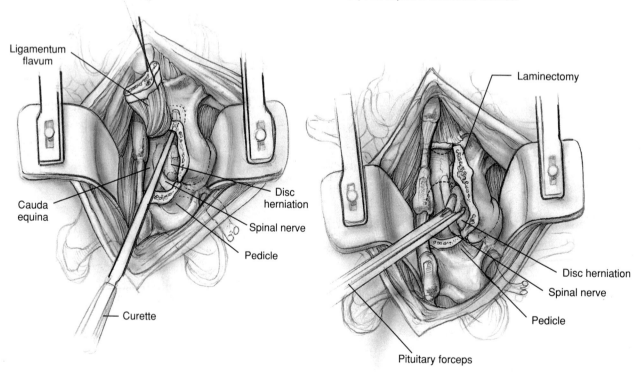

Figure 42–3 Unilateral flavectomy. The ligamentum flavum is excised. This can be accomplished with a Kerrosen, a #15 blade, or a curette.

Figure 42–4 Laminectomy. The herniated disc is removed with the appropriate size pituitary.

blade to protect the root from instruments at all times. Keep the retractor in gentle contact with the underlying disc and annulus to prevent the nerve from slipping under the retractor blade. Avoid pulling dorsally on the nerve root.

20. If adhesions are encountered, release can be accomplished with bipolar cautery and sharp dissection.

21. If ligaments such as the Hoffman ligament are encountered, incise these to free up the nerve root and dura.

22. When retraction is not needed, release tension on the retractor to minimize trauma to the nerve root.

23. Control bleeding with bipolar cautery and gelfoam impregnated in thrombin. Adequate suction expedites surgery. Have several suction tips available to allow for a quick exchange when a sucker tip becomes plugged.

24. Once the nerve root is retracted, identify the underlying annulus.

25. If a rent in the annulus with partial disc extrusion is encountered, use a #15 or #11 blade facing away from the nerve to extend the annular rent. This decreases the likelihood of nerve root damage.

26. Make a cruciate annular incision.

27. Place a blunt nerve hook through the incision. Free-up the disc material into the epidural space.

28. Remove the herniated disc with an appropriate size pituitary. Grasp additional small disc fragments within the intervertebral disc (Fig. 42–4). A discectomy limited to the herniated disc fragments is recommended.

29. Once the disc has been removed, pass a long ball-ended probe anterior to the dura and nerve root. This ensures the absence of extruded disc fragments. The nerve root should be easily retractable for a distance of about 1 cm. Commonly, nerve root pulsations are observed at this junction. Perform two valsalva maneuvers to 50 mm of Hg pressure with the field dry and the dura visualized. Absence of CSF fluid ensures that no occult dural tears have occurred.

Wound closure

30. Copiously irrigate the wound with antibiotic solution.

31. If possible, maintain a dry field to minimize postoperative scarring. Placement of a drain is not necessary if the field is dry.

32. Drape the preserved ligamentum flavum over the dura. If adequate ligamentum flavum is not available, place gelfoam impregnated in thrombin over the interlaminar defect.

33. Close the paravertebral fascia with 1-0 Vicryl. Close subcutaneous tissue with 2-0 Vicryl. Close the skin in a routine fashion.

34. Dress the wound with a sterile dressing.

Selected Readings

Abdullah AF, Wolper BG, Warfield JR, Gunadi IK. Surgical management of extreme lateral lumbar disc herniations: review of 138 cases. *Neurosurgery* 1988; 22:648–653.

McCullough JA. *Principles of Microsurgery for Lumbar Disc Disease.* New York, NY: Raven Press, 1989.

Spengler DM, Ouellette E, Battier M, Zeh J. Elective discectomy for herniation of a lumbar disc. *J Bone Joint Surg* 1990;72:230–237.

Weber H. Lumbar disc herniations: a controlled perspective study with ten years of observation. *Spine* 1983;8:131–140.

CHAPTER 43

Anterior Approach to the Cervical Spine

Discectomy, Fusion, and Vertebrectomy

Serena S. Hu

Indications

1. Patients with radiculopathy, pain, numbness or weakness in a dermatomal distribution, who require anterior discectomy and fusion; symptoms should correlate with the anatomic studies.
2. Vertebral corpectomy (i.e., a burst fracture with canal compromise, infection or tumor) **(Fig. 43–6A)**
3. Patients with cervical spondylosis who also have myelopathy, secondary to posterior osteophytes, or ossification of the posterior longitudinal ligament (OPLL); these patients may require anterior decompression via multiple level discectomies and fusion or corpectomy(ies).
4. In general, the standard anterior approach can be used to reach pathology from C4 to C7, although occasionally C3 or T1 can be reached in patients with long thin necks. Because of the mandible and collarbone, it is difficult to gain full anterior access to the ends of the exposure. Consequently, screw placement or other surgery at the incision ends can be difficult if not impossible.

Contraindications

1. In patients with greater than three levels of vertebral involvement, with adequate cervical lordosis, extensive OPLL is considered a relative contraindication. In these patients consider a posterior approach and laminaplasty.

Preoperative Preparation

1. Determine how many levels must be addressed surgically. Some surgeons feel that a partial vertebrectomy should be performed if multiple levels are involved. This allows a single bone graft to be placed in the trough, thereby requiring only two bony surfaces to heal to the host bone rather than the 4 or 6 that are needed if separate grafts are placed at each level. Others feel that with anterior plates, the fusion rate is acceptable even with three levels of bone graft.
2. Determine whether discectomies or corpectomies should be performed.
3. Determine if instrumentation is indicated. If so, the levels and construct to be utilized should be planned prior to surgery.

Special Instruments, Position, and Anesthesia

1. The surgery is performed under general anesthesia.
2. Either a left- or right-sided approach can be utilized. The left-sided approach is preferred by many surgeons because the recurrent laryngeal nerve has a more predictable distal course on the neck's left side. Conversely, others prefer the right-sided approach because it is technically easier for a right-handed surgeon to work on the patient's right side.

3. The endotracheal tube should be taped opposite to the side of the approach.

4. The patient is positioned with a small folded towel placed between the shoulder blades to allow the shoulders to fall back.

5. Consider stabilizing the patient's head on a horseshoe (Mayfield) headrest in light (5 to 15 pounds) head halter traction. If desired, additional traction can be applied during bone graft placement.

6. Pull the patient's shoulders distally and tape them to the end of the table to facilitate adequate X-ray localization. It can be difficult to balance the degree of shoulder traction needed to afford adequate X-ray visualization with the possibility of a traction injury to the brachial plexus.

7. The patient's anterior iliac crest can be elevated slightly on a sandbag or folded towel.

Tips and Pearls

1. One or two disc levels can be easily reached through a transverse incision; for greater numbers of levels, a longitudinal incision along the anterior aspect of the sternocleidomastoid muscle can be used.

2. Many patients have posterior osteophytes that encroach on the spinal canal. Some surgeons feel that after a fusion, these osteophytes will resorb over time; conversely others feel that osteophyte removal results in faster relief of symptoms. To remove osteophytes, they can be thinned with a high-speed burr and then the remaining cortical edge hooked and removed piecemeal with a small microcurette.

3. Graft measurement includes both the height and depth of the graft. Generally grafts for cervical discectomies are 6 to 7 mm in height and 1.5 cm in depth. In general, the minimum graft height for adequate compressive strength and appropriate neural foramen enlargement is 5 mm.

4. If a vertebrectomy has been performed, the graft harvest should take into account the additional length needed to key in the ends of the graft for maximum stability (see Fig. 43–5B). If greater than two levels of vertebra are removed, the iliac crest may not be of adequate length and fibula graft may be preferable.

5. When multiple levels of discectomy are performed, or if corpectomy has been performed for fracture or myelopathy, anterior plate fixation may be used for additional stability. While bicortical purchase is generally optimal for plate stability, the neurologic risk associated with it is not insignificant. Thus, most modern anterior cervical plate systems utilize unicortical purchase and lock the screws to the plate to prevent the screws from backing out. Halo fixation is also an alternative, although not as rigid a construct.

6. For patients with significant pre-existing neurologic deficits, particularly myelopathy, some surgeons prefer to use spinal cord monitoring.

7. Dural injury is more common with significant OPLL as the dura may be attenuated or adherent.

8. Deteriorating neurologic function needs to be investigated for cause, and oftentimes treated with steroids. MRI or CT scan may demonstrate hematoma or bony encroachment and should be promptly addressed.

What To Avoid

1. Attempt to avoid injury to the spinal cord, nerve roots or dura. Be especially wary of instrument penetration secondary to inadvertent deep placement (especially during posterior osteophyte removal), excessive depth of bone graft placement, or over distraction.

2. Protect the thyroid gland, trachea and esophagus by retracting the strap muscles medially. In particular, esophageal perforation can lead to abscess, fistula or mediastinal involvement.

3. Avoid injury to the sympathetic chain, which can result in Horner's syndrome. The sympathetic chain lies on the anterior aspect of the longus colli. Damage can be minimized by carefully dividing the longus colli in the midline and using the bipolar cautery rather than bovie cautery when possible.

4. Attempt to minimize airway problems particularly during prolonged procedures and in patients with cervical spinal cord injury. In these cases, consider prolonged intubation (2 to 3 days) to permit pharyngeal edema to decrease. Remember hoarseness may occur secondary to edema or retraction but

rarely occurs if the recurrent laryngeal nerve is injured.

Postoperative Care Issues

1. For postoperative immobilization use a Philadelphia collar or 4-poster brace, depending on the surgeon's preference.
2. Elevate the head of the bed to decrease postoperative swelling.

Operative Technique

Approach

1. Use surface landmarks to approximate the level of the incision. The thyroid cartilage is at the C4-5 disc space, and the cricoid cartilage is anterior to the C6 vertebra. Palpate Chassaignac's tubercle on C6; this is fairly easy to locate on thin patients but may be more difficult in a more muscular neck.
2. Once the approximate level of the incision is localized, tape a large-gauge needle or other metallic marker to the skin along the lateral aspect of the neck. Take a localizing X-ray to confirm the level of incision.
3. Prepare the neck past the midline. Ensure that the area prepped extends inferiorly to the clavicle, superiorly to the jawline, and posteriorly to the mid-coronal line. Prepare the iliac crest as well.
4. Make the incision along Langer's lines, adjusted as necessary based on the localizing X-ray. Begin at the neck's midline and extend the incision to the middle of the bulk of the sternocleidomastoid muscle (**Fig. 43–1**).
5. Incise the platysma muscle along the line of the incision with a needle-tipped bovie cautery. This muscle is more developed in men, and sometimes difficult to identify as a distinct muscle in women.
6. Undermine this layer with a metzenbaum scissors. Identify and develop the interval between the sternocleidomastoid and the strap muscles (**Fig. 43–2**).
7. If needed, ligate tributaries to the external jugular vein. Identify the carotid sheath by palpation of the artery's pulse. Do not dissect the sheath out (or risk damage to the carotid artery, internal jugular vein or vagus nerve).
8. Retract the carotid laterally. Develop the plane anterior to it with blunt dissection (a peanut or a gloved finger) until the prevertebral fascia lying on the anterior spine is palpated (**Fig. 43–2**).
9. Use hand held retractors to displace the strap muscles medially, protecting the thyroid gland, trachea and esophagus (**Fig. 43–3**). Avoid damage to these structures. Esophageal perforation can lead to abscess, fistula or mediastinal involvement. Above C4, the superior thyroid artery may be encountered; below C6, the inferior thyroid artery may be encountered. These should be ligated if the exposure requires it.
10. Identify the longus colli on the anterior aspect of the spine. Locate disc spaces by palpating the prominences ("hills"); the vertebral bodies are the concavities ("valleys") (**Fig. 43–4**).
11. Avoid damage to the sympathetic chain, which lies on the anterior aspect of the longus colli. Damage can be minimized by taking care to divide the longus colli in the midline and using the bipolar cautery rather than the bovie cautery when possible. Injury to the sympathetics can result in Horner's syndrome. Identify the midline as the area of thinnest muscle between the two defined bellies of the longus colli muscles. The longus colli muscle bellies run just lateral to the midline on both sides.
12. Use a key elevator to mobilize the longus colli laterally along the anterior aspect of the spine. Commonly, some vessels within the muscle will bleed and must be cauterized using bipolar cautery. Bleeding from the anterior vertebral bodies can be addressed using bone wax, applied using either a peanut or a Penfield elevator.
13. After one disc space has been identified, take a localizing X-ray with a spinal needle placed in the disc space. Bend or clamp the needle to prevent it from migrating in the disc or the field. In severely degenerated spines, anterior osteophytes may preclude needle placement into the disc space. If this occurs, use a ronguer to remove the osteophytes.
14. If the correct level is marked, proceed with the exposure. Otherwise, extend the exposure.
15. Expose the vertebral body laterally to just beyond the uncovertebral joints. These can be identified as

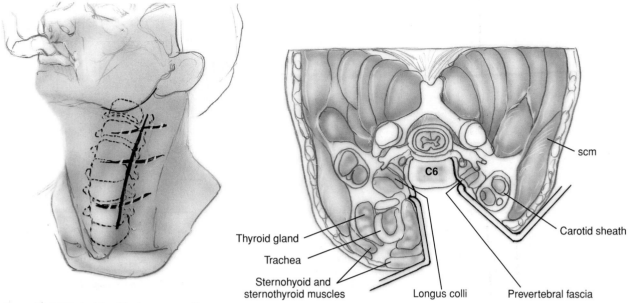

Figure 43–1 Skin incision. The transverse skin incision is made along Langer's lines. It is adjusted as necessary depending on the desired surgical level and the localizing radiograph. The incision should begin at the neck's midline and extend to the middle of the bulk of the sternocleidomastoid muscle. Also depicted is the position of a longitudinal incision that can be used for a multiple level corpectomy.

Figure 43–2 Cross-sectional anatomy. Note the plane of dissection between the sternocleidomastoid and the strap muscles. The carotid is retracted laterally.

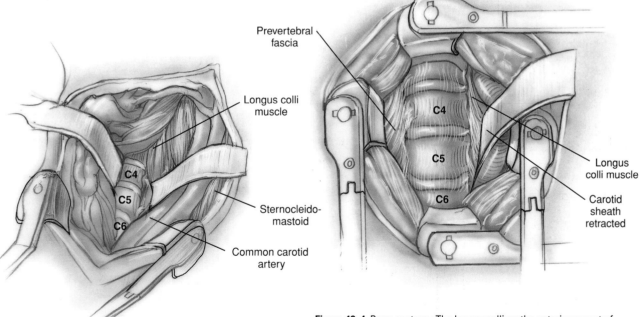

Figure 43–3 Deep dissection. Hand held retractors are used to displace the strap muscles medially. This helps protect the thyroid gland, trachea, and esophagus.

Figure 43–4 Bony anatomy. The longus colli on the anterior aspect of the spine is identified and the bony anatomy palpated. The disc spaces are the prominences ("hills") and the vertebral bodies are the concavities ("valleys").

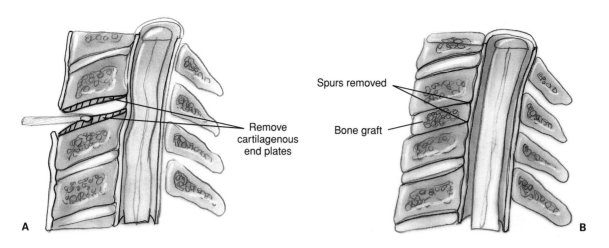

Figure 43–5 (A) Discectomy. As part of the discectomy, remove the cartilagenous endplates of the adjacent vertebral bodies to promote incorporation of the bone graft. If needed, posterior osteophytes can be removed by initially thinning with a high-speed burr and then hooking the remaining cortical edge and removing it piecemeal with a small microcurette. **(B)** Bone graft insertion. The bone graft is inserted with the disc space slightly distracted. This is accomplished either with the distractor or by applying additional traction through the head halter. In the standard Smith-Robinson style, the cortical side of the graft (the superior aspect of the iliac crest) faces anteriorly.

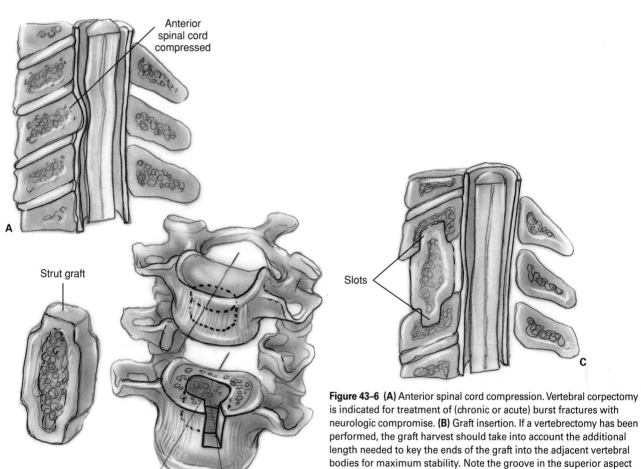

Figure 43–6 (A) Anterior spinal cord compression. Vertebral corpectomy is indicated for treatment of (chronic or acute) burst fractures with neurologic compromise. **(B)** Graft insertion. If a vertebrectomy has been performed, the graft harvest should take into account the additional length needed to key the ends of the graft into the adjacent vertebral bodies for maximum stability. Note the groove in the superior aspect of the adjacent inferior vertebral body to aid in introduction of the graft. **(C)** Graft in place. The graft should key into the adjacent vertebral bodies above and below the resected vertebral body.

the anterior body slants more posteriorly. If no instrumentation is planned, as with the majority of single level discectomies, only half the adjacent vertebral body above and below need be exposed. If plating is planned, as may be indicated for multiple level fusions, burst fractures, or corpectomies, the entire adjacent vertebral bodies should be exposed so that the margin of the adjacent disc space can be identified.

16. Place self-retaining Cloward retractors. Use the toothed blades to retract the longus colli muscle and the smooth blades for longitudinal exposure.

17. Incise the disc space with a 15-blade scalpel. Remove the disc material using a pituitary ronguer and curved and straight microcurettes.

18. Use magnification (lupes or microscope) after the initial stages of the discectomy even if they have not been used since the beginning of the case. If available, a distractor utilizing pins placed into the vertebral body above and below enhances exposure and graft placement. Avoid straying beyond or deeper than the vertebral body by ensuring that the curette is used against bone at all times.

19. Perform the discectomy into the uncovertebral joints, which can be identified as they angle cephalad relative to the endplate.

20. Palpate the posterior edge of the vertebral body with the curette or a small nerve hook. Identify the posterior longitudinal ligament. The longitudinally-running fibers are easily discernible from the more circumferentially-running annular fibers of the disc. It is not necessary to incise the PLL. However, if a soft disc protrusion was noted on the preoperative MRI or if a rent in the PLL is encountered, gently introduce a small nerve hook. This facilitates removal of the extruded fragment, or allows the rent in the PLL to be enlarged permitting direct view of the fragment for removal.

21. If desired, remove posterior osteophytes by initially thinning with a high-speed burr, and then hooking the remaining cortical edge and removing it piecemeal with a small microcurette (**Fig. 43–5A**).

22. If only discectomies are to be performed, proceed to the next disc or bone graft harvesting. Use gelfoam to slow slight endplate-oozing while working elsewhere.

Vertebrectomy (optional)

➢ Vertebral corpectomy is indicated for treatment of (chronic or acute) burst fractures with neurologic compromise (**Fig. 43–6A**).

   a. Identify and partially remove the two adjacent discs.

   b. Remove the anterior portion of the vertebral body with a ronguer.

   c. Use a high-speed burr to remove the posterior aspect of the vertebral body. Consider changing to a diamond-tipped burr, which is less likely to cut the dura, as dissection proceeds nearer to the denser cortical bone of the posterior vertebral body.

   d. Once the posterior cortex is thinned to a fine shell with a developed edge, use a microcurette to gently lift the shell away from the dura and spinal cord.

23. After the decompression has been completed, relax the self-retaining retractors.

Iliac crest bone graft harvest

24. Measure the defect to be filled using either calipers or a paper ruler. Harvest a tricortical graft (Smith-Robinson technique). Graft measurement should include both the height and depth of the graft. Commonly, grafts for cervical discectomies are 6 to 7 mm in height and 1.5 cm in depth. In general, the minimum graft height for adequate compressive strength and appropriate neural foramen enlargement is 5 mm. If a vertebrectomy has been performed, the graft harvest should take into account the additional length needed to key in the ends of the graft for maximum stability (**Figs. 43–6B and 6C**). If greater than two levels of vertebra are removed, the iliac crest may not support a graft of adequate length and a fibula graft may be preferable.

25. Exposed the iliac crest in a routine fashion.

26. Leave an adequate margin from the anterior superior iliac crest to minimize the risk of avulsion fractures (normally, at least 1 in) and harvest the structural graft using an oscillating saw.

27. If separate grafts are to be used in the disc spaces, it is usually easier to cut the pieces separately from the crest. After the first cut has been made, place a

narrow osteotome in the slot so that the second cut parallels the first. Make the deep transverse cut with a curved osteotome after all the vertical cuts have been completed. Hold the grafts before this last step to prevent inadvertent loss of the graft.

28. Pack this incision for later simultaneous closure. Prior to closure, smooth the sharp edges of the cut iliac crest with a ronguer and bone wax or gelfoam to decrease bleeding.

Bone graft placement

29. Respread the self-retaining retractors within the neck wound. Ensure that the sharp teeth are still nestled within the muscle substance of the longus colli.

30. Burr the endplates to bleeding bone (**Fig. 43–5A**).

31. Place the graft with the disc space slightly distracted, either using the distractor or by applying additional traction through the head halter. In the standard Smith-Robinson style, the cortical side of the graft (the superior aspect of the iliac crest) faces anteriorly (**Fig. 43–5B**).

32. Gently impact the graft into place and countersink it a couple of millimeters.

33. Obtain a lateral radiograph to assess graft position.

34. If a vertebrectomy has been performed, the graft harvest should take into account the additional length needed to key in the ends of the graft for maximum stability (**Figs. 43–6B and 6C**). If greater than two levels of vertebra are removed, the iliac crest may not have adequate length and a fibula is preferred.

Closure

35. Close the surgical site with interrupted sutures attempting to allow egress of blood to minimize the risk of hematoma formation. Rarely, airway or neurologic compromise occurs secondary to hematoma pressure. Consider placing a small Jackson-Pratt or Penrose-type drain overnight to decrease this risk.

36. Reapproximate the sternocleidomastoid muscle to the strap muscles with one or two sutures.

37. Close the platysma with interrupted sutures.

38. Close the skin with intracuticular sutures or staples. If intracuticular sutures are used, the suture should be able to slide in order to facilitate prompt removal if necessary.

Suggested Readings

Emery SE, Smith MD, Bohlman HH. Upper airway obstruction after multilevel cervical corpectomy for myelopathy. *J Bone Joint Surg* 1991;73A:544–551.

Flynn TB. Neurologic complications of anterior cervical interbody fusion. *Spine* 1982;7:536–539.

White A III, Jupiter J, Southwick WO, Panjabi MM. An experimental study of the immediate load bearing of three surgical constructions for anterior spine fusions. *Clin Orthop* 1973;91:21–28.

CHAPTER 44

Lumbar Spine Fusion

Srdjan Mirkovic

Indications

1. Incapacitating discogenic low back pain
2. Spinal stenosis with instability
3. Spondylolisthesis
4. Scoliosis or kyphosis
5. Pseudoarthrosis
6. Instability adjacent to a previous fusion
7. Re-do lumbar discectomy.

Contraindications

1. Spinal stenosis without deformity or known risk for deformity
2. Primary discectomy
3. Low back pain associated with multi-level degenerative disc disease

Preoperative Preparation

1. Medical and anesthetic evaluation
2. Anteroposterior (AP), lateral, oblique, and flexion extension X-rays
3. Lumbar imaging (MRI, CT myelography)
4. Consider electrodiagnostic studies.
5. Consider preoperative diagnostic studies (facet blocks, SI blocks, discograms, nerve root blocks).
6. Preoperative neurovascular assessment
7. Attempt to establish realistic expectations.

8. Encourage the patient to discontinue smoking. If possible, cessation of smoking should occur 6 months prior to the fusion.

Special Instruments, Position, and Anesthesia

1. The prone position is used for posterior spinal fusions.
2. Position the hips in neutral or slight extension. This helps maintain lumbar lordosis, which is imperative.
3. All pressure points should be carefully padded. The abdomen and genitalia (in males) should hang free. The arms must be placed in a 90/90 position to avoid brachial plexus traction injury. The ulnar nerve should be protected.
4. The lower extremities are placed in anti-embolic stockings and compression boots.
5. Spinal cord monitoring may be used.
6. X-rays and fluoroscopy should be available for verification of the appropriate level and in the case of instrumentation, to verify appropriate instrumentation placement.
7. If fluoroscopy is to be used, the undersurface of the table should be free to allow C-arm rotation.
8. Use specific instrumentation for planned spinal hardware.
9. In revision fusion surgery, determine prior to surgery which iliac crest(s) were harvested.

10. Surgery is done under general anesthesia.
11. Surgical instruments include: Cobb elevators, curettes, kerrosens, rongeurs, pituitaries, Penfields, osteotomes, and gauges.
12. Retractors should include: Hibbs, McCullough, Army-Navy, cerebellars, and deep Gulpies.
13. Bone wax, Cottonoids, gelfoam, and Thrombin should be available.

Tips and Pearls

1. Preoperative planning is paramount in determining the extent of fusion and the site for bone graft harvesting.
2. If instrumentation is to be used, preoperative planning allows determination of the levels of instrumentation and the site for purchase (pedicle, lamina, facet). If pedicle screws are planned, the sagittal and transverse orientation of the pedicles and their width, length, and height should be determined.
3. Imaging studies should be evaluated for the presence of any spinal anomalies.
4. The patient should be positioned in spinal lordosis. This is particularly important when long lumbar fusions are planned; it diminishes the possibility of postoperative flat back syndrome and spinal dysfunction.
5. Intravenous antibiotics are administered preoperatively. In the case of instrumentation, broad gram positive and gram-negative spectrum antibiotics are administered.
6. Paravertebral soft tissue dissection should proceed in a caudal-cephalad direction due to the caudal-cephalad orientation of the paravertebral muscle attachments.
7. The facet joint immediately cephalad to the fusion must be preserved to avoid iatrogenic instability.
8. Dissection should extend to the tips of the spinous processes bilaterally and to the lateral aspect of the facet joints. All soft tissue should be denuded to allow maximal surface area for bony fusion.
9. The majority of the decortication is carried out using sharp instruments such as osteotomes, curettes, and rongeurs.

10. Facet joints should be thoroughly cleared of all soft tissues and the intra-articular portion of the joint denuded of cartilage.
11. If a lumbar decompression has been performed prior to the fusion, the exposed dura should be protected with cottonoids to diminish the likelihood of an iatrogenic dural laceration.

What To Avoid

1. Avoid prolonged muscle retraction. Self-retaining retractors should be relaxed every hour and the wound re-irrigated. This allows re-perfusion of the paravertebral muscles and diminishes the possibility of infection. If there is excessive tension on the muscles, the incision can be lengthened.
2. Avoid using an inadequate amount of bone graft; occasionally harvesting of both iliac crests may be necessary and/or augmentation with allograft bone may be needed.
3. Avoid blood pooling, which occurs if the lordotic cephalad segments are decorticated first.
4. Avoid bony fragment extrusion into the spinal canal.
5. Avoid injury to the facet immediately cephalad to the fusion.
6. Avoid postoperative administration of nonsteroidal anti-inflammatories for 3 months.

Postoperative Care Issues

1. Suction drainage is used and removed 24 to 48 hours postsurgery (once drainage is below 20 cc per shift).
2. Consider using a PCA pump for initial postoperative analgesia and then switching to oral analgesics.
3. Consider using a stool softener to diminish the possibility of constipation.
4. The Foley catheter is removed as soon as the patient is able to stand at bedside.
5. Early mobilization with physical therapy and occupational therapy is encouraged.
6. Depending on the extent of fusion, either a LSO or a TLSO hard-shelled brace is used. Occasionally, a

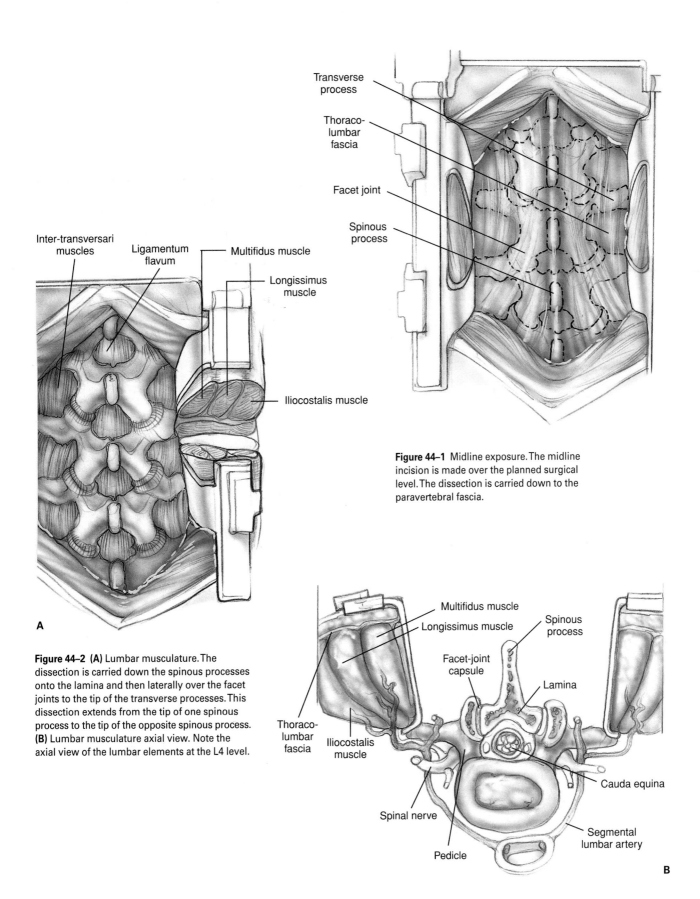

Figure 44–1 Midline exposure. The midline incision is made over the planned surgical level. The dissection is carried down to the paravertebral fascia.

Transverse process

Thoraco-lumbar fascia

Facet joint

Spinous process

Inter-transversari muscles

Ligamentum flavum

Multifidus muscle

Longissimus muscle

Iliocostalis muscle

Figure 44–2 (A) Lumbar musculature. The dissection is carried down the spinous processes onto the lamina and then laterally over the facet joints to the tip of the transverse processes. This dissection extends from the tip of one spinous process to the tip of the opposite spinous process. **(B)** Lumbar musculature axial view. Note the axial view of the lumbar elements at the L4 level.

A

Multifidus muscle

Longissimus muscle

Spinous process

Facet-joint capsule

Lamina

Thoraco-lumbar fascia

Iliocostalis muscle

Cauda equina

Spinal nerve

Pedicle

Segmental lumbar artery

B

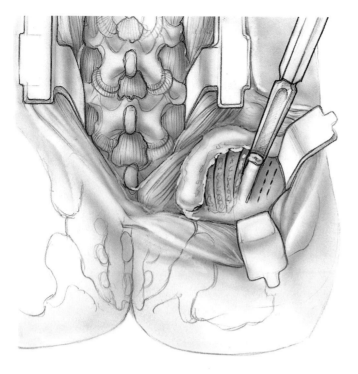

Figure 44–3 Iliac crest graft harvest. Bone graft is harvested from the iliac crest using osteotomes, curettes, and gauges.

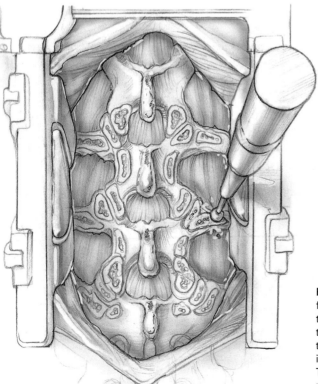

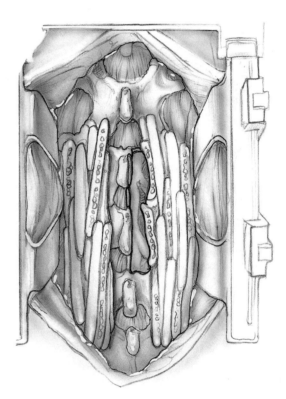

Figure 44–4 Decortication of posterior elements. The facet joints, laminae, and pars are decorticated with rongeurs, 1/4-in osteotomes, and curettes. A burr can be used to decorticate more dense cortical bone, such as the pars.

Figure 44–5 Fusion. The fusion should extend from the superior aspect of the superior transverse process to the inferior aspect of the inferior transverse process, and from the tip of the transverse process laterally to and including the lateral aspect of the superior facet. The harvested corticocancellous bone graft is packed into the facets and pars.

thigh cuff is added to the brace in cases where the fusion extends across L5-S1.

7. Barring medical contraindications, calcium intake of 1000 mg a day is encouraged in conjunction with a daily vitamin supplement.

8. Smoking is discouraged.

9. Neurovascular examination is performed frequently in the first 48 to 72 hours.

10. Patients are encouraged to donate two units of autologous blood.

Operative Technique

Approach

1. Administer preoperative antibiotics. After general anesthesia is administrated, insert a Foley catheter. Place compression boots and anti-embolic stockings over the lower extremities. Institute spinal cord monitoring.

2. Turn the patient prone on either chest rolls or a Jackson table. Carefully pad the extremities and protect the groin (males) and the breasts (females). Maintain the hips in neutral or slight extension while maintaining knee flexion. Allow the belly to hang free.

3. Prepare and drape the back and iliac crest in a sterile fashion.

4. Make a midline incision measuring about 4 in in length. Center it over the level of the planned surgery. The superior aspect of the iliac crest approximates the L4-L5 level and the posterior superior iliac spines approximates the L5-S1 level.

5. Carry the dissection down to the paravertebral fascia (**Fig. 44–1**).

6. Control bleeding with a Bovie cautery.

7. Use self-retaining cerebellar retractors.

8. Criss-crossing thoracolumbar fascial decussations serve as an additional guide to the L5-S1 level.

9. Incise the paravertebral fasciae insertion into the spinous processes. Bilaterally, carry the dissection down the spinous processes onto the lamina and then laterally over the facet joints to the tip of the transverse processes. This dissection should extend from the tip of one spinous process to the tip of the opposite spinous process.

10. Denude soft tissues off the facet joints, the pars, the lamina, and the transverse processes. Use a burr to denude some of the soft tissues.

11. Place deep self-retaining retractors. The author prefers the McCullough retractor either alone or in conjunction with an Overhill or Adson-Beckman retractor.

12. Control bleeding throughout the procedure using bipolar and Bovie cautery.

13. At this point, exposure should be adequate so that all posterior elements are clearly visualized (**Fig. 44–2A and 2B**).

14. If instrumentation is indicated, appropriate laminotomies for hook placement can be made, and anatomic landmarks are used to determine the pedicle entry point.

Iliac crest bone graft harvest

The iliac crest ipsilateral to the patient's most severe back and/or leg symptoms is chosen.

➤ If the fusion extends to S1, consider exposing the iliac crest from the same midline incision, by extending the dissection in the plane between the subcutaneous tissues and the lumbosacral fascia towards the iliac crest. Avoid excessive soft tissue retraction when performing the approach through the same incision.

➤ If the location of the iliac crest is too lateral or if the fusion extends to L5 or more proximally, a separate incision should be made over the iliac crest.

a. Incise the periosteum and reflect it off the inner and outer walls of the iliac crest. Dissect the outer wall by reflecting the gluteus muscles off of the posterior iliac crest. Carry the iliac crest dissection from the posterosuperior iliac spine medially for a distance of about 10 cm laterally. This diminishes the possibility of injury to the cluneal nerves.

b. After the iliac crest is exposed, place a deep self-retaining retractor such as an Overhill with assisted manual Hibbs retraction to provide adequate exposure.

c. Harvest bone from the iliac crest using osteotomes. Cut long longitudinal slivers of bone. Undercut them using a curved osteotome.

d. Harvest cancellous bone using curettes and gauges. Augment the volume of osteoprogenitor cells by aspirating bone marrow and placing it over the bone graft (**Fig. 44–3**).

e. Once ample bone graft has been harvested, copiously irrigate the wound with antibiotic solution.

f. Use bone wax to tamponade cancellous bleeders. A dry piece of gelfoam can be placed to maintain hemostasis. If the field is dry, a drain is not always necessary. Otherwise, tunnel a drain cephalad laterally to allow easy access postoperatively and to keep the drain away from the perianal area.

g. Approximate the paravertebral fascia with 1-0 Vicryl. Close the subcutaneous tissue with two layers of 2-0 Vicryl. Close the skin with either staples or vertical 3-0 nylon mattress sutures. In individuals with a small incision, a subcuticular 4-0 Vicryl can be employed.

h. Dress the wound with sterile dressing.

Fusion

15. Copiously irrigate the main lumbar incision with antibiotic solution. Use one or two Hibbs retractors to retract the soft tissues bilaterally over the transverse processes.

16. Copiously irrigate the lateral gutters with antibiotic solution. Avoid irrigation once decortication commences in order to preserve the decorticated bone, as well as the osteoprogenitor potential of the decorticated cancellous surfaces.

17. Denude the facet joints of cartilage and scrape them with a curette.

18. Continue decorticating in a cephalad-to-caudal direction. Avoid blood pooling, which occurs if the lordotic cephalad segments are decorticated first.

19. Split the transverse processes dorsally in the midline. Expose the cancellous surfaces by opening them like a book. Avoid fracturing the transverse processes.

20. Decorticate the facet joints, laminae, and pars using rongeurs, 1/4-in osteotomes, and curettes. In particular, the lateral aspect of the facet joint must be decorticated, augmenting the surface area for the fusion. Use a burr to decorticate more dense cortical bone, such as the pars (**Fig. 44–4**).

21. If the fusion extends to S1, perform an osteotomy of the superior sacral ala. Reflect the osteotomized bone in the L5-S1 intertransverse process interval.

22. Use a curette to scoop the exposed cancellous alar bone, thereby augmenting the fusion bed.

23. Place half of the harvested corticocancellous chips into the lateral gutters. Impact these using a tamp. The fusion should extend from the superior aspect of the superior transverse process to the inferior aspect of the inferior transverse process, and from the tip of the transverse process laterally to and including the lateral aspect ofthe superior facet.

24. Pack the facet joint intra-articularly with bone graft. Also place bone graft into the facets and pars (**Fig. 44–5**).

25. Drape the paravertebral muscles over the bone graft. Avoid medial displacement of the bone graft during retractor removal.

26. Repeat the same procedure on the opposite side.

Closure

27. Place a drain.

28. Approximate the deep paravertebral muscles to each other with #1 Vicryl. This helps obliterate the deep dead space.

29. Approximate the paravertebral fascia with #1 Vicryl in figure eight watertight fashion.

30. Close the superficial layers with 2-0 Vicryl; close the skin in a standard fashion.

31. Dress the wound with a compressive dressing.

Suggested Readings

Kurz LT, Samberg LC, Herkowitz HN. Spinal fusion: techniques and complications. In: Herkowitz HN, Garfin SR, Balderston RA, Eismont FJ, Bell GR, Wiesel SW, eds. *The Spine*. 3rd ed. Philadelphia, PA: W.B. Saunders, 1992, pp. 1756–1773.

CHAPTER 45

Spinal Lumbar Decompression

Srdjan Mirkovic

Indications

1. Spinal stenosis

    a. Failure to respond to nonoperative treatment with a predominance of lower extremity symptoms
    b. Unremitting pain and marked limitations of daily activities

2. Precipitous neurologic deterioration
3. Cauda equina syndrome

Contraindications

1. Low back pain in the presence of multi-level degenerative disc disease
2. Lack of confirmatory imaging study

Preoperative Preparation

1. Medical and anesthetic clearance
2. Clear identification of the exact location of spinal stenosis
3. If possible, cessation of smoking
4. Fitness education and weight reduction
5. Radiographic imaging (MRI, CT myelogram) including sagittal foraminal reconstruction

Special Instruments, Position, and Anesthesia

1. Position the patient in a prone kneeling position on chest rolls with the abdomen hanging free. The kneeling position is contraindicated in the presence of knee or hip disease.
2. Use spinal or general anesthesia for short segment, decompressive laminectomy without instrumentation. Use general anesthesia for long segment decompression or instrumentation. Consider hypotensive anesthesia to diminish epidural bleeding if there are no medical contraindications.
3. Special instruments: 45-degree angled Kerrosen rongeurs ranging in size from 1 to 4 mm.
4. Luksell rongeurs are used to debulk lamina, facet joints, remove spinous processes, and decorticate.
5. Use 4-mm and 5-mm burrs to thin lamina and facet joints.
6. Penfield elevators are used to palpate nerve roots and dura, and dissect surgical planes.
7. Different sized ball-ended probes are used to evaluate foraminal decompression.
8. Microscope or loop magnification and light augmentation
9. Angled curettes are used to free-up scar tissue and develop surgical planes.

10. Use gelfoam impregnated in thrombin to facilitate hemostasis.
11. Bipolar coagulation

Tips and Pearls

1. The interlaminar space may be completely obliterated in patients with severe spine degeneration. The superior aspect of the lamina can be difficult to identify due to severe shingling. Consider placing a laminar distractor between the spinous processes, thereby allowing distraction of the interlaminar space and delineation of the inferior border of the superior laminae, ligamentum flavum, and facet joints. This facilitates initiation of the laminectomy with kerrosens posterior to the ligamentum flavum. Once the ligamentum flavum plane is identified, the laminar spreaders can be removed and the spinous processes rongeured with a Luksell and removed with kerrosens. The laminectomy can then proceed in routine fashion.

2. The three common areas for significant nerve root compression are: the lateral recess secondary to facet joint hypertrophy; the central stenosis due to the hypertrophied ligamentum flavum; and the foraminal stenosis due to degenerative disc narrowing. Decompression of the superior aspect of the caudal lamina is facilitated by either partially or completely removing the spinous processes of the inferior vertebra. The underlying lamina is thick and should be thinned with a burr or with a rongeur.

3. In patients with one level spinal stenosis (e.g., the L4-L5 level), the inferior half of the lamina of L4 and the superior half of the lamina of L5 need to be removed.

4. Lateral recess stenosis due to dorsal compression from the overhanging hypertrophied facet is a common cause of surgical failure. Affected nerve roots need to be clearly decompressed with clear visualization of the medial aspect of the corresponding pedicle.

5. Check the foramina for impingement using ball-ended probes.

6. Consider concomitant spinal fusion in the presence of degenerative spondylolisthesis, scoliosis and/or kyphosis, greater than 50% excision of the facet bilaterally, as well as recurrent stenosis above a previous fusion.

7. If a kneeling position is used with a patient's back in kyphosis, ensure that adequate foraminal decompression has been performed to avoid postoperative stenosis when the patient resumes standing in the lordotic position.

What To Avoid

1. Avoid inadequate decompression.

2. If possible, avoid complete excision of the facet joints to minimize the incidence of postoperative instability.

3. Avoid dural tears. Minimize dural tears by carefully identifying the surgical planes (notably the plane between bone and ligamentum flavum, and between the ligamentum flavum and the epidural space). Cottonoids placed in the plane of dissection during laminectomy protect the dura and assist in hemostasis.

4. Avoid foregoing radiographs. Verify radiographically that the decompression has extended the extent of the desired surgery.

Postoperative Care Issues

1. The drain is commonly removed 24 to 48 hours after surgery when drainage is less than 20 mL per shift.

2. Physical therapy and occupational therapy are instituted on postoperative day one.

3. The Foley catheter is removed when the patient can sit or stand by the bedside.

4. Since spinal stenosis is a common condition in the elderly, prolonged immobilization particularly in these elderly patients leads to deconditioning and should be avoided. Patients are encouraged to sit by the bedside for as long as tolerated.

5. A soft corset is preferred in patients who do not undergo lumbar fusion. A rigid brace is recommended for patients who undergo lumbar fusion procedures.

6. Antibiotics are given for 48 hours postoperatively.

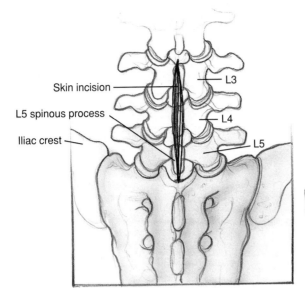

Figure 45–1 Midline incision. A midline incision is made directly over the spinous processes. The incision should be centered over the pathologic lumbar level(s).

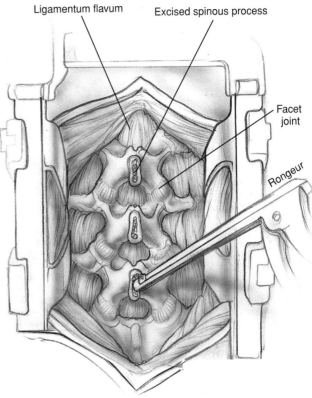

Figure 45–2 Spinous process excision. The spinous processes are excised with a large bone biter. The ligamentum flavum is exposed by removing any remaining soft tissues in the interlaminar space.

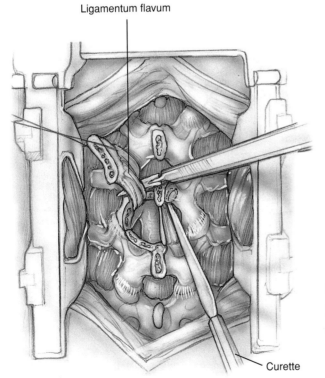

Figure 45–3 Ligamentum flavum excision. The plane between the lamina and the ligamentum flavum is developed using a curette. The curette is used to remove the superior portion of the ligamentum flavum from the lamina. The ligamentum flavum is excised by sharply dissecting the ligament with a #15 blade.

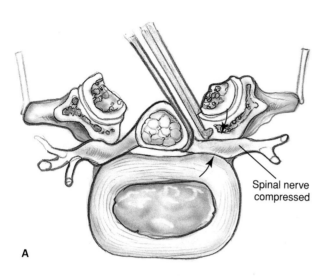

A

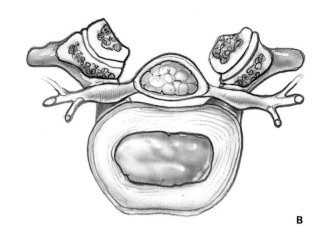

B

Spinal nerve
compressed

Figure 45–4 (A) Cross section-compressed spinal nerve. Note the nerve root is entrapped between the calcified degenerated disc, the pedicle, and the superior facet of the inferior vertebra. The facet should be undercut and then removed along with the ligamentum flavum using either a 2- or 3-mm Kerrosen. **(B)** Cross section-decompressed spinal nerve. The completed decompression should extend from pedicle to pedicle.

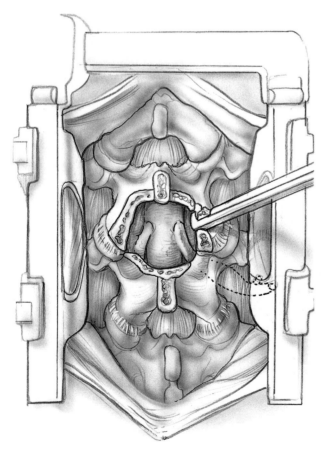

Figure 45–5 Complete laminectomy. The completed decompression should extend from pedicle to pedicle. The nerve root should be fully visualized as it exits around the pedicle. The nerve root should be followed into the foramina and further decompressed if there is stenosis at this level. Angled Kerrosens can be used to further decompress the spinal canal.

7. Judicious use of pain medication avoids confusion and disorientation in the elderly population.

8. Sutures are removed at 2 weeks. Patients are placed in a gentle cardiovascular-conditioning program at that time.

9. Low back exercises are begun 4 weeks postoperatively.

10. In the absence of fusion, the majority of patients can return to sedentary work 2 to 4 weeks after surgery. More demanding work is normally possible 6 to 12 weeks after surgery.

Operative Technique

Preoperative

1. Administer prophylactic antibiotics preoperatively.

2. Place the patient in the prone position. Consider using anti-embolic stockings, intermittent pneumatic compression, and spinal cord monitoring.

3. Insert a Foley catheter. Protect all extremities including the ulnar nerve, brachial plexus, genitalia in males, and breasts in females.

4. Prepare and drape the patient's back in the hospital's routine sterile fashion.

5. Determine the appropriate level for the spinal incision. Begin by examining the anteroposterior radiographs. Conventionally, these radiographs are positioned on the viewbox as if the examiner is facing the patient's back. Thus, the radiograph is positioned so the patient's right side is on the right side on the radiograph. Use the iliac crest as a landmark for the L4-L5 level and the posterior superior iliac spine as an L5-S1 landmark.

6. Place a spinal needle at the presumed pathological level. Use lateral radiographs and/or fluoroscopy to verify the position.

Approach

7. Infiltrate the paravertebral muscles with 1:500,000 epinephrine and saline solution.

8. Make a midline incision directly over the spinous processes (**Fig. 45–1**).

9. Dissect directly down through the soft tissues to the thoracolumbar fascia, which inserts into the spinous processes. Place self-retaining cerebellar retractors.

10. Dissect subperiosteally down the spinous processes to the laminae. Avoid violating the intramuscular

vessels and causing unnecessary hemorrhages. Coagulate all blood vessels that are encountered in order to optimize visualization.

11. Use the decussations of the lumbodorsal fascial fibers at the lumbosacral junction (L5-S1) as an additional intraoperative landmark.

12. Identify the paraspinal muscles which attach to the spinous processes. Dissect the paraspinal muscles with cautery by proceeding in a caudal-to-cephalad direction.

13. Use Cobb elevators to expose the laminae. Exposure should extend from the spinous processes medially to the facet joints laterally. Avoid stripping the facet joints unless a fusion is planned.

14. Remove the remaining soft tissues from the lamina and interlaminar space using curettes, pituitaries, or a burr. Place deep self-retaining retractors. The author prefers a McCullough retractor which allows flexibility with blades of different depth and width. Place the tips of the retractor blades over the facet joints to preserve the facet capsules, the muscular attachments, and innervation.

15. Re-check that the appropriate level has been exposed by placing a radiopaque marker at the interlaminar space and verifying its position on cross table lateral X-rays or fluoroscopy.

Decompression

➤ Minimize trauma to the soft tissues by removing the self-retaining retractors every hour for 5 minutes while copiously irrigating the wound with antibiotic solution.

➤ Control bleeding throughout the procedure using bipolar cautery on low intensity, thrombin impregnated gelfoam, and occasionally Avetene.

16. Remove the spinous processes with a large bone biter (**Fig. 45–2**). Control bleeding from the soft cancellous bone with bone wax. Expose the ligamentum flavum by removing any remaining soft tissues in the interlaminar space.

17. Thin the lamina of the involved segments with a rongeur or cutting burr. Bleeding from the bone can be controlled with bone wax. Clear visualization within the operative field facilitates subsequent laminectomy with kerrosens.

18. Develop the plane between the lamina and the ligamentum flavum using a 2-0 Epstein curette (**Fig. 45–3**). Place cottonoids in this plane, thereby protecting the underlying dura and ligamentum flavum.

19. Begin the decompression in the midline.

20. After the central decompression, proceed laterally excising the lateral aspect of the lamina. Do not extend the lateral decompression past the pars. Carefully protect the pars intra-articularis, thus minimizing the incidence of instability.

21. Decompress lateral recess stenosis by using a Kerrosen. A burr or a 1/4-in osteotome may also be used. The decompression should allow complete visualization of the ligamentum flavum.

22. Pass a ball-ended probe through the midline of the ligamentum flavum and split the ligamentum along its midline raphe.

23. Carry out a flavectomy by dissecting the ligament sharply with a #15 blade (**Fig. 45–3**). Laterally, the ligamentum flavum contributes to lateral recess stenosis and adheres to the undersurface of the hypertrophied degenerated facet joint. The nerve root is entrapped between the calcified degenerated disc, the pedicle, and the superior facet of the inferior vertebra. Commonly this is seen with severe disc degeneration with marked collapse of the intervertebral disc and overriding of the facet joints.

24. Undercut the facet and remove the ligamentum flavum using either a 2- or 3-mm Kerrosen. If the lateral recess is very tight, use a 1-mm Kerrosen. Remove the posterior aspect of the disc with sharp dissection. Alternatively, if the disc is markedly calcified use a small osteotome or less frequently a burr (**Fig. 45–4A**).

25. Fully visualize the nerve root exiting around the pedicle. If additional lateral recess stenosis is still present, further decompress the spinal canal by performing a foraminotomy. Follow the nerve root into the foramina. Remember that the dorsal root ganglion, which lies just inferior to the pedicle, is a significant source of pain mediators and should be thoroughly decompressed.

26. Carefully inspect the foramina using ball-ended probes up to 5 mm in diameter. If residual foraminal stenosis is present, further decompress the spinal foramina using an angled Kerrosen (**Fig. 45–4A**).

Severe stenosis

➤ The decompression once completed should extend from pedicle to pedicle (**Fig. 45–4B**). The possibility of an underlying disc herniation, contributing to the spinal stenosis should also be ruled out by inspecting the anterior aspect of the dura and nerve root. This is accomplished by carefully retracting the dura and the nerve root medially (**Fig. 45–5**).

Closure

27. Once the decompression is completed, copiously irrigate the wound with antibiotic solution.

28. Cover the length of the dura with gelfoam impregnated in thrombin.

29. Place a hemovac drain.

30. Approximate the paravertebral muscles with 1-0 Vicryl to diminish the dead space.

31. Close the paravertebral fascia with1-0 Vicryl and the subcutaneous tissue with 2-0 Vicryl.

32. Approximate the skin edges in routine fashion per surgeon's choice and apply a compressive dressing.

Suggested Readings

Garfin SR, Herkowitz HN, Mirkovic S. Spinal stenosis. *J Bone Joint Surg* 1999;81A(4):572–583.

Russell M, Hanley E. Indications, techniques and results of decompressive laminectomy. In: Herkowitz HN, Garfin SR, Balderston RA, Eismont FJ, Bell GR, Wiesel SW, eds. *The Spine*. 4th ed. Philadelphia, PA: W.B. Saunders, 1999, pp. 806F–806M.

Section Eight

Pediatrics

CHAPTER 46

Slipped Capital Femoral Epiphysis Hip Pinning

Kirk Aadalen and John F. Sarwark

Definitions

New terminology
Unstable slip: defined as clinical and radiographic evidence of slipped capital femoral epiphysis (SCFE) and inability to bear weight, even with assistive devices secondary to pain.
Stable slip: defined as clinical and radiographic evidence of SCFE and the ability to bear weight.

Indications

1. Mild, moderate, and some severe unstable (acute or acute-on-chronic) slipped capital femoral epiphysis (SCFE) **(Figs. 46–1A and 1B)**
2. Mild or moderate stable (chronic) SCFE

Contraindications

1. Severe acute on chronic SCFE
2. Severe chronic SCFE

Preoperative Preparation

1. Obtain hip radiographs including anteroposterior (AP) and true or cross table lateral views of the affected hip.

2. Appropriate medical and anesthesiology evaluation
3. Strict bed rest
4. Skin traction to affected limb for comfort

Special Instruments, Position, and Anesthesia

1. C-arm image intensifier fluoroscopy is required for percutaneous pinning.
2. A power driver with Kirshner wires and a 7.3-mm cannulated screw set is required.
3. The patient is placed supine on a radiolucent table or fracture table with the affected leg abducted 10–15 degrees and internally rotated moderately and without force **(Fig. 46–2)**.
4. Carefully pad all pressure points.
5. Place image intensifier between the patient's legs in order to obtain AP and lateral hip images by simply rotating around the arc of the C-arm machine.
6. General anesthesia is used during the procedure.

Tips and Pearls

1. Position the leg with 10–15 degrees of abduction and moderate internal rotation. This places the femoral neck as close as possible to a position parallel to the floor in order to obtain true AP and lateral views.

2. The starting point for the screw should be on the anterior surface of the femoral neck, not the lateral cortex of the proximal femur as in adult femoral neck fixation.

3. Commonly, as the proximal capital femoral epiphysis "slips" it rotates posteriorly. The more severe the slip, the more anterior the entry position of the guide pin on the femoral neck will need to be in order to achieve optimal, final, safe screw position (**Fig. 46–1B**).

4. The only safe location for screw placement is center-center with respect to the femoral head on the AP and lateral images. At least 5 mm of a margin from the femoral head surface should be seen.

5. A single larger 7.3-mm cannulated screw is technically easier and has better results than multiple screws.

What To Avoid

1. Avoid persistent joint penetration by the screw, which can lead to chondrolysis; however, transient penetration does not.

2. Avoid aggressive reduction maneuvers in order to decrease the risk of avascular necrosis.

3. Avoid placing the screw tip in the anterior and superior quadrant of the femoral head, as this can damage the terminal branches of the lateral cervical artery and lead to segmental collapse.

Postoperative Care Issues

1. A sterile occlusive dressing is placed over the wound.

2. Range-of-motion exercises are begun the first postoperative day.

3. Ambulation with crutches and partial weight bearing is begun on the first postoperative day.

4. Use of crutches is maintained until all signs of synovitis are gone and full painless range of motion is achieved (usually 6 weeks).

5. Vigorous sports and activities are restricted until demonstration of closure of the physis.

6. The screw can be left in place or removed after physeal closure in selected or symptomatic cases.

Operative Technique

1. Position the patient in the supine position on the fracture table or a radiolucent table. Without force, position the affected leg in 10–15 degrees of abduction and moderate internal rotation (**Fig. 46–2**).

2. Position the C-arm image intensifier between the patient's legs. Confirm that the entire proximal femoral epiphysis and joint space can be seen in the AP and lateral views.

3. Sterilely prepare and drape the entire anterior surface of the thigh as far medially as the pubis.

Determining screw insertion site

4. In the AP view, place a guide wire over the surface of the anterior thigh. Use the image intensifier to position the pin perpendicular to the physis and over the center of the femoral head. Draw a line on the skin along the pin.

5. In the lateral view, place a guide wire over the surface of the lateral thigh. Use the image intensifier to position the pin perpendicular to the physis and over the center of the femoral head. Draw a line on the skin along the pin.

6. The intersection of these two lines is the skin incision site for the guide pin (**Fig. 46–3**).

7. Make either a 1- or 2-cm incision or a simple puncture (stab) incision at the intersection of the two lines.

8. Advance the guide pin through a cannulated soft tissue protector. Push it through the soft tissues until the pin encounters the anterior lateral femoral neck.

9. Use the AP view to estimate the femoral neck axis, and the lateral view to confirm the degree of posterior angulation needed to cross the physis at a perpendicular angle and for the pin to achieve a center-center position in the femoral head (**Figs. 46–1A and 1B**).

10. Under fluoroscopic guidance, advance the guide pin to the level of the physis. Recheck the guide pin's position on the AP and lateral images.

11. After the correct pin position is confirmed, advance the guide pin in the center-center position to within 5 mm of the subchondral bone.

12. Remove the soft tissue protector. Use the depth guide to measure the length of the screw needed.

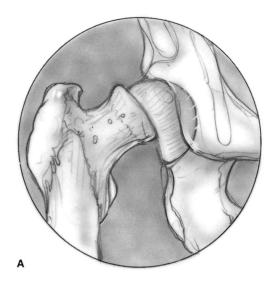

A

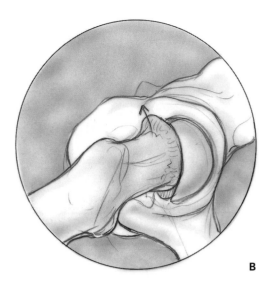

B

Figure 46–1 (A) Slipped capital femoral epiphysis (AP view). Note the inferior position of the slipped capital femoral epiphysis on the AP view. The AP view is used to estimate the femoral neck axis and the angle that the pin will need to achieve a center-center position in the femoral head. **(B)** Slipped capital femoral epiphysis (lateral view). Note the posterior position of the slipped capital femoral epiphysis on the lateral view. The lateral view is used to confirm the degree of posterior angulation that the pin will need to achieve a center-center position in the femoral head. The more severe the slip, the more anterior the entry position of the guide pin on the femoral neck will need to be in order to achieve optimal, final, safe screw position.

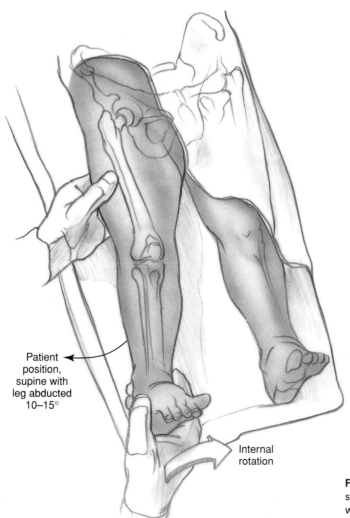

Patient position, supine with leg abducted 10–15°

Internal rotation

Figure 46–2 Patient position. The patient is placed supine on a radiolucent table or fracture table with the affected leg abducted 10–15 degrees and internally rotated moderately and without force.

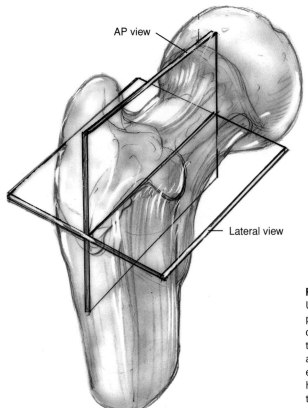

Figure 46–3 Fluoroscopic image intersection.
Using the AP image, a guide wire is positioned
perpendicular to the epiphysis and over the
center of the femoral head. A line is drawn on
the skin along the pin. Using the lateral image,
a guide wire is positioned perpendicular to the
epiphysis and over the center of the femoral
head. A second line is drawn on the skin along
the pin. The intersection of these two lines is the
skin incision site for the guide pin.

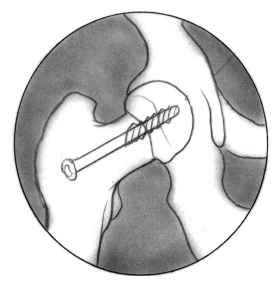

Figure 46–4 Screw placement. A single 7.3-mm
cannulated, partially-threaded screw is placed
perpendicular to the fracture line. The screw is
advanced to within 5 mm of the subchondral
bone.

13. Insert a single 7.3-mm cannulated, partially-threaded screw over the guide pin. Advance it to within 5 mm of the subchondral bone. Remove the guide pin **(Fig. 46–4)**.
14. Remove the leg from the fracture table leg holder. Run the hip through a range of motion while observing under AP and lateral image control to assure that the screw has not violated the joint space.
15. Close the wound with a subcuticular stitch.

Suggested Readings

Aronson DD, Carlson WE. Slipped capital femoral epiphysis. *J Bone Joint Surg (Am)* 1992;74:810–819.

Canale ST, Beaty JH. Fractures and dislocations. In: *Operative Pediatric Orthopaedics*. 2nd ed. New York, NY: Mosby, 1995, pp. 982–1004.

Jacobs B. Diagnosis and natural history of slipped capital femoral epiphysis. *Instr Course Lect* 1972;21:167–173.

Loder RT, Richards BS, Shapiro PS, et al. Acute slipped capital femoral epiphysis: the importance of physeal stability. *J Bone Joint Surg (Am)* 1993;75:1134–1140.

Morrisey RT. Slipped capital femoral epiphysis technique of percutaneous in situ fixation. *J Pediatr Orthop* 1990;10:347–350.

Morrisey RT, Weinstein SL. Slipped capital femoral epiphysis. In: *Lovell and Winter's Pediatric Orthopaedics*. 4th ed. Philadelphia, PA: Lippincott-Raven, 1996, pp. 993–1022.

Southwick W. Osteotomy through the lesser trochanter for slipped capital femoral epiphysis. *J Bone Joint Surg (Am)* 1967;49:807–835.

Ward WT, Stefko J, Wood KB, et al. Fixation with a single screw for slipped capital femoral epiphysis. *J Bone Joint Surg (Am)* 1992;74:799–809.

Wilson PD, Jacobs B, Schecter L. Slipped capital femoral epiphysis: an end-result study. *J Bone Joint Surg (Am)* 1965;47:1128–1145.

CHAPTER 47

Clubfoot Surgery

Posteromedial and Posterolateral Releases

Michael Kuczmanski and John F. Sarwark

Indications

1. Rigid clubfoot
2. Foot unresponsive/partially responsive to casting correction

Contraindications

1. If the patient is older than 6 years, correction usually requires bony procedures in addition to soft tissue releases.
2. Revision surgery in severe rigid syndromic clubfeet; in these cases talectomy may be a better option.

Preoperative Preparation

1. Attempt manipulation and corrective casting during the first 6 to 8 weeks of life. First correct adductus, then hindfoot varus, and then equinus.
2. Casting allows soft tissue stretching prior to reconstruction even if casting fails.
3. X-rays: weight-bearing anteroposterior (AP) and forced dorsiflexion lateral to assess AP talocalcaneal angle, AP talo-first metatarsal angle, and lateral talocalcaneal angle.
4. Incision options: Cincinnati circumferential incision or Carroll technique with curvilinear medial and longitudinal posterolateral incisions. Both procedures allow access to medial, lateral, and posterior aspects of the foot. The Cincinnati incision is described in the text.
5. The goal of the procedure is to achieve a pain-free, plantigrade foot with near-normal range of motion and function.

Special Instruments, Position, and Anesthesia

1. Place the patient prone
2. Tenotomy scissors
3. Vessel loops
4. K-wires
5. Plain radiography
6. Loop magnification
7. Limb tourniquet

Tips and Pearls

1. Use vessel loops to isolate and protect the neurovascular bundle medially and sural nerve laterally.
2. The degree of deformity dictates the extent of releases necessary (i.e., perform tendoachilles lengthening and posterior capsule release for isolated equinus deformity).
3. Consider releasing the tourniquet if the neurovascular bundle is difficult to identify.

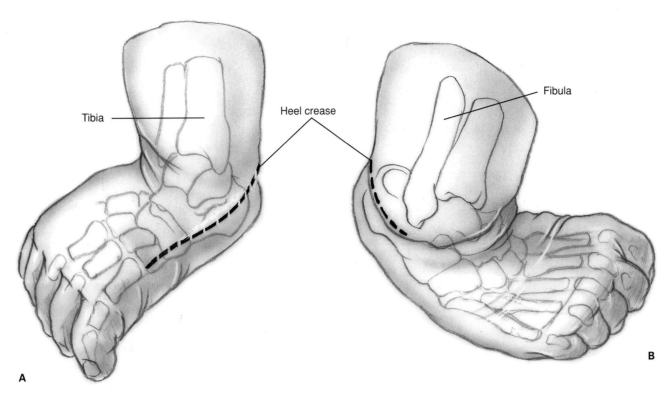

Figure 47–1 (A) Skin incision—medial view. Make a transverse incision. This should start at the base of first metatarsal medially. Stay in the dorsal skin, 0.5 cm proximal to the heel crease. **(B)** Skin incision—lateral view. The transverse incision should extend to the base of the fibula laterally. Stay in the dorsal skin, 0.5 cm proximal to the heel crease.

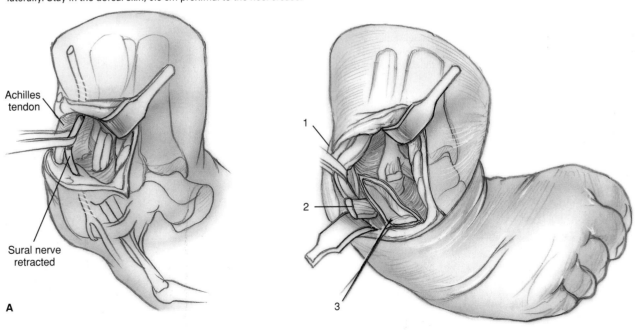

Figure 47–2 (A) Lateral release. (1) The peroneal tendon sheath is elevated and retracted anteriorly. (2) The calcaneofibular ligament is incised close to the fibula. (3) The lateral subtalar joint is identified and a capsulotomy performed up to the calcaneocuboid joint.

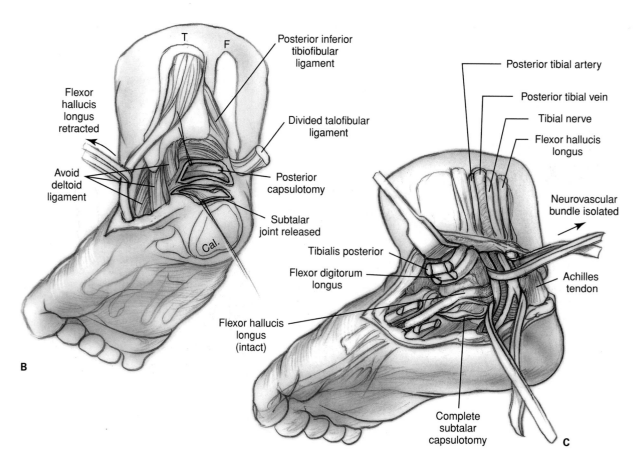

Flexor hallucis longus retracted

Avoid deltoid ligament

Posterior inferior tibiofibular ligament

Divided talofibular ligament

Posterior capsulotomy

Subtalar joint released

Cal.

B

Posterior tibial artery

Posterior tibial vein

Tibial nerve

Flexor hallucis longus

Neurovascular bundle isolated

Tibialis posterior

Flexor digitorum longus

Flexor hallucis longus (intact)

Achilles tendon

Complete subtalar capsulotomy

C

Figure 47–2 *(Continued)* **(B)** Posterior release. Sequential capsulotomies of the posterior ankle joint are performed by the subtalar joint. **(C)** Capsulotomies of the talonavicular and subtalar joints. Identify and perform capsulotomies of the talonavicular joint (superior, inferior, medial, and lateral). Complete the capsulotomy of the subtalar joint.

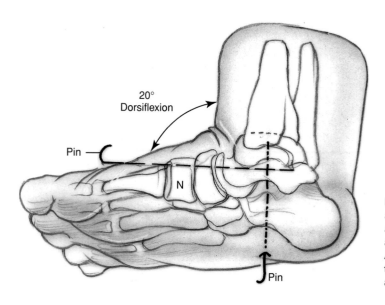

20° Dorsiflexion

Pin

N

Pin

Figure 47–3 K-wire placement. Smooth K-wires are placed from the posterolateral corner of talus across the talonavicular joint. The first wire is aimed so it exits dorsally at the first web space. A second smooth K-wire is placed from calcaneus to talus (plantar to dorsal) without entering the ankle joint.

4. To avoid wound problems (dehiscence), the foot can initially be casted or splinted in equinus and then recasted at 2 weeks.

What To Avoid

1. Avoid injury to neurovascular bundle and sural nerve with careful dissection medially and laterally.
2. Avoid aggressive dissection around talus to decrease risk of avascular necrosis.
3. Avoid injury to distal tibial physis during capsulotomies.
4. Avoid overlengthening of tendoachilles to prevent recurrence.
5. Avoid overcorrection of deformity (results in valgus heel).
6. Avoid incisions in the plantar skin.

Postoperative Care Issues

1. Place the foot in a well-padded, well-molded long leg posterior mold or cast. If skin is under tension place the foot in equinus.
2. If necessary perform a cast change at 2 weeks.
3. Remove pins at 6 weeks.
4. Brace with corrective ankle-foot orthosis (AFO) for 1 year.

Operative Technique

1. Place the patient prone at the end of the operating table. Put a tourniquet on the proximal thigh. Prepare and drape the leg to the midthigh. Place a bump under the contralateral hip to present the medial aspect of the operative foot.
2. Make a transverse incision from the base of first metatarsal medially to the base of the fibula laterally. Stay in the dorsal skin, 0.5 cm proximal to the heel crease **(Fig. 47–1)**.
3. Use sharp dissection to isolate the Achilles tendon. Carefully isolate the sural nerve laterally and protect it with a vessel loop.

4. Elevate the peroneal tendon sheath and retract it anteriorly. Incise the calcaneofibular ligament close to the fibula. Identify the lateral subtalar joint and perform a capsulotomy up to the calcaneocuboid joint **(Fig. 47–2A)**.
5. Perform a "Z" lengthening of the tendoachilles. Incise proximal/lateral and distal/medial with a lengthening of at least 2.5 cm.
6. Expose the posterior capsule, divide the posterior talofibular ligament, retract the flexor hallucis longus (FHL) tendon medially and the peroneal tendons laterally. Plantarflex and dorsiflex the ankle to determine the level of the joint line. Perform sequential capsulotomies of the posterior ankle joint followed by the subtalar joint. Take care not to injure the deep fibers of the deltoid ligament **(Fig. 47–2B)**.
7. Medially, using the FHL muscle as a guide, carefully expose the neurovascular bundle and isolate it with two vessel loops. Dissect the medial and lateral plantar branches of the nerve and artery into the arch of the foot. Preserve the calcaneal branch of the nerve.
8. Incise the posterior tibial (PT) tendon sheath and perform a "Z" lengthening proximal to the medial malleolus. Incise the tendon sheath of the flexor digitorum longus (FDL) to the Master Knot of Henry, and perform a "Z" lengthening. Identify and free the FHL. An intramuscular lengthening of the FHL may be performed at the conclusion of the procedure.
9. Identify and perform capsulotomies of the talonavicular joint (superior, inferior, medial, and lateral). Complete the capsulotomy of the subtalar joint **(Fig. 47–2C)**.
10. Release the abductor hallucis (adductor hallucis recession) from its origin along with its fascial attachments if needed.
11. Reduce the talonavicular, calcaneocuboid, and subtalar joints. If necessary, partially incise the interosseous talocalcaneal ligament to allow derotation of subtalar joint.
12. Assess need for calcaneocuboid joint capsulotomy and plantar fasciotomy.

13. Place a smooth K-wire from the posterolateral corner of talus across the talonavicular joint. Aim the wire to exit dorsally at the first web space. Place a second smooth K-wire from calcaneus to talus (plantar to dorsal) without entering the ankle joint **(Fig. 47–3)**.

14. Release the tourniquet prior to taking films. Achieve hemostasis.

15. Assess the correction with plain films (AP and lateral). The lateral is the most useful.

16. Suture the tendons with foot in 20 degrees of dorsiflexion. Ensure that the peroneal tendons are located and stable.

17. Close the wound with interrupted or running subcuticular suture.

Suggested Readings

Beaty JH. Congenital anomalies of the foot and lower extremity. In: Canale ST, Beaty JH, eds. *Operative Pediatric Orthopaedics*. St. Louis, MO: C.V. Mosby, 1995, pp. 72–134.

Crawford AH, Marxen JL, Osterfeld DL. The Cincinnati incision: a comprehensive approach for surgical procedures of the foot and ankle in childhood. *J Bone Joint Surg* 1982;64A:1355–1358.

Sullivan JA. The child's foot. In: Morrissy RT, Weinstein SL, eds. *Lovell and Winter's Pediatric Orthopaedics*. Philadelphia, PA: Lippincott-Raven, 1996, pp. 1077–1135.

CHAPTER 48

Distal Humerus Supracondylar Fracture

Reduction and Pinning

John J. Grayhack

Indications

1. Distal humerus supracondylar fractures with significant displacement or angulation
2. Minimally or nondisplaced distal humerus supracondylar fractures with associated trauma or injury (i.e., neurovascular compromise, compartment syndrome, associated fractures or soft tissue loss)

Contraindications

➤ Avascular/ischemic distal upper extremity before or after attempted reduction (relative)

Preoperative Preparation

1. Physical examination to include

   a. Evaluation of skin integrity and examination of soft tissues
   b. Assessment of any impingement of fracture fragments in muscle
   c. Analysis of distal pulses (palpation and/or Doppler) and capillary return
   d. Distal neurological evaluation (all nerves and nerve branches—motor and sensory)
   e. Assessment of any evidence of a compartment syndrome

2. Appropriate medical and anesthesiology evaluations
3. Elevation and splinting (avoid significant elbow flexion) of involved limb
4. Close observation with intermittent re-examination of distal motor, sensory, and vascular status
5. Elbow radiographs including true anteroposterior (AP) and lateral views; if needed, contralateral elbow radiographs may be helpful.

Special Instruments, Position, and Anesthesia

1. Inverted C-arm fluoroscopy is necessary.
2. A power drill and Kirschner wire set are required.
3. Sterile Doppler ultrasound probe may be required for certain cases.
4. The patient is positioned supine on the operating room table with ipsilateral shoulder at table edge and abducted 60 to 90 degrees. The patient's arm is placed over (or upon) the inverted C-arm. This is utilized as the operating surface. The elbow should rest at the center of the C-arm surface.
5. General anesthesia is preferred for this procedure. The anesthesiologist should be made aware of the force necessary for appropriate traction during reduction.

Tips and Pearls

1. A preoperative detailed neurovascular assessment is essential. Pay particular attention to pulses, capillary refill, and function of the anterior interosseous nerve branch.
2. If the patient is too small to allow the elbow to be centered on the C-arm, place a radiolucent arm table securely as a lateral table extension and move the patient laterally.
3. If the vascular examination deteriorates after attempted reduction, release the reduction. Either delay intervention or proceed with open reduction.
4. If swelling obscures bony landmarks, consider making a small dermal skin incision followed by blunt dissection to bone. The elbow should be kept in extension to help protect the ulnar nerve.

What To Avoid

1. Avoid compromising vascular blood flow to achieve bone reduction.
2. Avoid the ulnar nerve during pin placement.
3. Avoid placing pins that do not engage the contralateral cortex.
4. If placing medial and lateral pins, avoid placing them so they cross at the level of the fracture site on the AP view. Preferably they should cross proximal to the fracture to enhance stability.

Postoperative Care Issues

1. Splint or cast the extremity with the elbow flexed 90 degrees or less.
2. Hand elevation above the elbow and elbow elevation above the heart should continue for 12 to 48 h after surgery unless vascular compromise is noted. Frequent, detailed neurovascular examinations are essential. Direct your attention toward changes of neurovascular compromise and/or a developing compartment syndrome. If such changes are noted, consider extending the elbow and/or releasing the dressing.
3. If ulnar nerve signs are noted, consider removing the medial pin and/or extending the elbow.

Operative Technique

1. Position the patient supine on the operating room table. Drape the injured arm over an inverted C-arm. The elbow should rest at the center of the C-arm surface. This is utilized as the operating surface. Do not apply a tourniquet.
2. Document the distal neurovascular examination prior to attempting a reduction.
3. Attempt a closed reduction prior to sterile preparation of the extremity.
4. Stabilize the proximal humerus taking care not to place pressure or traction at the axilla. Attempt to reduce the fracture.

Fracture reduction

a. Align the distal fragment in the medial-lateral plane. Apply traction to the extremity so the fragments are distracted "out to length" (**Fig. 48–1A**).
b. Flex the elbow, translating the distal fragment anteriorly as desired (**Fig. 48–1B**). If the distal fragment is anterior, reverse this final maneuver.
c. If the proximal fragment is impinged in the anterior musculature, "milk" the fragment out.
d. Repeat the vascular examination (palpable or Doppler pulses and capillary return) with the fracture in the reduced position and the elbow flexed 90 degrees. If any deterioration in the vascular examination is noted, release the reduction and re-evaluate the vascular examination.
e. Assess the reduction radiographically in both the AP (often by slightly obliquing the view) and lateral planes. The best lateral view is usually obtained by *external* rotation of the shoulder.
f. If open reduction is anticipated, apply the tourniquet at this time.

5. Prepare and drape the arm from shoulder to hand in the hospital's standard sterile fashion. Drape the C-arm base with a half-sheet. Secure the sheet with a Penrose drain that is stretched and clamped beneath the rim of the C-arm.

Lateral pin

a. After reducing the fracture and flexing the elbow, percutaneously place the lateral pin. An appropriate size smooth pin (usually 0.062 in) is used.

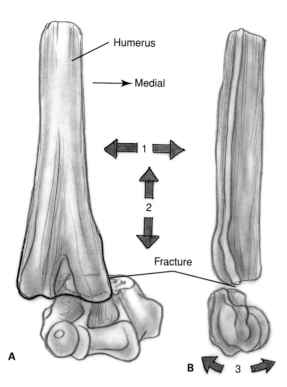

Figure 48–1 (A) Distal humerus fracture—AP view. (1) The first step is to align the distal fragment in the medial-lateral plane. (2) Next traction is applied so the distal fracture fragment is distracted "out to length." **(B)** Distal humerus fracture—lateral view. (3) The final step in the reduction requires translating the distal fracture fragment anteriorly by flexing the elbow. If the distal fragment is anterior, reverse this final maneuver.

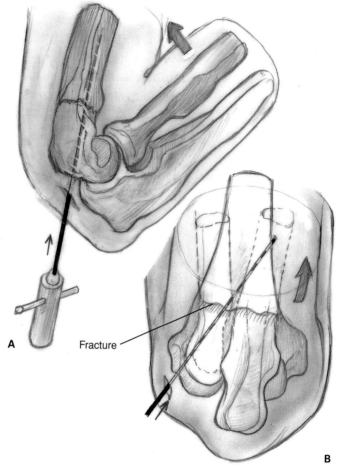

Figure 48–2 (A) Lateral pin insertion—lateral view. Insert the lateral pin with the patient's elbow flexed. Insert the pin by placing it against the bone distal to the lateral epicondyle. The pin should be angled obliquely and aimed medially and proximally. **(B)** Lateral pin insertion—AP view (with elbow flexed). The pin is across the fracture line. It is fully seated when it is advanced into the contralateral cortex of the proximal bone.

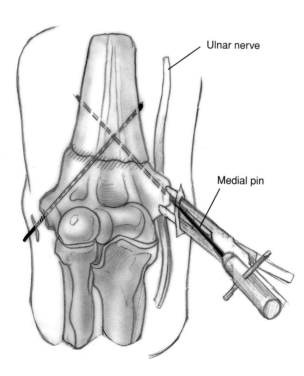

Figure 48–3 Medial pin insertion—AP view. The medial pin is inserted with the elbow extended. The lateral pin maintains the reduction. The medial pin can be inserted through a small dermal incision slightly distally to the medial epicondyle. A small clamp is bluntly advanced down to bone and the pin inserted between the clamp's arms into the distal fragment. Note the elbow is *flexed* prior to advancing the pin into the proximal fragment and contralateral cortex (not pictured).

b. Insert the pin by starting distal to the lateral epicondyle. Angle the pin obliquely. Aim medially and proximally.

c. First advance the pin through the distal fragment and then across the fracture line. Continue advancing the pin into the contralateral cortex of the proximal bone (**Figs. 48–2A and 2B**). There is no consensus on the optimal number of lateral pins to be placed (one or two) or whether a medial pin should be inserted. If you insert a second lateral pin, place it parallel to the initial pin. Some surgeons believe two lateral pins are sufficient, while others believe a medial pin should supplement lateral pin fixation. In general, lateral pins minimize risks to the ulnar nerve, however, biomechanically they may not achieve equivalent fixation to crossed pins (medial and lateral pins).

Medial pin

Take care while inserting the medial pin to avoid injury to the ulnar nerve. Crossed pins (medial pin in conjunction with lateral pin(s)) may optimize stability.

a. Extend the elbow partially or fully. Maintain the reduction with the lateral pin.

b. Palpate and protect the ulnar nerve.

c. If swelling is significant, make a 4-mm dermal incision slightly distally to the medial epicondyle. Bluntly dissect down to the medial epicondyle.

d. Advance an appropriate size smooth pin (usually 0.062 in) to the bone between the arms of a mosquito clamp (**Fig. 48–3**).

e. Advance the pin into the distal fragment with the patient's elbow extended.

f. Flex the elbow and advance the pin into the proximal fragment and contralateral cortex. The medial and lateral pins must not cross at the level of fracture site on AP view. Commonly, they cross proximal to the fracture site.

6. Perform a final assessment of the reduction, fixation, and vascular status.

7. Bend the pins over, being careful not to pull these back from the contralateral cortex. Cut them off outside the skin. However, ensure that the ends of the pins protrude sufficiently so that they do not recede beneath the skin.

8. Apply a sterile dressing.

9. Apply a splint or cast with the elbow flexed not more than 90 degrees. Assess elbow radiographs for reduction and pin placement.

Suggested Readings

Canale ST. Fractures and dislocations. In: *Operative Pediatric Orthopaedics*. 2nd ed. St. Louis, MO: Mosby-Year Book, 1995, p. 1043.

Green NE. Fractures and dislocations about the elbow. In: *Skeletal Trauma in Children*. Vol. 3. 2nd ed. Philadelphia, PA: W.B. Saunders, 1998, pp. 271–274.

CHAPTER 49

Hip Aspiration

Roger Dunteman and John F. Sarwark

Indications

1. Evaluation of infectious, inflammatory, or metabolic disorders
2. Assessment of reduction and morphology of the cartilaginous femoral epiphysis in hip dysplasia
3. Decompression of significant joint effusions due to septic arthritis, hemarthrosis, or inflammation
4. Injection of therapeutic agents into the joint

Contraindications

1. Soft tissue cellulitis in the path of needle placement
2. Tumor tissue in the path of needle placement
3. Uncontrolled bleeding tendency

Preoperative Preparation

1. Obtain anteroposterior (AP) pelvis and lateral hip radiographs.
2. If infection is suspected, send blood for culture, complete blood count (CBC), differential, erythrocyte sedimentation rate (ESR), and C-reactive protein (CRP) prior to initiation of antibiotics.
3. Obtain vials for cell count, Gram stain, culture (aerobic, anaerobic, acid-fast bacteria, and fungal), crystal analysis, and chemistry (glucose and protein).

Special Instruments, Position, and Anesthesia

1. Monitored intramuscular or intravenous sedation (preferred) or general anesthesia
2. For local anesthesia, 1% lidocaine can be injected subdermally. Remember lidocaine is bacteriostatic. Do not inject it into the joint.
3. Fluoroscope or fluoroscopy
4. Sterile preps, drapes, and gloves
5. 18 to 20-gauge lumbar puncture needle with stylet to prevent inadvertent breaking or needle plugging
6. Sterile saline (nonbacteriostatic)
7. Two 10-cc syringes
8. Two intravenous extension tubes
9. Cell count and culture tubes (as above)
10. Use diatrizoate sodium (Renograffin) diluted to half-strength as a contrast medium.

Tips and Pearls

1. Use air instead of contrast media to prove that the needle tip needle is in the joint. Extra-articular contrast media will obscure the field.
2. Most contrast media is bactericidal and will reduce the culture's sensitivity if injected prior to obtaining an adequate fluid sample.
3. Do not judge the presence or absence of infection based on the aspirated fluid's appearance.

4. The hip joint cavity extends distal to its capsular insertion at the cervicotrochanteric line.

What To Avoid

1. Avoid injecting the femoral vessels. Consider marking the vessels with a pen prior to the procedure. Remember the nerve, artery, and vein lie from lateral to medial in the femoral triangle.
2. Avoid injecting the round ligament or the articular cartilage. Using the anterior approach may reduce this possibility.
3. Avoid injecting or traumatizing the physis, especially when using the anterior or lateral approach.
4. Avoid injecting the bone or cartilage when using contrast dye. This problem can be minimized by slowly rotating and withdrawing the needle while simultaneously injecting the dye.

Postoperative Care Issues

1. Some patients develop an acute, painful, sterile effusion after aspiration usually within 12 h. Reaspiration is not usually necessary, but normally reveals no organisms.
2. Mild allergic reactions consisting or urticaria and pruritis can occur within 15 min of contrast dye injection.
3. Joint infection is extremely rare following arthrograms (one infection in 25,000 arthrograms).

Operative Technique

Three approaches are commonly used: medial (adductor), anterior, and lateral.

1. Position the patient as described below depending on the approach chosen.
2. Prepare and drape the patient in a standard fashion. Allow for later manipulation of the hip joint.
3. Fill and label one syringe with saline and the other with contrast.

Adductor medial approach

a. Position the hip in maximum abduction, maximum external rotation, and 60 to 90 degrees of hip flexion (**Fig. 49–1**).
b. Insert the needle into the skin posterior to the adductor longus. Confirm placement with fluoroscopy. Incline the needle 20 degrees posterior and advance it toward the ipsilateral axilla.
c. Continue advancing the needle until the femoral neck is encountered. A "pop" may be felt as the hip capsule is pierced.
d. Confirm needle position by moving the thigh. The needle head should move in the opposite direction of the hip. The tip may be felt scratching the cartilage.
e. Confirm needle position utilizing radiographs or fluoroscopy. The image should show the needle directed at the upper portion of the femoral neck.

Anterior approach

a. Position the hip in neutral rotation and in the maximal extension tolerable to the patient.
b. Insert the needle into the skin one to two fingerbreadths lateral to the femoral artery pulse and one fingerbreadth below the middle of inguinal ligament. Confirm placement with fluoroscopy.
c. Incline the needle 20 degrees medially and posteriorly and advance it. Keep the bevel facing the femoral neck to minimize physeal trauma (**Fig. 49–2**).
d. A "pop" maybe felt as the hip capsule is pierced.
e. Confirm needle position by moving the thigh. The needle head should move in the opposite direction of the hip. The tip may be felt scratching the cartilage.
f. Confirm needle position utilizing radiographs or fluoroscopy. The image should show the needle tip in the upper portion of the femoral neck, distal to the femoral physis.

Lateral approach

This approach is useful when the full length of the needle needs to be visualized. It is not a useful approach in obese patients.

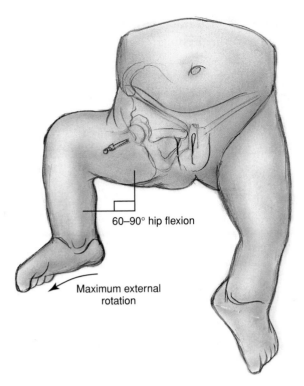

Figure 49–1 Patient position. Position the hip in maximum abduction, maximum external rotation, and 60 to 90 degrees of hip flexion.

60–90° hip flexion

Maximum external rotation

Figure 49–2 Anterior approach. The needle is inserted one to two fingerbreadths lateral to the femoral artery and one fingerbreadth below the middle of inguinal ligament. The needle is inclined 20 degrees medially and posteriorly and advanced. A "pop" may be felt when the hip capsule is pierced.

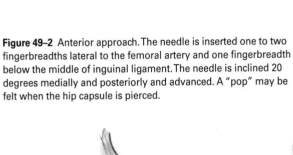

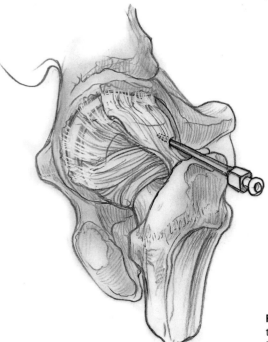

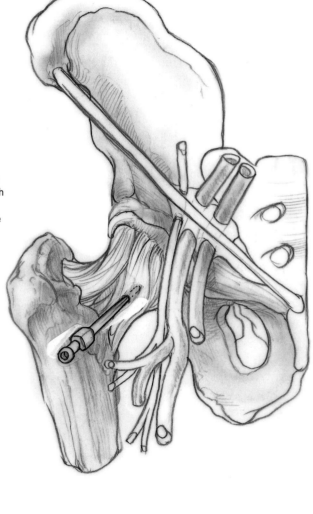

Figure 49–3 Lateral approach. Advance the needle perpendicular to the lateral thigh. Enter the lateral joint capsule medially. A "pop" may be felt when the hip capsule is pierced.

a. Position the hip in neutral rotation.

b. Insert the needle into the skin just proximal to the tip of the greater trochanter. Confirm placement with fluoroscopy.

c. Advance the needle perpendicular to the lateral thigh. Enter the lateral joint capsule medially **(Fig. 49–3)**. A "pop" may be felt when the hip capsule is pierced.

d. Confirm needle position by moving the thigh. The needle head should move in the opposite direction of the hip. The tip may be felt scratching the cartilage.

e. Confirm needle position utilizing radiographs or fluoroscopy. The image should show the needle directed at the center of the femoral head.

4. Reconfirm needle position with fluoroscopy.

5. Consider injecting air into the joint to make fluoroscopic detection easier.

6. Inject 1 to 3 cc of sterile saline (nonbacteriostatic). If the saline is difficult to inject the needle is probably inside the articular cartilage.

7. Attempt to withdraw the sterile saline. If the saline is difficult to withdraw, the needle is probably extra-articular.

8. Draw samples for culture and analysis when needle is believed to be correctly positioned.

9. After fluid is aspirated, but not prior to this time, inject radio-opaque dye. This procedure outlines the joint surface and confirms that the needle position is extra-articular.

10. Apply gentle pressure to obtain hemostasis.

11. Apply sterile dressing.

Suggested Readings

Aliabadi P, Baker ND, Jaramillo D. Hip Arthrography, aspiration, block, and bursography. *Radiol Clin North Am* 1998;36:673–690.

Blake MP, Halasz SJ. Effect of X-ray contrast media on bacterial growth. *Australas Radiol* 1995;39:10–13.

Freiberger RH. Introducing arthrography. In: Freiberger RH, Kaye JJ, eds. *Arthrography*. Norwalk, CT: Appleton-Century-Crofts, 1979, pp. 1–3.

Kasser JR. *Bone and Joint Infections*. In: Canale ST, Beatty SH, eds. *Operative Pediatric Orthopaedics*. 2nd ed. St. Louis, MO: Mosby-Year Book, 1995, pp. 1128–1129.

Kilcoyne RF, Kaplan P. The lateral approach for hip arthrography. *Skeletal Radiol* 1992;21:239–240.

Sponseller PD, Stevens HM. *Handbook of Pediatric Orthopedics*. Boston, MA: Little, Brown, 1997.

Tachdjian MO. *Pediatric Orthopedics*. 2nd ed. Philadelphia, PA: W.B. Saunders, 1990.

Towers JD. Radiographic evaluation of the hip. In: Callaghan JJ, Rosenberg AG, Rubash HE, eds. *The Adult Hip*. Philadelphia, PA: Lippincott-Raven, 1998, pp. 338–372.

CHAPTER 50

Idiopathic Scoliosis

Posterior Spinal Instrumentation and Fusion

Erik C. King and John J. Grayhack

Indications

1. Thoracic curve greater than 50 degrees
2. Thoracolumbar curve greater than 40 degrees
3. Progressive curve greater than 40 degrees in a skeletally immature patient that is associated with significant spinal imbalance or that cannot be controlled with a brace
4. Cosmetically unacceptable spinal deformity

Contraindications

1. Active infection or sepsis (absolute)
2. Anemia
3. Cardiac, pulmonary, or other medical comorbidities that have not been optimally managed

Preoperative Preparation

1. Comprehensive physical examination including neurologic testing if indicated
2. Full-length (14 in × 36 in) standing coronal anteroposterior (AP) and sagittal (lateral) radiographs of the thoracic-lumbar-sacral spine. If desired by the surgeon, preoperative supine right and left side-bending radiographs to assist in the selection of spinal levels for fusion.
3. The planned instrumentation pattern (hooks, wires, screws, and rods) is drawn on the coronal radiograph.

4. Two to four units of autologous or directed donor blood should be cross-matched. Intraoperative blood salvage (cell-saver) may also be utilized.
5. Pulmonary function tests if indicated
6. Discussion of indications, goals, perioperative care, and common potential risks with the patient and family

Special Instruments, Position, and Anesthesia

1. Spinal components and techniques are selected preoperatively.
2. Prone positioning device, such as the Hall-Relton or Wilson frame, which cushions pressure points and permits free expansion of the thorax and abdomen; minimizing abdominal pressure decreases venous pressure, and aids in reducing intraoperative bleeding.
3. Multiple self-retaining retractors such as Weitlaner, Gelpi, and Adson-Beckman retractors
4. Somatosensory-evoked potential (SSEP) monitoring; motor-evoked potential (MEP) monitoring is also used by some spine surgeons.
5. Headlamp
6. Bone graft substitute and/or bone graft extender products
7. Gelfoam and thrombin
8. The procedure is performed under general anesthesia.

Tips and Pearls

1. Carefully document the preoperative neurologic examination (motor, sensory, and reflexes) so that a comparison can be made in the event that a neurologic deficit is detected during the postoperative period.
2. Prepare and drape the surgical area widely in case surgical extension is required.
3. Scrutinize preoperative radiographs for:

   a. Anatomic anomalies that may predispose the patient to unexpected neurologic injury (e.g., spina bifida occulta, hemivertebra)
   b. Sagittal imbalance
   c. Anatomic relationships that will aid intraoperative decision making (e.g., apex of deformity, relationship of iliac crest to lower vertebral bodies)

4. Intravenous antibiotics should be administered prior to the skin incision and repeated at appropriate intervals. Because of blood loss and fluid shifts, the dosing interval is shorter than in nonoperative situations.
5. Ensure that the anesthesiologist monitors the patient's coagulation status. Baseline health status, duration of procedure, intraoperative blood loss, and temperature influence coagulation.
6. A separate skin incision to harvest iliac crest bone may be used if the caudal end of the planned fusion ends in the upper lumbar spine. Alternatively, the crest may be approached through the spine incision by subcutaneous dissection and a separate fascial incision directly over the iliac crest.

What To Avoid

1. Avoid straying from the subperiosteal plane when exposing the spine.
2. Avoid incorrect placement of instruments in the vicinity of the dura and/or nerve roots.
3. Avoid inserting implants at unintended levels. Do not accept a less than adequate intraoperative scout radiograph when identifying vertebral levels. If necessary, repeat the radiograph.

4. Avoid ending the implanted construct in the apices of secondary coronal or sagittal curves. Chronic instability and late deformity progression may result from partially fusing a curve.
5. Avoid imprecise use of instrumentation implants (e.g., stripping or cross-threading screws/nuts).

Postoperative Care Issues

1. A suction drain is optional. If a drain is used, a closed suction drain should be placed superficial to the deep fascial closure.
2. Neurologic examination should be performed immediately after termination of general anesthesia and repeated frequently during the postoperative period. If a significant neurologic deficit develops, consider removal of the implanted instrumentation.
3. Consider patient controlled anesthesia (PCA) for postoperative analgesia. Alternatively, epidural anesthesia can be used if adequate pain control can be obtained without motor blockade.
4. Postoperative immobilization is not mandatory. However, some surgeons may elect to use a brace if they are concerned with the quality of the internal fixation.
5. The patient is allowed to sit up and take a few steps with assistance on the day after surgery.
6. The surgical dressing is changed on the second postoperative day. It is discontinued on the fifth postoperative day if there is no wound drainage.

Operative Technique

This chapter describes basic surgical techniques for performing a selective thoracic fusion for an idiopathic thoracic curve, King–Moe type II or III curve. There are several alternative techniques to those described. Successful techniques have in common the following principles: meticulous subperiosteal dissection, clear understanding of the biomechanics of spinal deformity, precise technical handling of spinal implants, and thorough decortication of posterior elements. Several spinal instrumentation systems are available for selection.

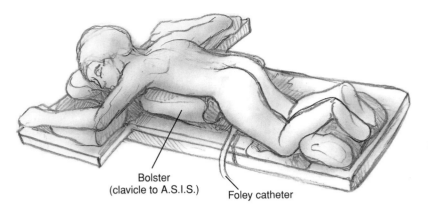

Figure 50–1 Patient position. The patient is positioned prone on a positioning device or on longitudinal bolsters. The abdomen and genitalia should not be compressed.

Bolster (clavicle to A.S.I.S.)

Foley catheter

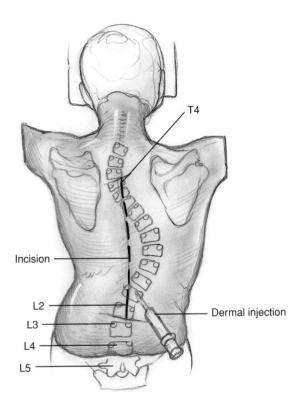

T4

Incision

L2

L3

L4

L5

Dermal injection

Figure 50–2 Skin incision. Plan the skin incision so it is straight in the midline. It should extend from the spinous process proximal to the most cephalad-planned instrumented vertebra to the spinous process of the most caudal-planned instrumented vertebra. A solution of 1:500,000 epinephrine in normal saline is injected into the dermis and subdermal tissues along the planned incision.

Figure 50–3 Subperiosteal infiltration. A solution of 1:500,000 epinephrine in normal saline is injected subperiosteally over each lamina at the desired surgical levels. Take care to avoid penetrating the interlaminar space.

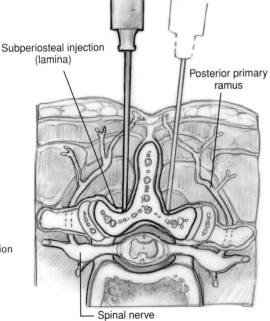

Subperiosteal injection (lamina)

Posterior primary ramus

Spinal nerve

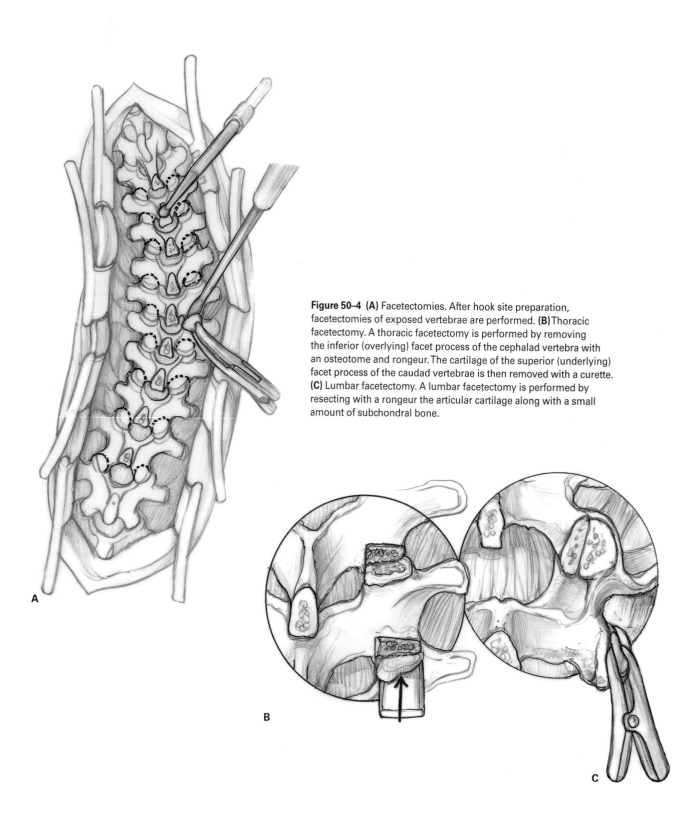

Figure 50–4 (A) Facetectomies. After hook site preparation, facetectomies of exposed vertebrae are performed. **(B)** Thoracic facetectomy. A thoracic facetectomy is performed by removing the inferior (overlying) facet process of the cephalad vertebra with an osteotome and rongeur. The cartilage of the superior (underlying) facet process of the caudad vertebrae is then removed with a curette. **(C)** Lumbar facetectomy. A lumbar facetectomy is performed by resecting with a rongeur the articular cartilage along with a small amount of subchondral bone.

A

B

C

Positioning and anesthesia

1. Initiate general anesthesia while the patient is supine on the transportation cart.

2. Place a radial arterial line and a central venous line.

3. Insert a Foley catheter.

4. Secure the endotracheal tube and intravenous/arterial lines.

5. Turn the patient to the prone position on top of the padded positioning device. Ensure free expansion of the abdomen and support of the hips. Remember that the amount of hip flexion affects the amount of lumbar lordosis (**Fig. 50–1**).

6. Take care to insure that the axilla is not compressed.

7. Pad the legs so that pressure is distributed as widely as possible.

Incision and exposure

8. Prepare and widely drape the back and posterior iliac crest. Cover the entire operative field with a self-adhering povidone-iodine drape (Ioban).

9. Plan the skin incision. The incision is straight in the midline. It should extend from the spinous process proximal to the most cephalad-planned instrumented vertebra to the spinous process of the most caudal-planned instrumented vertebra (**Fig. 50–2**).

10. Infiltrate the intradermal and subdermal tissues with a solution of 1:500,000 epinephrine in normal saline to minimize bleeding. If desired, infiltrate subperiostally over the lamina utilizing a spinal needle on both sides of the posterior spinous processes of the levels to be dissected. Take care not to penetrate the interlaminar space (**Fig. 50–3**).

11. Incise the skin with a scalpel. Use an electrocautery to dissect the deeper tissues. Divide the avascular median raphe (interspinous ligaments) in the midline. The raphe can be visualized as a thin white line between the paraspinal muscles. Use 3 or 4 Weitlaner retractors to retract the tissue.

12. Identify the apophysis of each posterior spinous process. After they have all been identified, split each with a scalpel or electrocautery.

13. Expose the lamina, facet joint, and transverse process of each vertebral level. This should be done in a subperiosteal fashion to minimize bleeding. Use a Cobb elevator to dissect off the cartilaginous apophysis. Continue in a subperiosteal plane by sliding the elevator onto the lamina and the trans-verse process. Paraspinal muscles attach to the caudal edge of the lamina and must be divided with a scalpel or electrocautery. This is best done while placing the tissue under traction with an elevator. The anatomy of the lumbar spine differs from that of the thoracic spine. In the lumbar spine, divide the capsule of the facet joint and then expose the facets with an elevator.

14. After completing the dissection at a vertebral level, pack that level with a surgical sponge to minimize bleeding and proceed to the next level. Repeat this procedure until both sides of the spine are adequately exposed. Do not expose the facets distal to the most caudal vertebra to be included in the fusion.

15. Place a radiopaque marker (towel clip) onto a spinous process and take an AP radiograph to confirm the vertebral level. When interpreting the radiograph, remember that in the lower thoracic spine, the cephalad aspect of a spinous process coincides or is slightly distal to the caudal edge of its associated vertebral body.

Bone graft procurement

Iliac crest bone graft harvesting techniques are described in Chapter 44. Consider harvesting the iliac crest bone graft while awaiting development of radiographs for level confirmation.

16. In skeletally immature patients, the cartilaginous apophysis over the crest is usually split with a scalpel or electrocautery.

17. Bone is then harvested as in adults.

18. Irrigate the wound and obtain hemostasis. If necessary, use Gelfoam or Surgicell.

19. Close the apophysis and fascia tightly with heavy absorbable suture; then close the subcutaneous tissue in layers.

20. If desired, place a closed suction drain superficial to the fascia.

Instrumentation

Based on the preoperative plan, prepare hook sites on both the concave and convex sides of the curve. After the hooks are placed, the concave rod is secured and manipulated. Next, the convex rod is secured. In order to increase torsional stability, the two rods are connected by transverse cross-links.

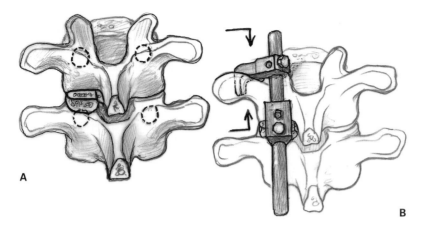

Figure 50–5 **(A)** Thoracic claw preparation. Note the anatomy showing the location of the pedicle and transverse process. **(B)** Thoracic claw. A thoracic claw consists of a caudal-facing transverse process hook and a cephalad-facing pedicle hook.

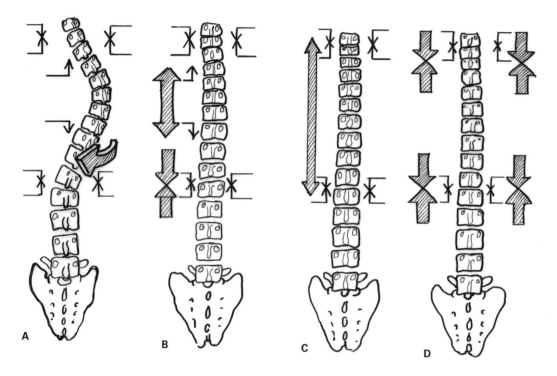

Figure 50–6 A typical maneuver sequence to treat a right thoracic scoliotic curvature. Hook positions are designated by up-going and down-going thin arrows. Compression forces and distraction forces that are applied by the surgeon are designated by thick arrows. **(A)** After placing the hooks, the left concave rod is secured and then slowly rotated dorsally and toward the midline. Normal thoracic kyphosis is re-established. **(B)** The caudad claw is compressed together and tightened. The intermediate hooks are then distracted and tightened. **(C)** The cephalad and caudad claws are distracted away from each other. **(D)** The right convex rod is placed, and then the cephalad and caudad claws of both rods are compressed and tightened. Transverse cross-link connectors are then placed.

Transverse process hook preparation (caudad-facing or down-going)

a. Expose the transverse process of the vertebra to receive the hook. Transverse process hooks are usually placed on the most cephalad vertebra instrumented as part of a claw construct spanning one or two levels.

b. Pass the laminar hook starter or pedicle hook starter over the cephalad edge of the selected vertebra. Ensure that the hook starter is placed around the transverse process since this structure can be easily broken.

c. Remove the hook starter.

Pedicle hook preparation (cephalad-facing or up-going)

a. Make a transverse osteotomy on the inferior edge of the lamina (and inferior articular process) of the vertebra. Position the osteotomy so that the tips of the bifid pedicle hook will engage the pedicle as the shoulder of the hook touches the bone of the osteotomized inferior facet.

b. Remove the full thickness of bone at the osteotomy site with a rongeur. This should expose the articular surface of the superior facet of the next caudal vertebra.

c. Remove the articular cartilage of the superior facet with a curette.

d. Insert the trial pedicle hook (pedicle finder) into the prepared site and seat it gently with a mallet. Make sure that you do not split the tables of the lamina. Great care must be taken not to allow the tips of this instrument to slip into the spinal canal. This is best accomplished by directing the trial pedicle hook in a cephalad and lateral direction.

e. Remove the pedicle hook trial.

Supralaminar hook preparation (caudad-facing or down-going)

a. Using a rongeur, remove the spinous process cephalad to the vertebra to receive the supralaminar hook. Continue removing bone until the instraspinous space and the ligamentum flavum are exposed.

b. Create a 3-mm opening in the midline portion of the ligamentum flavum with a narrow rongeur or a #15 scalpel. Bulging epidural fat signals successful entrance into the spinal canal.

c. Excise the ipsilateral ligamentum flavum using narrow rongeurs and kerrison rongeurs.

d. Perform a laminotomy by using kerrosen rongeurs to remove the inferior lamina of the next cephalad vertebra. Remove as little bone as possible from the superior edge of the lamina of the selected vertebra. Excess bone removal will compromise purchase of the caudally facing hook.

e. Place the laminar hook starter into the prepared space.

f. Remove the hook starter.

Infralaminar hook preparation (cephalad-facing or up-going)

a. Using a laminar elevator, elevate the ligamentum flavum from the undersurface of the caudal edge of the vertebra. Stay close to the midline.

b. Insert the laminar hook starter along the tract that has just been created underneath the caudal edge. Preserve the interspinous ligament distal to the spinous process of the most caudal instrumented vertebra.

c. Remove the hook starter.

Facetectomy and decortication

21. Remove all trial hooks and perform facetectomies (**Fig. 50–4A**).

22. There are several facetectomy techniques, all of which share the goal of promoting arthrodesis of the facet joint. In the thoracic spine, remove the inferior facet with a straight or curved osteotome (**Fig. 50–4B**) and then curette the articular cartilage of the superior facet of the caudal vertebra. In the technique popularized by Moe, corticancellous bone graft is impacted into the defect of the facet joint. In the lumbar spine, resect with a rongeur the articular cartilage along with a small amount of subchondral bone (**Fig. 50–4C**). Remember the locations of the previously prepared hook sites, as any further bone removal could impair the integrity of these sites.

23. Decorticate the spinous process, the laminae, and the transverse process with an osteotome or a power burr.

Implantation

24. Measure, cut, and contour the metal rods. The concave rod should conform to the normal sagittal

contour of the spine segment to be fused. Some surgeons contour the convex rod with less thoracic kyphosis than normal (i.e., flatter). The purpose of this under-contouring is to place an anterior directed corrective force against the rib prominence.

25. Place appropriate size hooks into the previously prepared hook sites (**Figs. 50–5A and 5B**).
26. Place bone graft over the decorticated bone surfaces.
27. Place the concave rod and secure it to the hooks. The assistant should stabilize the hooks and aid in the assembly of the components of the construct.
28. Seat the hooks by segmental distraction using a rod holder, vise grip, distraction device, and compression device. The exact sequence varies among spine surgeons.
29. Rotate the rod slowly and gently. The direction of rotation is such that the scoliotic (coronal) contour is converted to a kyphotic (sagittal) contour (**Fig. 50–6A**). The rod should be rotated no more than 90 degrees. Check SSEP and MEP signals prior to and throughout rod rotation. In some cases, the assistant can facilitate rotation by applying anterior-directed pressure over the rib prominence.
30. Check the seating of the hooks and the integrity of the bone-hook and hook-rod interfaces.
31. Compress together and then tighten the caudal claw (**Fig. 50–6B**).
32. Distract the intermediate hooks and then tighten (**Fig. 50–6B**).
33. Distract the cephalad and caudad claws away from each other (**Fig. 50–6C**).
34. Insert the convex rod and secure it to the hooks. Compress the hooks enough to seat them firmly.
35. Compress and tighten the cephalad and caudad claws of both rods (**Fig. 50–6D**).
36. Perform a final tightening of all components.
37. Connect the rods with two transverse cross-links, one near each end.
38. Irrigate the wound thoroughly.
39. Place the remainder of the bone graft over exposed bone surfaces and metal implants.

Closure

40. Re-approximate the apophyses and myofascial layers with a heavy absorbable suture.
41. If desired, place a suction drain superficial to the fascial closure.
42. Close the subcutaneous tissue and skin in layers.
43. Apply a sterile dressing.
44. Carefully turn the patient to the supine position and transfer to the transportation cart.
45. Take a long cassette AP radiograph of the spine.
46. Review the radiograph for curve correction, hardware position, and pneumothorax. Conclude general anesthesia if the radiographic findings are satisfactory.
47. Perform a brief neurologic examination.
48. Transfer the patient to the recovery room.

Suggested Readings

Asher MA. Isola instrumentation. In: Bradford DS, ed. *The Spine*. Philadelphia, PA: Lippincott-Raven, 1997, pp. 407–434.

Cotrel Y, Dubousset J, Guillaumat M. New universal instrumentation in spinal surgery. *Clin Orthop* 1988; 227:10–23.

Johnston CE II, Ashman RB, Richards BS, Herring JA. TSRH universal spine instrumentation. In: Bradford KH, Bridwell RL, eds. *The Textbook of Spinal Surgery*. Philadelphia, PA: Lippincott-Raven, 1997, pp. 535–567.

King HA, Moe JH, Bradford DS, Winter RB. The selection of fusion levels in thoracic idiopathic scoliosis. *J Bone Joint Surg* 1983;65A:1302–1313.

Shufflebarger HI. Theory and mechanisms of posterior derotation spinal systems. In: Weinstein SI, ed. *The Pediatric Spine: Principles and Practice*. New York, NY: Raven Press, 1994, 1515–1543.

Section Nine

Miscellaneous

CHAPTER 51

Femoral and Tibial Traction Pin Placement

Bradley R. Merk

Indications

1. Ipsilateral pelvic, acetabular, or femoral fracture as a definitive or temporary treatment
2. Preoperative soft tissue relaxation prior to limb lengthening reconstruction
3. Adjunctive aid to fracture reduction in the operative treatment of femoral or acetabular trauma

Contraindications

1. Active local infection
2. Significant local wound contamination
3. Inadequate soft tissue envelope
4. Polyligamentous knee injury or tibia fracture (avoid tibial traction)

Preoperative Preparation

1. If necessary, initial stabilization per ATLS protocols.
2. Obtain appropriate biplanar radiographs to allow for the identification and classification of the skeletal injury.
3. Document preoperative neurovascular and soft tissue examination.

Special Instruments, Position, and Anesthesia

1. Supine position
2. Place a bump under the knee to allow for free access to the limb.
3. If available, fluoroscopy may be helpful in minimizing the risk of physeal injury and/or to mark the knee joint axis in the coronal plane.
4. The procedure is generally performed under local anesthesia. The anesthetic is injected into the subcutaneous and subperiosteal tissues on both the medial and lateral sides of the extremity.
5. A minor surgical tray, a threaded Steinmann pin set, a hand drill, a Steinmann pin holder or Kirschner wire bow, and a bolt cutter are required.

Tips and Pearls

1. Don't be distracted by the obvious injury. Be sure to fully assess the entire skeletal system.
2. If the skeletal injury allows, assess the ligamentous knee integrity prior to placement of a tibial traction pin.
3. The Steinmann pin must be placed orthogonal to the long axis of the limb in all three planes. This is the most important if traction is to be used for the

maintenance of alignment over an extended period or as definitive treatment.

4. In a patient with good bone stock, a power drill may generate excessive heat and result in bone necrosis.

5. The ends of the Steinmann pin should be trimmed with a bolt cutter and capped to avoid inadvertent lacerations to the contralateral limb or healthcare personnel.

6. In older patients with osteopenic bone, consider placing the pins in a more diaphyseal location to improve fixation.

7. If femoral rodding is anticipated, femoral traction pins should be placed anterior in the femur to allow for nail passage. Alternatively, use tibial traction.

What To Avoid

1. Minimize injury to soft tissues and/or neurovascular structures by bluntly dissecting to bone.

2. Avoid oblique pin placement in any plane.

3. Avoid inserting the femoral traction pin from lateral to medial because this increases the chance of injury to the superficial femoral artery in the adductor canal.

4. Avoid inserting the tibial traction pin from medial to lateral because this increases the chance of injury to the common peroneal nerve.

5. Avoid tension at the pin/skin interface.

6. Avoid physeal injury in children.

Postoperative Care Issues

1. Place vaseline gauze over the pin sites followed by a rolled cotton dressing.

2. Place the limb in the appropriate form of skeletal traction as required by the skeletal injury.

3. Take postprocedure radiographs to assess pin orientation and fracture alignment.

Operative Technique

Femoral traction pin

1. Place the patient supine on the emergency room cart or the operating room table.

2. Place a bump under the knee. The degree of knee flexion should correlate with the amount of flexion anticipated for treatment (i.e., 20 to 30 degrees for balanced skeletal traction and 90 degrees for 90-90 traction).

3. If available, consider using a portable fluoroscopy unit to mark a line parallel to the knee joint. This aids orientation and helps minimize physeal injury.

4. Prepare the leg widely with antiseptic solution. Drape the relevant area with sterile towels.

5. Infuse local anesthetic into the subcutaneous and subperiosteal tissue on both the medial and lateral sides (**Figs. 51–1 and 51–2**).

6. Make a vertical stab incision on the medial side of the leg approximately one to two fingerbreadths above the superior pole of the patella at the adductor tubercle (**Fig. 51–3**).

7. Bluntly dissect to the medial femoral cortex using a hemostat.

8. Place a large threaded Steinmann pin (3/16 in for adults or 3/32 in for children) using a Jacob's chuck and a hand drill through a soft tissue protection sleeve (**Fig. 51–4**).

9. Palpate the pin as it exits the far lateral cortex. Make a stab incision in the skin to allow final pin passage.

10. Apply a vaseline dressing followed by a rolled cotton wrap (**Fig. 51–5**).

11. Trim the ends of the pin with a bolt cutter.

12. Attach a Steinmann pin holder or Kirschner wire holder to the traction pin.

13. Place the patient into traction as required by the fracture.

Operative Technique

Tibial traction pin

1. Place the patient supine on the emergency room cart or the operating room table.

2. Place a bump under the knee. The degree of knee flexion should correlate with the amount of flexion anticipated for treatment (commonly about 20 to 30 degrees of flexion).

3. If available, consider using a portable fluoroscopy unit to mark a line parallel to the knee joint. This aids orientation and helps minimize physeal injury.

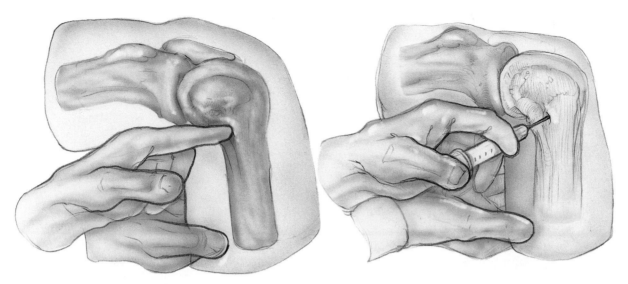

Figure 51–1 Palpation of the entry point. Palpate the entry point for the traction pin on the distal medial femur at the level of the adductor tubercle.

Figure 51–2 Local anesthetic. Local anesthetic is injected at the level of the adductor tubercle.

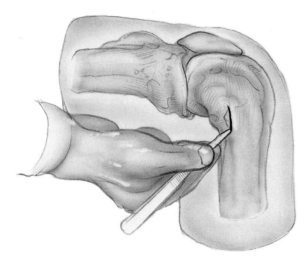

Figure 51–3 Stab incision. Make a vertical stab incision on the medial side of the leg approximately one to two fingerbreadths above the superior pole of the patella at the adductor tubercle.

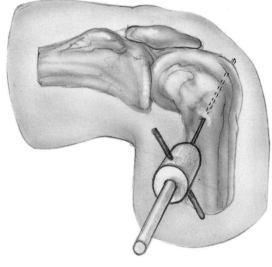

Figure 51–4 Insertion of the traction pin. Insert a large threaded Steinmann pin using a hand drill.

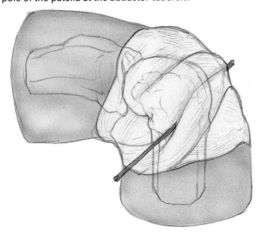

Figure 51–5 Dressing. Cover the traction pin with a vaseline dressing followed by a rolled cotton wrap.

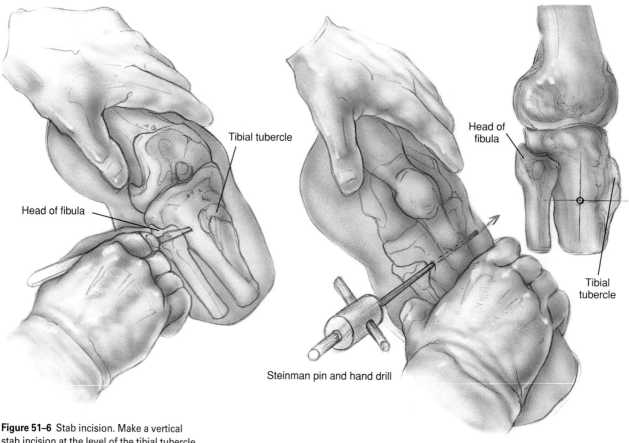

Figure 51–6 Stab incision. Make a vertical stab incision at the level of the tibial tubercle approximately 1 to 2 cm anterior to the anterior border of the fibular head.

Figure 51–7 Insertion of the traction pin. Insert a large threaded Steinmann pin using a hand drill. Note the desired position of the traction pin.

Head of fibula

Tibial tubercle

Head of fibula

Tibial tubercle

Steinman pin and hand drill

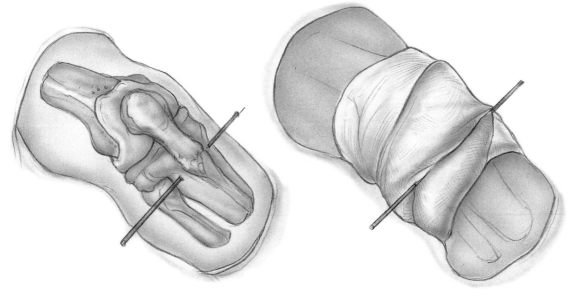

Figure 51–8 Traction pin after insertion. Note the desired position of the traction pin.

Figure 51–9 Dressing. Cover the traction pin with a vaseline dressing followed by a rolled cotton wrap.

4. Prepare the leg widely with antiseptic solution. Drape the relevant area with sterile towels.

5. Infuse local anesthetic into the subcutaneous and subperiosteal tissue on both the medial and lateral sides.

6. Make a vertical stab incision at the level of the tibial tubercle approximately 1 to 2 cm anterior to the anterior border of the fibular head (**Fig. 51–6**).

7. Bluntly dissect to the lateral tibial cortex using a hemostat.

8. Place a large threaded Steinmann pin (3/16 in for adults or 3/32 in for children) using a Jacob's chuck

and a hand drill through a soft tissue protection sleeve (**Fig. 51–7**).

9. Palpate the pin as it exits the far medial cortex. Make a stab incision in the skin to allow final passage of the pin (**Fig. 51–8**).

10. Apply a vaseline dressing followed by a rolled cotton wrap (**Fig. 51–9**).

11. Trim the ends of the pin with a bolt cutter.

12. Attach a Steinmann pin holder or Kirschner wire holder to the traction pin.

13. Place the patient into traction as required by the fracture.

Index

Note: Illustrative material is represented with an "i" following the page on which it appears.